Atlas of

Male Sexual Dysfunction

Atlas of

Male Sexual Dysfunction

Editor

Tom F. Lue, MD

Professor and Vice Chairman
Department of Urology
University of California, San Francisco
San Francisco, California

With 27 Contributors

Developed by Current Medicine LLC, Philadelphia

CURRENT MEDICINE LLC

400 Market Street, Suite 700 • Philadelphia, PA 19106

Developmental Editor . . . . *Elise M. Paxson*
Editoral Assistant . . . . *Annmarie D'Ortona*
Cover Design . . . . *William C. Whitman, Jr.*
Design and Layout . . . . *William C. Whitman, Jr. and Christine Keller-Quirk*
Illustrators . . . . *Marie Dean, Wieslawa Langenfeld, Maureen Looney, and John McCullough*
Assistant Production Manager . . . . *Margaret La Mare*
Indexing . . . . *Holly Lukens*

Library of Congress Cataloging-in-Publication Data

Atlas of male sexual dysfunction / editor, Thomas F. Lue; with 26 contributors.
p. ; cm.
Includes bibliographical references and index.
ISBN 1-57340-207-9 (alk. paper)
1. Impotence–Atlases. 2. Sexual disorders–Atlases. I. Title: Male sexual dysfunction.
II. Lue, Tom F.
[DNLM: 1. Sex Disorders–pathology–Atlases. 2. Impotence–therapy–Atlases. 3.
Penile Diseases–pathology–Atlases. WJ 17 A8816 2004]
RC889.A875 2004
616.6'9–dc22

2003067485

ISBN 1-57340-207-9

Although every effort has been made to ensure that drug doses and other information are presented accurately in this publication, the ultimate responsibility rests with the prescribing physician. Neither the publishers nor the author can be held responsible for errors or for any consequences arising from the use of the information contained therein. Any product mentioned in this publication should be used in accordance with the prescribing information prepared by the manufacturers. No claims or endorsements are made for any drug or compound at present under clinical investigation.

Printed in Thailand by Imago LLC

10 9 8 7 6 5 4 3 2 1

For more information please call 1 (800) 427-1796 or (215) 574-2266

www.current-science-group.com

PREFACE

The past three decades have seen a drastic change in the diagnosis and treatment of male sexual dysfunction. The implantable penile prosthesis, developed in the 1970s, provided the first effective medical treatment for erectile dysfunction (ED) outside the realm of psychosexual therapy. The dramatic introduction of penile injection in the Annual Meeting of the American Urological Association in Las Vegas in 1983 demonstrated that drug therapy can also be a highly effective alternative. In the ensuing years, vacuum erection devices and transurethral prostaglandin E1 also became available. In 1998, another new era was ushered in with the approval of sildenafil, a specific oral phosphodiesterase type 5 inhibitor, by the US Food and Drug Administration (FDA). Two more type 5 phosphodiesterase inhibitors, vardenafil and tadalafil, were approved by the FDA in 2003. These revolutionary changes have benefited millions of men and their partners. The phenomenal success of the oral phosphodiesterase inhibitors and the media blitz regarding these "potency pills" have also changed the attitudes of physicians, patients, partners, insurance companies, and government agencies toward sexual dysfunction. Innovative research in the past two decades has also greatly improved our understanding of penile physiology and pathophysiology of ED. In this Atlas, I have invited experts to present state-of-the-art information from basic physiology to diagnosis and treatment of male sexual dysfunction.

Drs. Leung, Christ, and Melman elegantly update the understanding of the functional anatomy, pharmacology, and neurophysiology of penile erection as well as the pathogenesis of various causes of ED. The chapter by Drs. Montague and Lakin thoroughly address the questions asked most frequently by physicians: How much evaluation is necessary? Which test should be performed in a particular patient? How valid are the current tests? Dr. Broderick expands the discussion on diagnostic evaluation and discusses in detail the usage of color Doppler ultrasound, cavernosometry and cavernosography, and arteriography in the work-up of ED, Peyronie's disease, and priapism. Drs. Morales and Heaton, with their special knowledge in pharmacology and andrology, present a comprehensive review of the hormones and their unique place in male sexual dysfunction. They also introduce the work-up and therapy related to androgen deficiency as recommended by the International Consultation on Sexual Medicine. Normal sexual function requires a harmonic relationship between mind and body. With multiple effective treatments now available, it has become more obvious that a successful treatment, defined as restoration of a satisfactory sexual relationship, cannot be achieved by just giving the patient a rigid erection. Dr. Levine's chapter wonderfully discusses the changing view of psychogenic ED and the practical aspect of managing the patient with mixed psychogenic and organic ED.

Oral phosphodiesterase type 5 inhibitors (PDE5Is) are currently the mainstay of medical therapy for ED. Drs. Kuan and Brock present the extensive world-wide experience of sildenafil and discuss the similarities and differences between sildenafil and the two new PDE5Is as well as other medical treatments, intracavernous injection, transurethral suppository, and vacuum constriction devices, which are effective second-line therapies when PDE5Is are ineffective or contraindicated. Penile prosthesis, although the most invasive treatment, is still the most successful for ED, especially with the newly improved prosthetic devices now available. Dr. Mulcahy shares his vast experience in implanting prostheses and managing complications. His results in salvage operations for penile prosthesis infection are so far the most impressive in the field. Penile revascularization is one of the rare cause-specific curative treatments for ED, and is quite successful in young men whose arterial insufficiency is a result of injury. Drs. Palese, Mulhall, and Goldstein have perfected the diagnostic and surgical approach to this condition and their suggestions should be followed closely to achieve the best result.

Ejaculatory disorder, especially premature ejaculation, is one of the most frequent complaints among men. Ironically, the concept of currently used medical treatment such as selective serotonin uptake inhibitors (SSRI) and local anesthetics are derived from side effects of the medications. Drs. Perelman, McMahon, and Barada discuss the pathogenesis as well as psychosexual and medical therapy of this frequent complaint.

The treatment of both ischemic and nonischemic priapisms has also been revolutionized thanks to the better understanding of their pathogenesis. Dr. Nehra reviews the world literature on priapisms and introduces the Practice Guideline of the American Urological Association on Priapism to the management of this condition.

Peyronie's disease is another common cause of ED. Drs. Rajfer, Gonzalez-Cadavid, and Jalkut have investigated the pathogenesis of Peyronie's disease with modern molecular biologic techniques and present a comprehensive review of the current understanding of the condition. Drs. Bochinski, Carrion, Rahman, and I discuss various medical and surgical treatments and illustrate our simplified surgical techniques for the correction of the deformed penis secondary to Peyronie's disease.

Overall, I believe this is an excellent reference book skillfully presented by authorities in the fields of ED, priapism, and Peyronie's disease. Readers will not only appreciate the tremendous advances in male sexual dysfunction research and management but will also learn of rational and cost-effective approaches to these conditions.

Tom F. Lue

CONTRIBUTORS

JAMES H. BARADA, MD, FACS
Clinical Assistant Professor of Surgery (Urology)
Albany Medical College;
Director, Center for Male Sexual Health
Albany, New York

DEREK BOCHINSKI, BSC, MD, FRCSC
Fellow
Department of Urology
University of California, San Francisco
School of Medicine
San Francisco, California

GERALD B. BROCK, MD, FRCSC
Associate Professor
Department of Urology
University of Western Ontario School of Medicine
London, Ontario
Canada

GREGORY A. BRODERICK, MD
Professor
Department of Urology
Mayo Medical School
Jacksonville, Florida

RAFAEL CARRION, MD
Urology Fellow
Department of Urology
University of California, San Francisco
School of Medicine
San Francisco, California

GEORGE J. CHRIST, PHD
Professor
Department of Urology and Physiology & Biophysics
Ben Marden Distinguished Scholar in Urology;
Director, Institute of Smooth Muscle Biology
Albert Einstein College of Medicine
Bronx, New York

IRWIN GOLDSTEIN, MD
Professor
Departments of Urology and Gynecology;
Director
Institute for Sexual Medicine
Boston University School of Medicine
Boston, Massachusetts

NESTOR GONZALEZ-CADAVID, PHD
Professor
Department of Urology
University of California at Los Angeles
School of Medicine
Los Angeles, California

JEREMY HEATON, MD
Professor of Urology
Department of Urology
Kingston General Hospital
Kingston, Ontario
Canada

MARK JALKUT, MD
Chief Resident
Department of Urology
University of California at Los Angeles
School of Medicine
Los Angeles, California

JAMES K. KUAN, MD
Chief Resident
Department of Urology
University of Western Ontario School of Medicine
London, Ontario
Canada

HALUK KULAKSIZOGLU, MD
Consultant Urologist
Department of Urology
SSK Istanbul Teaching Hospital
Istanbul, Turkey

MILTON M. LAKIN, MD
Head, Section of Medical Urology
Glickman Urological Institute
Cleveland Clinic Foundation
Cleveland, Ohio

ALBERT C. LEUNG, MD
Resident
Department of Urology
Albert Einstein College of Medicine
Montefiore Medical Center
Bronx, New York

STEPHEN B. LEVINE, MD
Clinical Professor of Psychiatry
Case School of Medicine;
Co-director, Center for Marital and Sexual Health
Beachwood, Ohio

TOM F. LUE, MD
Professor and Vice Chairman
Department of Urology
University of California, San Francisco
San Francisco, California

CHRIS G. McMAHON, MB, BS (MONASH), FACSHP
Director
Australian Centre for Sexual Health
New South Wales, Australia

ARNOLD MELMAN, MD
Professor and Chairman
Department of Urology
Albert Einstein College of Medicine
Montefiore Medical Center
Bronx, New York

DROGO K. MONTAGUE, MD
Head, Section of Prosthetic Surgery
and Genitourethral Reconstruction
Glickman Urological Institute
Cleveland Clinic Foundation
Cleveland, Ohio

ALVARO MORALES, MD
Professor of Urology and Oncology
Department of Urology
Kingston General Hospital
Kingston, Ontario
Canada

JOHN J. MULCAHY, MD, PHD, FACS
Professor
Department of Urology
Indiana University School of Medicine
Indianapolis, Indiana

JOHN P. MULHALL, MD
Associate Professor
Department of Urology
University College
Dublin, Ireland;
Director, Sexual Medicine Program
New York Hospital
Cornell University Weill Medical Center
New York, New York

AJAY NEHRA, MD
Professor of Urology
Department of Urology
Mayo Clinic College of Medicine
Rochester, Minnesota

MICHAEL A. PALESE, MD
Assistant Attending
Department of Urology
Cornell University Weill Medical Center
New York, New York

MICHAEL A. PERELMAN, PHD
Co-Director, Human Sexuality Program
Clinical Associate Professor of Psychiatry
Department of Reproductive Medicine & Urology
The New York Presbyterian Hospital
Weill Medical College of Cornell University
New York, New York

NADEEM RAHMAN, MD
Resident
Department of Urology
University of California, San Francisco
School of Medicine
San Francisco, California

JACOB RAJFER, MD
Professor
Department of Urology
University of California, Los Angeles
School of Medicine
Los Angeles, California

CONTENTS

Physiology of Penile Erection and Pathophysiology of Erectile Dysfunction

1

Albert C. Leung
George J. Christ
Arnold Melman

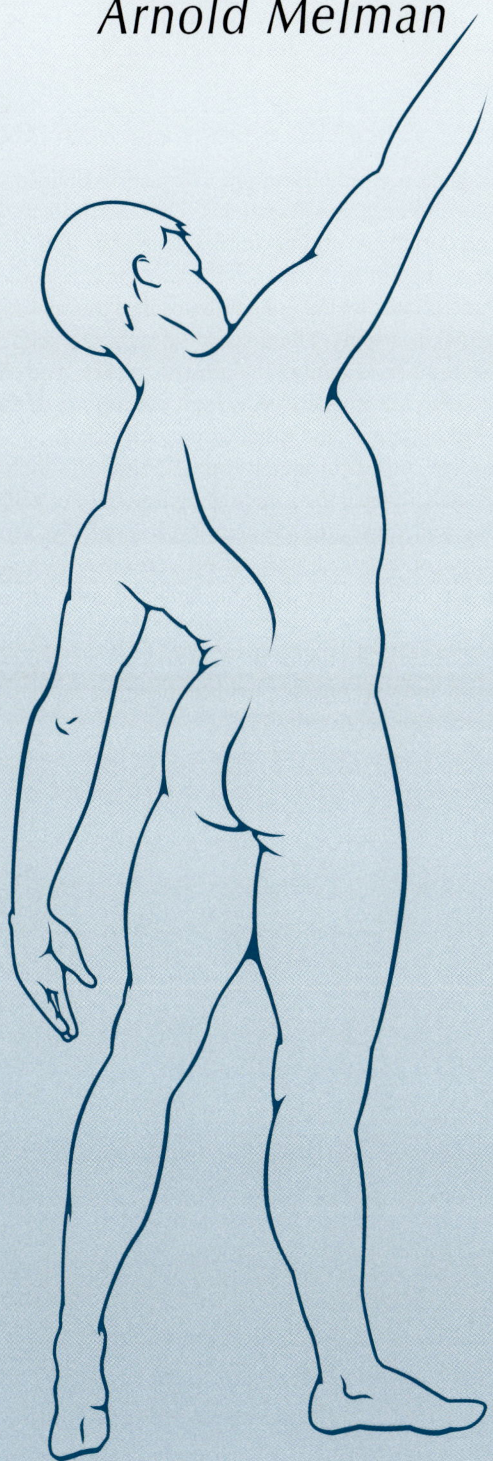

Until recently, erectile dysfunction (ED) was treated by either sexual counseling or penile prosthesis implantation. The advent of intracavernous and transurethral agents has expanded the number of therapeutic options available to ED patients. Furthermore, the approval of oral sildenafil for the treatment of ED in 1998 has prompted an increased awareness of the disease process. With ED now amenable to pharmacologic solutions, research is continuously underway to elucidate the mechanisms underlying the pathophysiologic basis of ED. The hemodynamic changes associated with each erectile event require the integrity of the penile vasculature and neural pathways. Studies that scrutinize the pathophysiology of ED have revealed various modulators or agents that may play a significant role in penile erection. These agents have been demonstrated to mediate their effects through modulation with gap junctions and potassium channels. These findings are facilitated through studies on animal models, specifically aged and diabetes-induced rats. There also appears to be a central control of the cardiac, respiratory, and penile functions that ultimately effects penile tumescence via an intricate cascade of coordinated events. With investigators striving to shed light on the pathophysiologic process of ED, the future does look bright for ED patients as more therapeutic agents, such as new oral agents and gene therapy, are on the horizon.

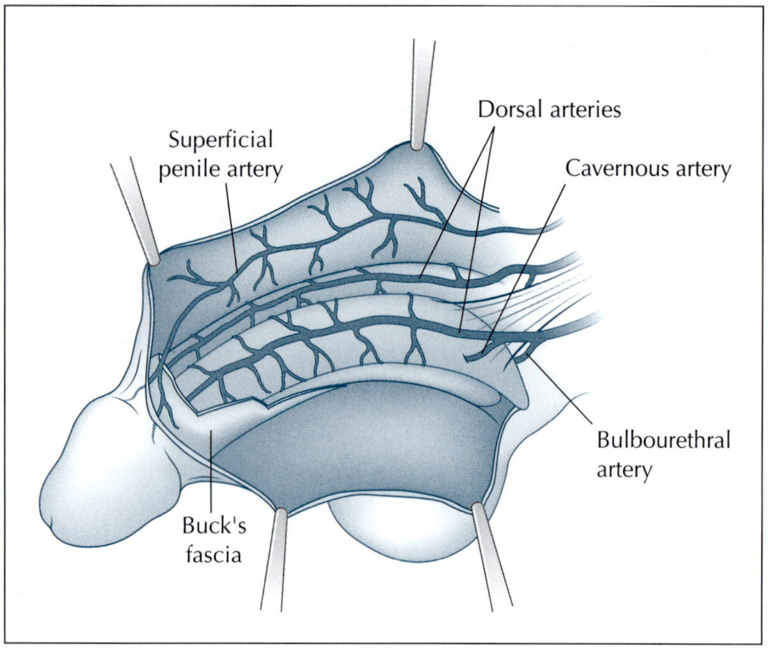

FIGURE 1-1. Penile anatomy: arterial supply. The arterial inflow to the penis is the end terminal of the internal pudendal artery, a branch of the hypogastric or internal iliac artery. After passing through the Alcock's canal, the internal pudendal artery gives rise to the common penile artery, which further subdivides into three branches: the bulbourethral artery, urethral artery, cavernous artery and ultimately terminates as the dorsal artery of the penis. The cavernous arteries of the penis are responsible for flow to the corporal bodies and give off multiple helicine arteries that are tortuous and contracted in the flaccid state while becoming straight and larger during erection. The dorsal artery passes anterior to the crus and courses distally along the dorsum of the penis under Buck's fascia to the glans penis medial to the dorsal nerve and lateral to the dorsal vein. Circumflex branches to the mid-dorsal corpora cavernosa arise from the dorsal artery of the penis. An accessory internal pudendal artery that may be jeopardized during surgery resulting in arteriogenic erectile dysfunction may branch off from the obturator, inferior vesical, or superior vesical artery. The superficial arterial supply to the penis derives from the superficial penile arteries, branches of the external pudendal artery. These superficial arteries then subdivide into the dorsolateral and ventrolateral branches.

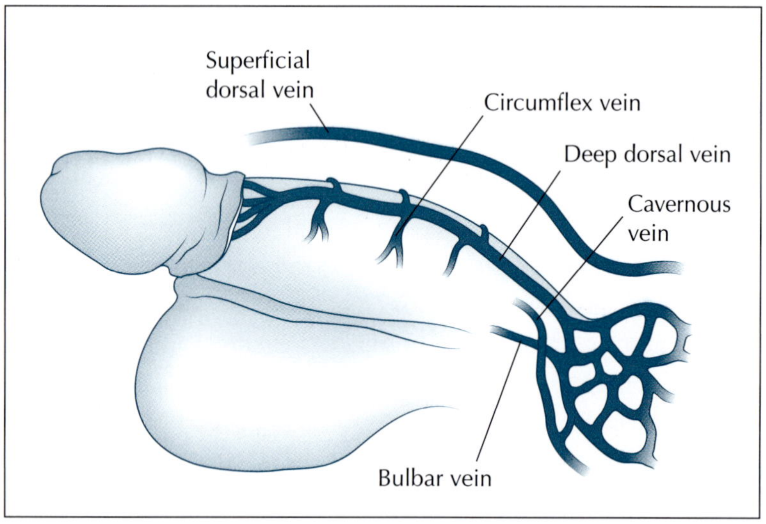

FIGURE 1-2. Penile anatomy: venous supply. The penis is drained via the superficial, intermediate, and deep venous systems. The intermediate system is composed of the deep dorsal vein and circumflex veins. The deep dorsal vein runs in the groove at the junction between the two corporal bodies and empties into the prostatic plexus, which in turn drains into the vesical plexus and ultimately the internal iliac veins. The deep dorsal vein may connect with the superficial system prior to joining the prostatic plexus. The circumflex veins communicate with the emissary veins from the corpora to drain the glans penis, corpus spongiosum, and distal corpora cavernosa.

The deep venous system consists of the cavernous, crural, and bulbar veins. The emissary veins that pierce the tunica albuginea drain directly into the cavernous veins, which in turn drain into the internal iliac veins. Crural veins arise from the dorsolateral aspect of each crus that drain into the internal iliac veins. The bulbar veins drain the bulb and empty into the prostatic plexus.

Finally, the superficial dorsal vein drains the skin and subcutaneous tissue superficial to Buck's fascia and may receive blood supply from the scrotum prior to emptying into the saphenous veins [1].

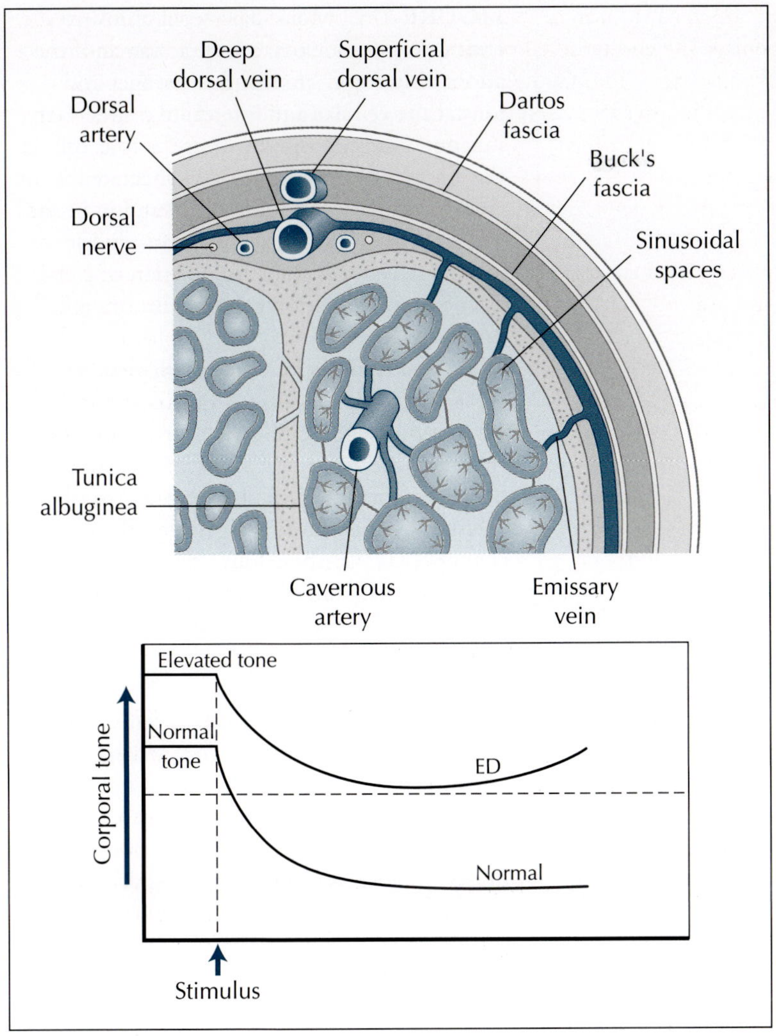

FIGURE 1-3. Corporal ultrastructure and elevated corporal tone in erectile dysfunction (ED) patients. The corpora cavernosa are enclosed in a thick fibrous sheath, the tunica albuginea, whose fibers unite medially to form a perforated septum that allows the two bodies to function as a single unit. Cavernosal tissue is spongelike and contains a meshwork of interconnected cavernosal spaces known as sinusoidal or lacunar spaces, which are lined with vascular endothelium and separated by trabeculae composed of bundles of smooth muscles fibers intertwined with an extracellular matrix of collagen (predominantly type I and IV), elastin, and fibroblasts. Collagen and elastin are crucial in permitting increases in penile girth and length during tumescence. Alterations in the relative quantities and structure of the cytoskeleton and contractile proteins may contribute to changes in the penile smooth muscle and results in incomplete relaxation thereby leading to ED. Ultrastructural analysis of penile smooth muscle cells reveals filamentous structures composed mainly of actin, myosin, desmin, and vimentin [2].

Penile erection and detumescence are hemodynamic events regulated by corporal smooth muscle relaxation and contraction, respectively. In the flaccid state, sympathetic influence predominates and the corporal smooth muscle, helicine arterioles, and cavernous sinusoids are tonically contracted, thereby permitting only small amount of blood to enter the penis at 5 mL/min. Upon sexual stimulation, parasympathetic activity causes a decrease in peripheral resistance secondary to vasodilatation and increased blood flow through the cavernous and helicine arteries. Relaxation of the trabecular smooth muscle causes increased compliance of the cavernosal spaces leading to penile erection. In the full erection state, increased blood volume and compression of the relaxed trabecular smooth muscle against the fibroelastic tunica albuginea lead to venous outflow reduction. With competent flap-valve mechanism between the trabecular smooth muscle and tunica albuginea, the corporal bodies become noncompressible cylinders from which indwelling blood cannot be expressed. Detumescence ensues secondary to increased sympathetic activity, which leads to contraction of the smooth muscle. Arterial inflow resumes while venous outflow channels reopen and the veno-occlusive mechanism is inactivated, ultimately returning the penis to the flaccid state. A delicate balance between the sympathetic and parasympathetic effects on the corporal smooth muscle tone as well as a threshold amount of relaxation are required to effect penile erection. In ED patients with heightened corporal tone as illustrated in the lower part of the figure, the corporal tone fails to relax adequately and the intracavernosal pressure thus cannot rise enough to induce penile erection on sexual stimulation [3].

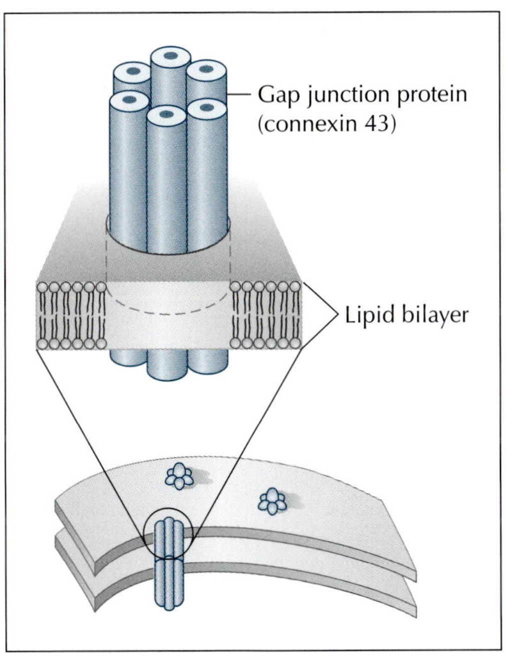

FIGURE 1-4. Gap junctions. Neural signals sent upon sexual stimulation cause release of neurotransmitters that promote smooth muscle relaxation leading to dilation of cavernosal arteries. These signals arrive at the penis and spread rapidly through the corporal tissues via *gap junctions.* Gap junctions are hexamer protein–lined aqueous intercellular channels that connect the smooth muscle cells of the corpora cavernosa into a syncytial network and provide cytoplasmic continuity between adjacent cells. These channels allow the intercellular passage of current-carrying ions and crucial second messenger molecules such as cAMP, cGMP, and calcium ions that have been shown to diffuse between cultured corporal smooth muscle cells. Gap junction protein (connexin43) appears to modulate α1-adrenergic and endothelin-1–induced contractility as well as nitric oxide–induced relaxation responses of corporal smooth muscle [4–6].

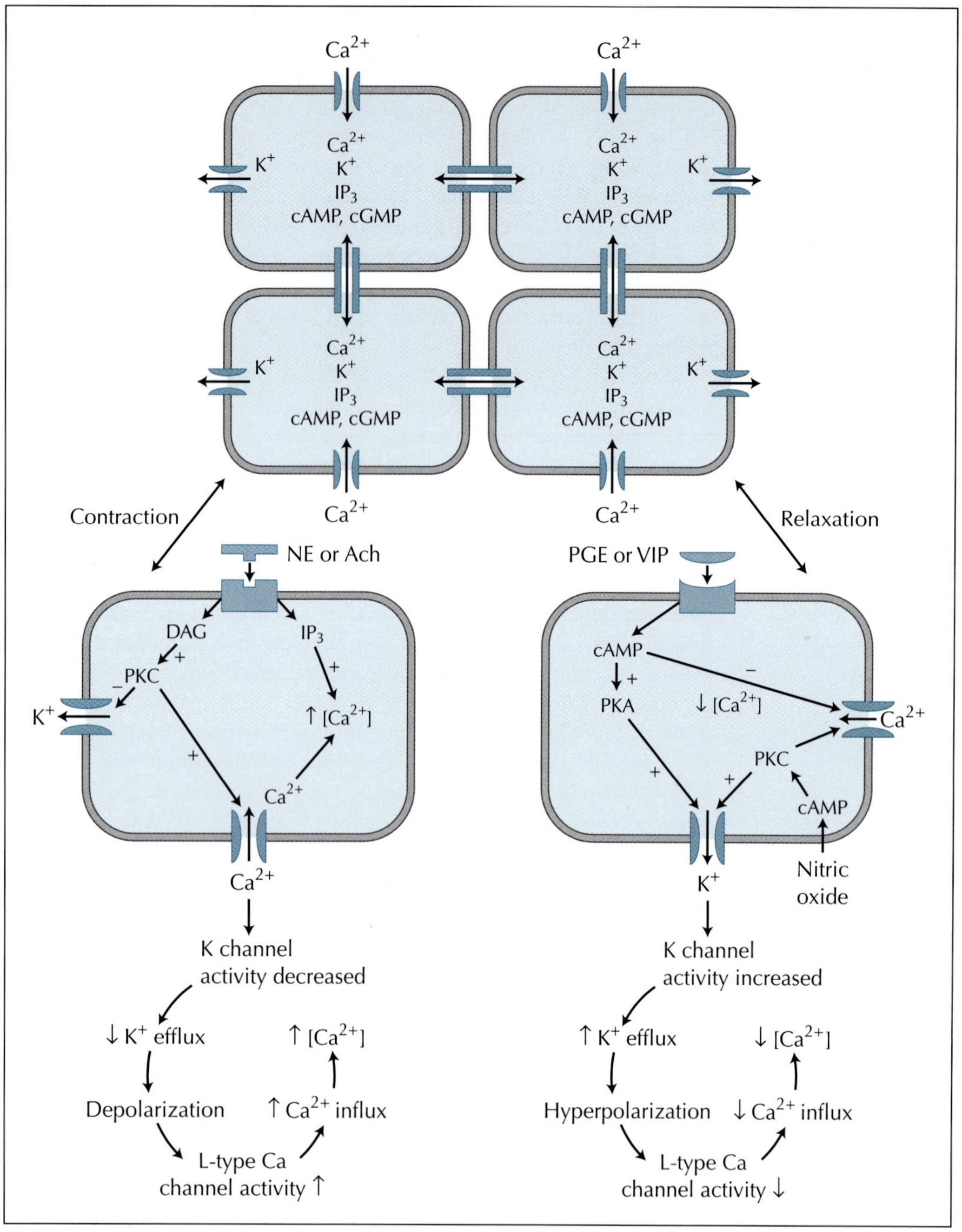

FIGURE 1-5. Molecular mechanisms governing corporal myocyte contraction and relaxation: interaction of second messenger and ions at the cellular and intercellular sites. Gap junction channels interconnect the four cells in the *top* part of this image. Also illustrated is the basis for the integral roles, direct and indirect, played by gap junctions and potassium ion channels (*middle*) in the modulation of contraction and relaxation responses in smooth muscle cells [7].

At least four distinct potassium channel subtypes have been identified in the corporal smooth muscle: calcium-sensitive potassium channels (maxi-K or KCa); ATP-dependent potassium channel (KATP); inwardly rectifying channel (Kir); and voltage-gated potassium channel (Kv). Of these four subtypes, the KATP and maxi-K channels are the most thoroughly studied and represent a crucial convergence point for modulating cellular function. Sustained contractions of corporal smooth muscle are dependent on continuous transmembrane calcium flux through voltage-dependent calcium channels, and hyperpolarization of corporal smooth cells via potassium channels may represent an important mechanism for corporal muscle tone regulation [8]. Ca^+—calcium ion; IP_3—inositol triphosphate; K^+—potassium ion; NE—norepinephrine; PGE1—prostaglandin E1; PKA—protein kinase A; PKC—protein kinase C.

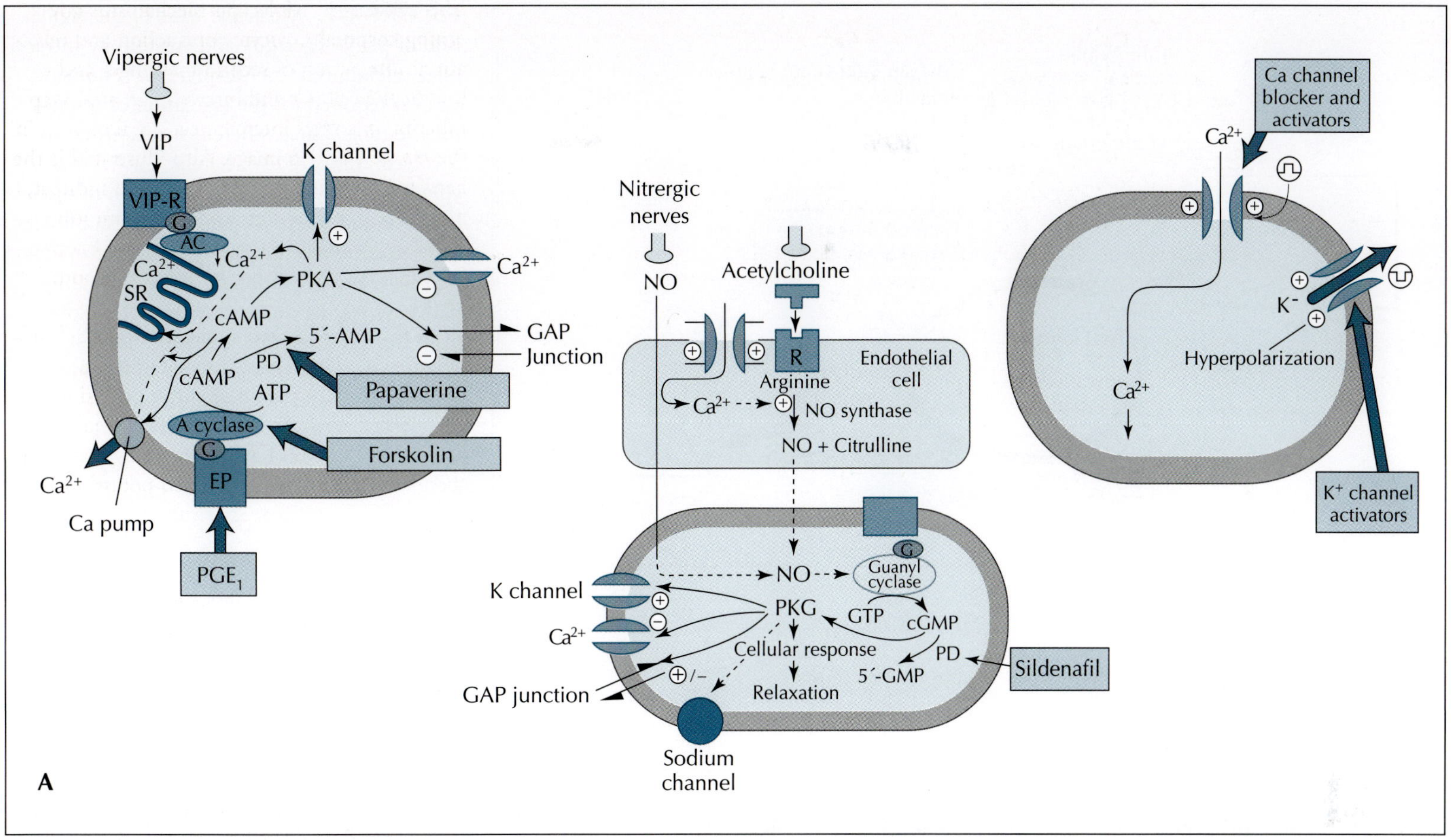

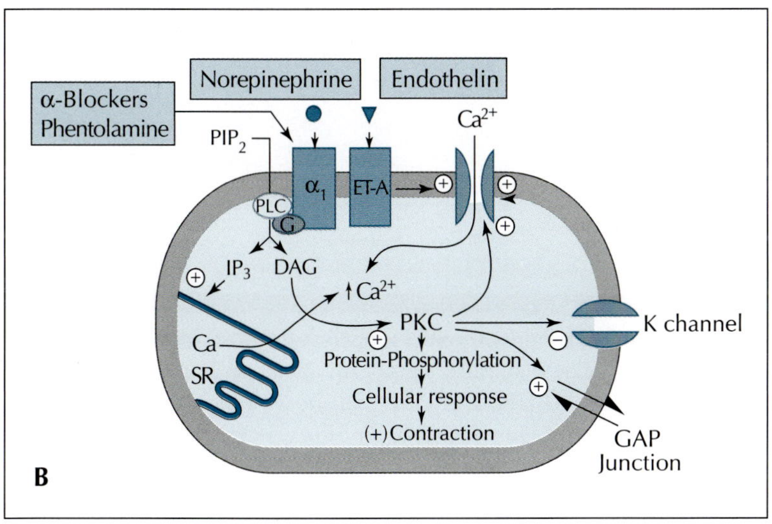

FIGURE 1-6. Signal transduction in corporal smooth muscle during penile erection and flaccidity. **A,** Penile erection. Elevations in both cyclic guanosine monophosphate and cyclic adenosine monophosphate are thought to be important [9–14]. **B,** Penile flaccidity. Intracellular events linked to corporal smooth muscle contraction following activation of the α-adrenergic receptor by norepinephrine or by endothelin are illustrated. Also shown are drugs acting at different sites. AC—adenyl cyclase; AMP—adenosine monophosphate; ATP—adenosine triphosphate; Ca^{2+}—intracellular calcium; cAMP—cyclic adenosine monophosphate; cGMP—cyclic guanosine monophosphate; DAG—diacyl glycerol; ETA—endothelin-A receptor; EP—prostaglandin E1 receptor; G—G protein; IP_3—inositol 1,4, 5-triphosphate; NO—nitric oxide; PD—phosphodiesterase; PGE—prostaglandin E; PIP—phosphatidylinositol 4-phosphate; PKA—protein kinase A; PKC—protein kinase C; PKG—protein kinase G; PLC—phospholipase C; SR—sarcoplasmic reticulum; VIP—vasoactive intestinal polypeptide.

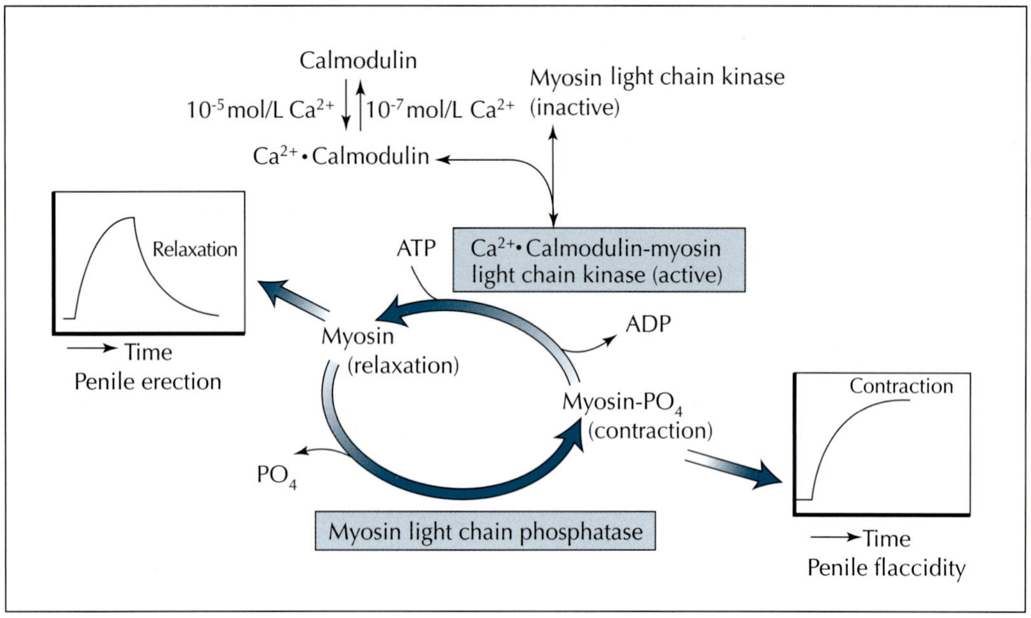

FIGURE 1-7. Molecular basis of the regulation of penile flaccidity and erection by intracellular calcium (Ca^{2+}). Adequate Ca^{2+} homeostasis is required for the regulation of smooth muscle tone. Three different mechanisms are involved: influx of extracellular Ca^{2+} through voltage-regulated channels; activation of membrane-bound receptors that allow extracellular Ca^{2+} to enter the cell through receptor-operated channels; and activation of specific signaling pathways relying on intracellular release of Ca^{2+} from sarcoplasmic reticulum [15]. ADP—adenosine diphosphate; ATP—adenosine triphosphate; PO_4—phosphorus.

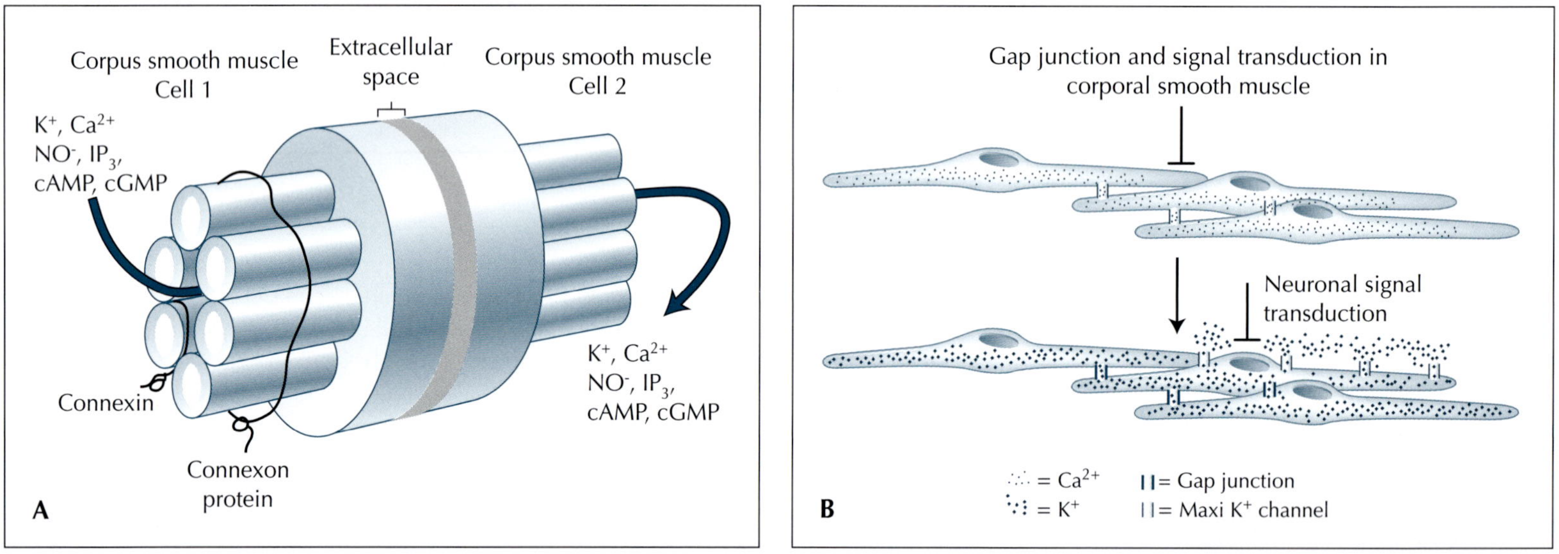

FIGURE 1-8. The role of gap junctions in signal coordination and propagation in corporal smooth muscle cell during penile erection (**A** and **B**). Despite the relatively sparse neuronal innervation of the corporeal parenchyma, electromyographic studies in patients with normal erectile function show that cavernous electrical activity is synchronous throughout the entire corpus cavernosum. Corporal neurotransmitters transmit electrical or chemical signals through gap junctions, and the whole penis acts as syncytium. Gap junctions are made up of six homologous membrane-spanning proteins from each cell (connexins) that join in the extracellular space. Age or disease may cause significant alteration in gap junction protein (Cx43 mRNA) expression in patients with organic erectile dysfunction [15–17]. Downregulation of the gap junctions has been shown to exist in diabetic and aging men. cAMP—cyclic adenosine monophosphate; cGMP—cyclic guanosine monophosphate; IP_3—inositol 1,4,5-triphosphate; NO—nitric oxide.

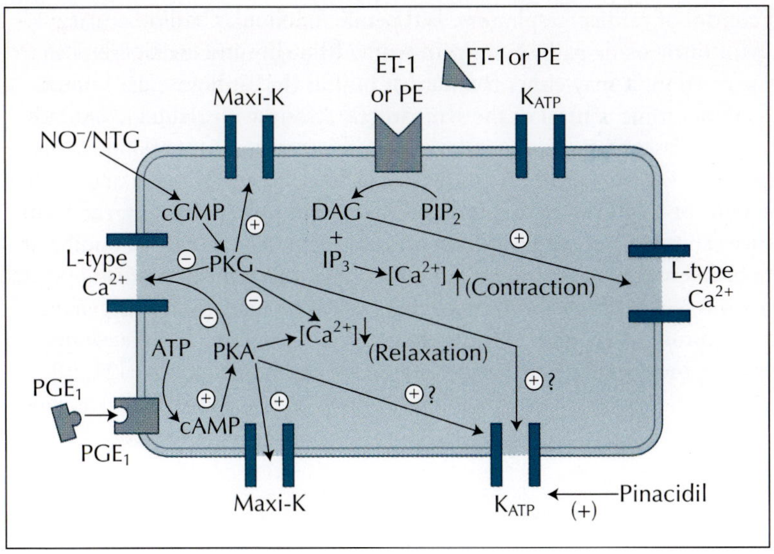

FIGURE 1-9. Role of calcium and potassium channels in penile erection and flaccidity. Stimulation of potassium channels causes hyperpolarization (relaxation) of corporal smooth muscle cell, which prevents the voltage-dependent calcium channels from opening [18]. Because sustained contractions of corporal smooth muscle depend on continuous transmembrane calcium flux through voltage-dependent calcium channels, potassium channel activity inhibits calcium influx. Penile corpora consist of four distinct potassium channels: the calcium-sensitive potassium channel (maxi-K), the metabolically regulated potassium K channel (K_{ATP}), the delayed rectifier, and the fast transient A current (IA) [4,19]. The maxi-K channel mediates most commonly in corporal smooth muscle cells. Alteration of the maxi-K^+ channel in cells from impotent patients has been found, suggesting that impairment in the function or regulation of potassium channels may contribute to decreased hyperpolarizing ability, altered calcium homeostasis, and impaired smooth muscle relaxation in impotence [16]. ATP—adenosine triphosphate; Ca^{2+}—intracellular calcium; cAMP—cyclic adenosine monophosphate; cGMP—cyclic guanosine monophosphate; DAG—diacyl glycerol; ET-1—endothelin-1; IP_3—inositol 1,4,5 triphosphate; NO—nitric oxide; NTG—nitroglycerine; PE—phenyl ephrine; PGE—prostaglandin E; PIP—phosphatidylinositol 4-phosphate; PKA—protein kinase A; PKG—protein kinase G.

Neurochemical Control of Penile Erection and Flaccidity

Neurotransmitter	*Source*	*Receptor*	*Second Messenger*	*Corporal Smooth Muscle Cell Ca^{2+}*	*Corporal Smooth Muscle Cell Response*
Neurogenic					
Norepinephrine	Adrenergic neurons	α-Adrenergic	IP_3/diaglycerol/Ca^{2+}/PKC	Increased	Contraction
Acetylcholine	Cholinergic neurons	Muscarinic	Nitric oxide/guanylate cyclase/cGMP/PKG	Decreased	Relaxation
Nitric oxide (neuronal)	Noradrenergic, noncholinergic (nitrergic)	Guanylate cyclase, K channel	Guanylate cyclase/cGMP/PKG	Decreased	Relaxation
VIP	Noradrenergic, noncholinergic (vipergic)	Vasoactive intestinal polypeptide	Adenylate cyclase/cAMP/PKA	Decreased	Relaxation
Endothelial					
Endothelin-1	Endothelial cells	Endothelin-A, endothelin-B	IP_3/diaglycerol/Ca^{2+}/PKC	Increased	Contraction
Nitric oxide (endothelial)	Endothelium	Guanylate cyclase, K channel	Guanylate cyclase/cGMP/PKG	Decreased	Relaxation
PGE_1	Endothelial cells	Prostaglandin receptor	Adenylate cyclase/cAMP/PKA	Decreased	Relaxation

FIGURE 1-10. Neurochemical control of penile erection and flaccidity. In cholinergic mechanisms, adrenergic nerves in the corpus cavernosum receive inhibitory interneuronal regulation from cholinergic nerves (cross-talk). Cholinergic nerves also may facilitate noradrenergic, noncholinergic relaxation. For nitrergic noradrenergic, noncholinergic mechanisms, the nitric oxide is produced by 1) activation of cholinergic receptors on endothelial cells [20–22]; 2) direct noradrenergic/noncholinergic neurotransmission; and 3) mechanical deformation of the endothelial cells (shear stress). In vipergic noradrenergic, noncholinergic mechanisms, vasoactive intestinal polypeptide is a co-neurotransmitter in corporal smooth muscle cells [23]. Intracorporeal injection of exogenous vasoactive intestinal peptide alone has failed to produce erections in many impotent men, indicating that other modulators must be involved in corporal smooth muscle relaxation [24,25]. In adrenergic mechanisms with noradrenaline, adrenergic fibers outnumber cholinergic fibers in the penis. Injection of the α-blockers phenoxybenzamine and phentolamine causes erection, whereas the α-agonist causes shrinkage of both the erect and flaccid penis [26]. These findings suggest that the tone of corporal smooth muscle in the flaccid penis is maintained by continuous α-adrenoceptor stimulation. Endothelin-1 (ET-1), also used for noradrenergic mechanisms, is synthesized by the human corpus cavernosum endothelium and elicits strong, sustained contractions of corpus cavernosum smooth muscle. Endothelin may contribute to the maintenance of penile flaccidity by providing sustained tone to the corporal smooth muscle. Noradrenergic mechanisms also use prostaglandins (PG), including PGF_2-α, PGE_2, and PGI_2, as well as thromboxane, which are synthesized in the endothelium of the corpus cavernosum. PGE_1 is the only endogenous prostaglandin that appears to elicit relaxation of human corporal smooth muscle. During erection, there is a state of blood stasis in the corpora. The antiplatelet aggregating effects of PGI_2, together with those of nitric oxide, both released by the endothelium, may be important in preventing coagulation of blood during erection. PGE_1 produces dose-dependent corporal smooth muscle relaxation and also inhibits the α-adrenergic mechanism that tonically contracts this muscle and maintains the flaccid nonerect state of the penis [24]. cAMP—cyclic adenosine monophosphate; cGMP—cyclic guanosine monophosphate; IP_3—inositol 1,4,5-triphosphate; PKA—protein kinase A; PKC—protein kinase C; PKG—protein kinase G; VIP—vasoactive intestinal polypeptide.

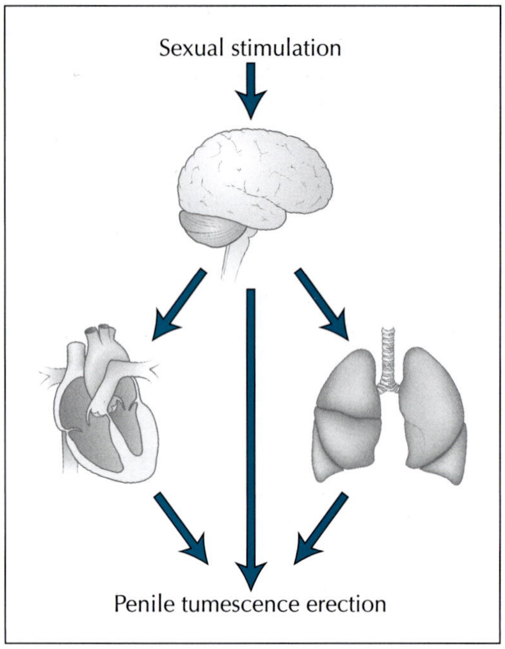

FIGURE 1-11. Central control of cardiac, respiratory, and penile functions. Cardiovascular risk factors are associated with nitric oxide pathway impairment. Although nitric oxide exerts an excitory effect during penile erection, it may either facilitate or inhibit the cardiovascular system. Similarly, while the penis is under tonic control of the sympathetic system with resultant vasoconstriction and flaccidity, the cardiovascular system is under tonic parasympathetic predominance, and activation of the sympathetic system contributes to increased blood pressure, pulse, and respiratory rate. When the fight-or-flight response is induced by the sympathetic system, the concomitant penile flaccidity cannot be reversed by pharmacotherapy, perhaps a natural bodily adaptation to prioritize life or safety over copulation. Common nuclei that regulate cardiac, respiratory, and penile functions have been discovered through transneuronal labeling and viral injection [27]. Sexual behavior prompts changes in the cardiorespiratory system, and the central nervous system helps coordinate the overall physiologic response via autonomic activity [28,29].

Neural Origin of Penile Erection

Mode	*Afferent*	*Central*	*Efferent*
Reflexogenic (spinal) Tactile stimuli Friction of genitalia	Dorsal nerve of the penis, pudendal nerve	Spinal (spinal reflex pathways are also modulated by brain [*eg,* tactile stimuli → (spinothalamic tract) → thalamus → (somatic sensory nerves) → postcentral gyrus])	Pelvic nerve, cavernous nerve
Psychogenic (central) Special sensory Visual Auditory Olfactory Psychic Memory Fantasy	Thalamic (somatosensory, visual) Rhinencephalon (olfactory) Limbic (temporal and frontal lobe) for emotion and memory	Supraspinal Medial preoptic area of hypothalamus Paraventricular area of hypothalamus	Pelvic nerve, hypogastric nerve, cavernous nerve
Sleep Erection	Endogenous neurotransmitters	Reticular activating system → ? reticulospinal or ? spinothalamic	Pelvic nerve, hypogastric nerve, cavernous nerve

FIGURE 1-12. Neural origin of penile erection. Penile erections are elicited by local sensory stimulation of the frenulum, glans penis, and penile skin (reflexogenic erections) and by central psychogenic stimuli received by or generated within the brain (psychogenic erections). Reflexogenic erections are mediated by a spinal reflex pathway in which the afferent limb consists of sensory receptors in the penile skin and glans, carried through the dorsal nerve that joins the pudendal nerve to reach the sacral spinal cord. Entirely reflex erection can be observed in men with complete spinal cord lesions above the sacral segments. In these men there is obviously no sensation, and erection depends on a sacral cord mechanism in isolation from the rest of the central nervous system. Psychogenic erection in response to sexual thoughts or auditory, olfactory, imaginative, or visual stimuli only, without tactile stimulation, occurs in most normal men [30–32]. Sleep erection happens in 95% of rapid eye movement sleep and lasts 30 to 60 minutes per episode, occurring, on the average, three to five times per night.

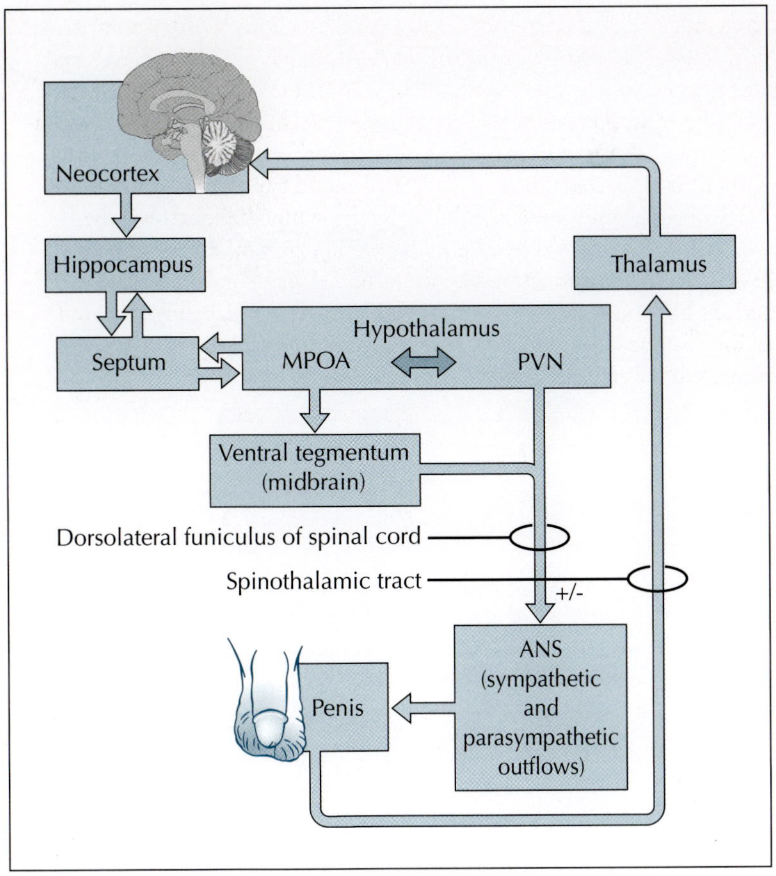

FIGURE 1-13. Central nervous system pathways involved in penile erection and flaccidity. In cerebral mechanisms, the cortex receives sensory information derived from the penis. Thalamic and cortical areas associated with somatomotor pathways elicit sexual feelings and genital sensations when stimulated, but do not elicit penile erection. In the medial preoptic area (MPOA), sexual behavior depends on neural mechanisms involving the brain and spinal cord. The MPOA is the important component of the neural circuitry underlying the expression of male copulatory behavior in mammals. Destruction of the nerve cell bodies of the MPOA by a neurotoxin, which spares axons passing through the region, seriously disrupts the male animal's ability to copulate. MPOA also contains a high density of receptors for testosterone. The paraventricular nucleus of the hypothalamus (PVN) has been determined to be the sexual response center [33–35]. Oxytocin is released into the circulation during sexual activity [36]. The hormone reaches maximum plasma levels at the time of ejaculation and then rapidly disappears from the circulation. Oxytocin in the circulation may, therefore, play a role in ejaculation or the refractory period, rather than erection. ANS—autonomic nervous system; MPOA—medial preoptic area; PVN—paraventricular nucleus.

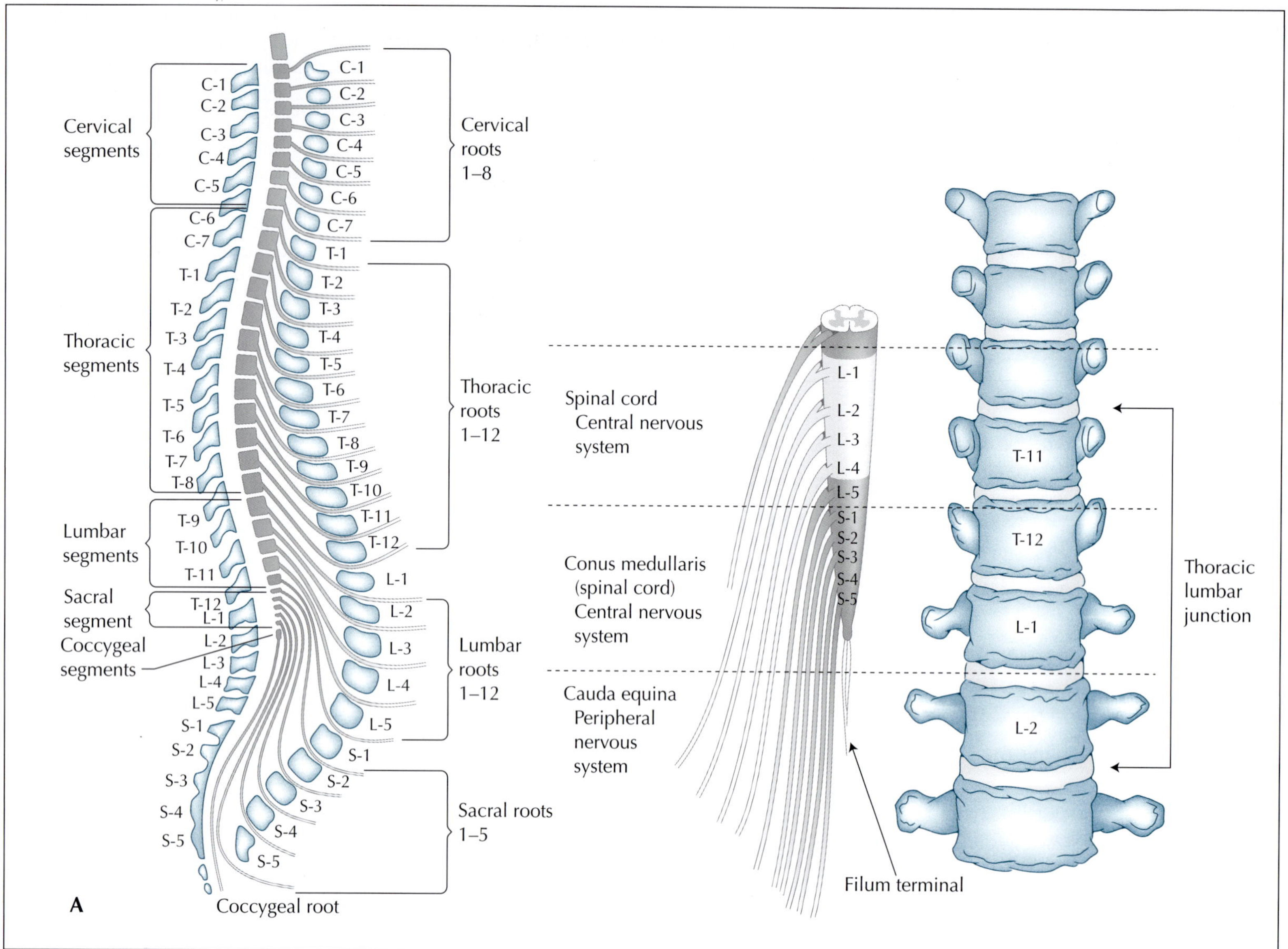

FIGURE 1-14. Neural control of penile erection. **A,** Spinal cord segments and their corresponding vertebral column levels. The spinal cord and vertebral column grow asynchronously in the fetus such that the cord initially terminates at the sacral and then lumbar levels. In a newborn, the spinal cord terminates at the L3 vertebra. From 2 months of age through adulthood, the cord usually ends at the L1-L2 vertebrae.

(*Continued on next page*)

B. Effects of Neurogenic Lesions on Penile Erection

Level of Lesion	*Alteration of Sexual Function*
Cortical	Perception of sexual input signal is gone. Inhibitory or facilitatory output on supraspinal sex centers (MPOA and PVN) is abolished. Normally, release of inhibition is needed for erection.
Bilateral anterolateral cordotomy	Complete loss of erection, loss of orgasm sensation
Bilateral anterolateral cord stimulation (brain stem level)	Erection and ejaculation
Complete cord lesion, spinal tract pathway, ? spinothalamic, ? reticulospinal	Prolonged reflex erection (priapism secondary to interruption of vasoconstrictor pathway) may occur for 2 to 3 days. Erection and ejaculation lost for weeks or months, areflexic, atonic, nonresponsive to plantar stimulation. Bulbocavernous reflex returns early but reflex ejaculation seldom returns. The return of normal erectile function coincides with the return of deep tendon and visceral reflexes.
Cord lesion (above T6, UMN lesion), sympathetic fibers in cord involved	Autonomic dysreflexia, psychogenic erection absent
Cord lesion (above T12, UMN lesion), sympathetic route involved	Psychogenic erection absent
Cord lesion (below T12, UMN lesion), sympathetic route escaped	Psychogenic erection present
Sacral cord lesion (S2,3,4, UMN + LMN lesion)	Reflexogenic erection disappears, psychogenic erection persists
Conus medullaris lesion (UMN + LMN lesion)	Mixed pattern depending on fibers involved; mostly absent erection
Cauda equina lesion (LMN lesion)	Loss of genital sensation, reflex erections, and ejaculation (psychogenic erection may be retained)
Dorsal nerve of penis (no efferent input to keep the neurogenic impulse going and to secrete neurotransmitters)	Inability to sustain erection

FIGURE 1-14. ***Continued*** **B**, Effects of neurogenic lesions on penile erection. The spinal cord is a major site for the regulation of erectile and antierectile outflows and the coordination of autonomic with somatic pathways. In patients with spinal cord injuries above sacral segments, stimulation of penile receptors triggers erection through the sacral spinal reflex. Lesions of the sacral segments of the spinal cord, the sacral roots, or the pelvic or pudendal nerves abolish reflexogenic erections. Psychogenic erections occur in men with complete lesions of the cord as high as T12, suggesting that they are mediated by the sympathetic pathway. Reflex erection involves the corpus cavernosum and spongiosum if the lower level of injury is above T10 to T12; it involves only the corpus cavernosum if the lesion is caudal to T10 to T12. All lesions proximal to S2–S4 produce an upper motor neuron type of bladder and striated sphincter. Lesions at multiple levels or mixed with incomplete lesions can give variable patterns. Erections in spinal cord injury are usually short-lived, only partial, and lack the rigidity due to lack of control of supraspinal erection centers. These erections cannot be used for satisfactory sexual intercourse. LMN—lower motor neuron; MPOA—medial preoptic area; PVN—paraventricular nucleus; UMN—upper motor neuron.

Central Neurotransmitters Involved in Penile Erection and Flaccidity

Transmitters	*Receptor*	*Secondary Mediator*	*Pharmacologic Effect on Sexual/Erectile Behavior*
Dopamine	D_1	Activate adenylate cyclase (↑ cAMP → excitatory)	Facilitate
(Antipsychotic block, D_2 receptor)	D_2	Inhibit adenylate cyclase (↓ cAMP → inhibitory)	?
Epinephrine Found in small neuronal clusters in brain stem, especially medulla Norepinephrine Highest in locus ceruleus, rich in β1 and β2 receptors that activate adenylate cyclase (excitatory)	α1 (postsynaptic)	(↑ intracellular Ca)	Inhibit
	α2 (pre- and postsynaptic)	Inhibit adenylate cyclase (↓ cAMP)	Inhibit (activation of α_2 adrenoreceptor in the MPOA is associated with decrease in sexual behavior)
Serotonin Found in high concentrations in raphe nuclei. Certain antidepressants increase 5HT availability by reducing its uptake	$5HT_{1A}$	↓ cAMP	Both facilitatory and inhibitory
	$5HT_{1B}$	↓ cAMP	Both facilitatory and inhibitory
	$5HT_{1C}$	↑ Phostidylinositol turnover	Facilitatory (direct stimulation of $5HT_{1C}$ causes erection
	$5HT_{1D}$	(similar to 5HT1-B)	
	$5HT_2$	Similar to 5HTC1-C and linked phosphatidyl turnover	Inhibit/facilitate (agonists inhibit erection but facilitate seminal emission and ejaculation)
	$5HT_3$	(↑ inflow of Na and Ca)	Facilitate/inhibit
Acetylcholine (Somatic and visceral nuclei)	ACh Nicotinic Muscarinic (M_1–M_3)	Act via G-protein	Facilitate
Enkephalins			Inhibit (inhibitory control on central oxytocinergic transmission)
GABA	$GABA_A$ $GABA_B$	Open C1 channel, ↓ release of other neurotransmitters	Inhibit
Oxytocin			Facilitate
Prolactin			Inhibit (inhibition of dopaminergic activity in the MPOA)

FIGURE 1-15. Central neurotransmitters involved in penile erection and flaccidity. Sexual drive results from the action of dopaminergic and adrenergic receptors and is inhibited by serotoninergic receptors in the supraspinal erection centers (medial preoptic area and paraventricular nucleus) and possibly at the sacral erection center. Clinical observation suggests that dopaminergic stimulation increases libido and produces erection. Drugs that increase central serotonergic neurotransmission depress sexual activity. Serotonin agonists, on the other hand, induce erection. Serotonergic compounds appear to have an inhibitory effect on sex drive centrally but an erectogenic effect peripherally. These effects may contribute to the induction of priapism in patients treated with the antidepressant trazodone [37]. Noradrenergic pathways in the brain may exert a stimulatory influence on penile erection. The most distinct group of noradrenergic neurons is the locus ceruleus, found in the pons. The neurons project through the dorsal noradrenergic bundles to innervate the cortex, cerebellum, and hippocampus. Other groups of noradrenergic neurons project through the ventral noradrenergic bundle to the hypothalamus, hippocampus, cerebellum, and spinal cord. Endogenous opioid peptides and gamma aminobutyric acid (GABA) have been implicated as inhibitory transmitters in sexual pathways. Administration of opioid or GABA receptor agonists to the central nervous system inhibits male animal copulatory behavior, whereas the administration of antagonists for either transmitter facilitates copulatory behavior. In humans, intrathecal administration of opiate drugs (*eg*, morphine) inhibits ejaculation but not erection. Loss of ability to achieve or maintain erection is a commonly noted side effect in heroin- or methadone-addicted patients. Spontaneous erections are reported as side effects during treatment with the opiate antagonists naloxone and naltrexone [38]. Ca—calcium; cAMP—cyclic adenosine monophosphate; HT—hydroxytryptamine (serotonin); MPOA—medial preoptic area; Na—sodium.

Penile flaccidity

Corporal smooth muscle contracted
Noradrenaline release from sympathetic system
Endothelin comodulator with noradrenaline
Minimal blood flow (5 mL/min)

↓

Sexual desire/erotic stimuli/tactile stimuli (neuronal signal generated)

Reflexogenic (spinal) route
Psychogenic/cortical (limbic, MPOA, PVN) route
Nocturnal erection (RA system)

Release of central inhibition (release of central neurotransmitters)

↓

Neuronal signal propagation

Signal from supraspinal centers travels through spinal cord to sacral sex center (S2, 3, 4), hypogastric, pelvic nerve, and via cavernous nerve to penis

↓

Release of local corporal vasorelaxants (peripheral neurotransmitters)

Parasympathetic (Ach) inhibition of adrenergic system
Parasympathetic (Ach)-mediated release of endogenous NO
NANC nerves–release of neuronal NOS
Vipergic nerves–release of VIP

↓

Relaxation of corporal smooth muscle (final common pathway of erection)

Arterial dilation and rapid inflow of blood
Sinusoidal expansion and sinusoidal filling (capacitor)

↓

Occlusion of penile outflow (blood trapping)

Subtunical venous plexus compression due to:
Sinusoidal expansion
Differential stretching of inner and outer layer of tunica, leading to elongation and compression (passive veno-occlusive mechanism)

Increased ICP reaching MAP leading to elongation and increase of girth → indistensibility → rigidity

FIGURE 1-16. Normal sexual function in men involves initiating and maintaining erection, emission, ejaculation, and orgasm. Male sexual response can be divided into behavior, erectile, and ejaculatory phases. Functional impairment of arterial inflow (failure to fill) or inadequate restriction of venous outflow (failure to store), or both, may result in erectile dysfunction [9]. The local control mechanisms that regulate the relaxation and contraction of the corporal smooth muscle may be significantly abnormal in the majority of men with erectile dysfunction. Ach—acetylcholine; ICP—intracorporal pressure; MAP—mean arterial pressure; MPOA—medial preoptic area; NANC—nonadrenergic noncholinergic; NO—nitric oxide; NOS—nitric oxide synthase; PVN—paraventricular nucleus; RA—reticulating activating system; VIP—vasoactive intestinal polypeptide.

Classification of Erectile Dysfunction

Etiology
- Neurogenic
- Endocrinologic
- Arteriogenic
- Venogenic
- Psychogenic
- Pharmacologic
- Iatrogenic

Function classification
- Failure to initiate (neurogenic, psychogenic, endocrinologic)
- Failure to fill (arteriogenic)
- Failure to store or maintain (corporal veno-occlusive dysfunction)
- Failure to achieve rigidity/penetration
- Failure to detumesce (priapism)

FIGURE 1-17. Classification of erectile dysfunction (ED). ED may be categorized by its etiology or functional effects.

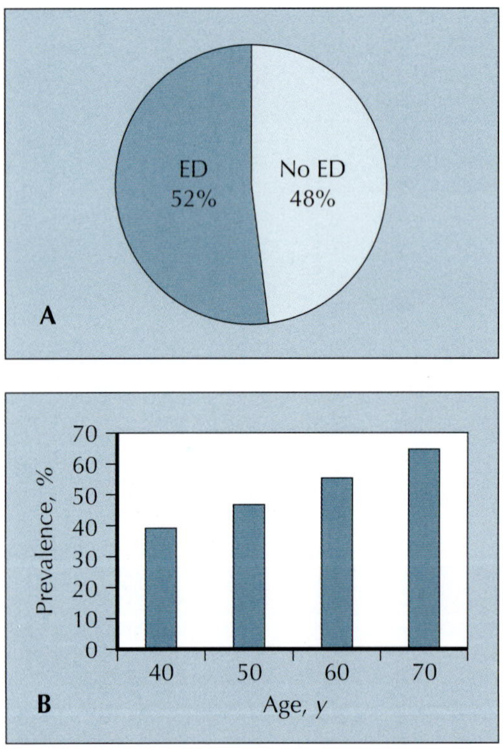

FIGURE 1-18. Prevalence (**A**) and association between age and erectile dysfunction (ED) (**B**). The overall prevalence (minimal, moderate, severe) of ED is estimated to be 52% in men 40 to 70 years of age (based on the Massachusetts Male Aging Study). Using these data and United States population projections for the year 2005, of more than 50 million men 40 to 70 years of age, ED will affect more than 25 million men, and millions more over the age of 70. The projected worldwide prevalence of ED for the year 2025 will be a staggering 322 million men. However, variations have been noted pertaining to ED prevalence. Such discrepancy can be explained by variations in definitions, methodology, and study populations. European studies demonstrate a prevalence of 5% to 19% for moderate to severe ED, versus 35% as reported by Feldman *et al.* [39].

PSYCHOGENIC ERECTILE DYSFUNCTION

A. Psychologic Determinants of Erectile Dysfunction

Predisposing Factors	***Etiologic Factors***	***Pathogenetic Factors (Precipitating)***	***Maintaining Factors***
Psychophysiologic vulnerability of the sexual response system	Intrapsychic factors	Psychoeffective mechanisms	Performance anxiety
Ego-structural deficits		Cognitive mechanisms	Phobic avoidance Fear of intimacy
Traumatic early sexual experiences	Partnership problems	Psychophysiologic mechanisms	Depression and anxiety, withdrawal, or impaired self-image
Restrictive upbringing		Infidelity	
Disturbed family relationships		Aging or random failure	Loss of desire or restricted foreplay
Early insecurity in psychosexual role		Reaction to organic factors	Guilt, sexual myths, or inadequate sexual information
Poor sexual information		Discord in the general relationship	Performance anxiety and anticipation of failure
Socially withdrawn		Unreasonable and high expectations	Loss of attraction between partners
		Dysfunction in the partner	Poor communication between partners
		Traumatic sexual experience	Discord in the general relationship

B. Psychologic Subtypes Predisposed to Erectile Dysfunction

Actual Neurotic	***Psychoneurotic***	***Psychosomatic***	***Functional***
Psychic conflict	Deep-rooted conflicts and anxiety concerning sexuality and partnership	Primary psychosomatic constellation	No psychopathologic attributes
↓	↓	↓	↓
No repression, no working over	Sexuality → unconscious threat to coherence or identity	Somatization, affective repression, "somatic communication"	Life events or other situation for which no coping program is available
↓	↓	↓	↓
Direct somatic manifestation of tension and anxiety	Neurotic defense mechanisms, inhibition of sexual arousal	Specific releasing conflict, ego regression	Alarm reaction, panic, acute stress result in sexual dysfunction
↓	↓	↓	↓
Erectile dysfunction = anxiety	Erectile dysfunction	Resomatization, sexual dysfunction	Maintained and exacerbated by performance anxiety

FIGURE 1-19. Psychologic determinants of erectile dysfunction. **A,** Psychogenic stimuli can inhibit penile erection by either direct inhibition of the spinal erection center by the brain as an exaggeration of the normal suprasacral inhibition [32] or excessive sympathetic outflow or elevated peripheral catecholamine levels, which may increase penile smooth muscle tone, preventing the relaxation necessary for erection. **B,** Psychologic subtypes predisposed to erectile dysfunction. Recently, predisposing personality types have been described [40]. Clinically, psychogenic dysfunction can be suspected in the presence of sudden onset, diminished libido, and preservation of masturbation and morning erection. (*Adapted from* Hartmann [40].)

Neurogenic Erectile Dysfunction

Neurologic Cause	*Erectile Dysfunction*
Neurologic injury	
Suprasacral lesion	5% to 8%. Lesions proximal to cord segments S2–S4 (*ie,* vertebrae T10–L1) produce a UMN type of bladder, external sphincter dysfunction, intact BC reflex, and preserved reflexogenic erections.
Sacral lesion	60% to 80%. Lesions of S2–S4 cord or sacral roots of pelvic nerve and pudendal nerve result in mixed lesions. Neurologic injury to the conus medullaris and cauda equina results in LMN lesions with loss of BC reflex and reflexogenic erections but preservation of psychogenic erections (possibly through preserved sympathetic route).
Spinal shock	Return of erections parallels return of other reflexes. Of returning erections, 80% occur by 1 year. Erections return in 75% of paraplegics but only 25% of these are rigid enough for penetration.
Central nervous system disorders	
Parkinson's disease	60%. Degeneration of the peripheral and autonomic systems results in erectile dysfunction. Efferent pathways that travel through the ventrolateral part of the pons and medulla into the anterolateral tracts in the spinal cord are affected.
Multiple sclerosis	70%. There is a high association between erectile dysfunction and bladder dysfunction (76% have hyperreflexia).
Other cortical lesions	One third of patients with cerebrovascular accidents have erectile dysfunction.
Temporal lobe epilepsy	
Head trauma	
Stroke	
Peripheral neuropathy	
Dorsal nerve pathology	These patients have difficulty maintaining an erection. The NPT may be normal, with the only abnormality being biothesiometry and evoked response.
Diabetes	Neuropathy involving somatic, peripheral, and autonomic neurons
Alcoholism	Autonomic neuropathy (can reverse with abstinence from alcohol)
Aging	Loss of pressure, touch, and vibration sense
Chronic renal failure	Autonomic neuropathy and hormonal abnormalities
Other peripheral neuropathies	
Scleroderma	
Lupus	
Hypothyroidism	
Vitamin B_1, B_2, and B_6 deficiencies	
Amyloidosis	
Industrial toxins	
AIDS (via autonomic neuropathy)	
Neuronal injury secondary to surgery or pelvic trauma	
Aortoiliac vascular bypass	30%
Abdominoperineal resection	60%
Transurethral resection of the prostate	4%
Internal urethrotomy	1%
Pelvic fracture	50%

FIGURE 1-20. Neurogenic erectile dysfunction (ED). Central or peripheral neurologic lesions account for 20% of causes of organic erectile dysfunction. The central lesions that affect the motor parasympathetic sacral spinal cord or the peripheral efferent autonomic fibers to the penis cause partial or complete erectile dysfunction as a result of the inability of these nerves to cause relaxation of penile smooth muscle. Erections in spinal cord injury are usually short-lived, only partial, and lack rigidity due to lack of control of supraspinal erection centers. These erections cannot be used for satisfactory sexual intercourse. The degree of erectile function that persists in the patient with a spinal cord lesion depends largely on the nature, location, and extent of the spinal lesion. Reflexogenic erection is preserved in 95% of patients with complete upper cord lesions, but only in about 25% of those with complete lower cord lesions [41]. Peripheral lesions include those produced by neuropathy and radical pelvic surgery. Polysensory neuropathies occasionally cause subtle erectile dysfunction. BC—bulbocavernosus; LMN—lower motor neuron; NPT—nocturnal penile tumescence; UMN—upper motor neuron.

Endocrinologic Erectile Dysfunction

States causing hypogonadotropic hypogonadism (decreased luteinizing hormone and follicle-stimulating hormone)
- GnRH deficiency
  - Hypothalamic lesions (*eg,* tumors, encephalitis, granulomas, craniopharyngioma)
  - Isolated GnRH deficiency (idiopathic; associated with Kallmann syndrome or fertile eunuch syndrome)
  - Prader-Willi syndrome
  - Laurence-Moon-Biedl syndrome
  - Alstrom's syndrome
  - Familial cerebellar syndrome
  - Hyperprolactinemia
  - Hemochromatosis
  - Neurosarcoid
  - Myotonic dystrophy
- Pituitary disorders (gonadotrophin deficiency)
  - Isolated luteinizing hormone deficiency (*eg,* Pasqualini syndrome; eunuchoidism, absent secondary sexual characteristics, oligospermia)
  - Tumors (functional and nonfunctional)
  - Pituitary infarction
  - Pituitary apoplexy
  - Empty sella syndrome
  - Hemochromatosis

States causing hypergonadotropic hypogonadism (increased luteinizing hormone and follicle-stimulating hormone)
- Testicular disorders (primary gonadal failure)
  - Undescended testes
  - Acquired bilateral torsion of testes
  - Orchitis
  - Seminiferous tubule dysgenesis (Klinefelter's syndrome)
  - Pure gonadal dysgenesis (46XX and 46XY)
  - Sweyer's syndrome; phenotypic female with gonads and genitalia identical to gonadal dysgenesis
  - Noonan (Bonnevie-Ullrich) syndrome
  - Hemochromatosis
  - Impaired Leydig cell activity
    - Inborn errors of testosterone biosynthesis
      - P-450c 3β-hydroxysteroid dehydrogenase (male or female pseudohermaphroditism and adrenal insufficiency)
      - P-450c 17α-hydroxylase (male pseudohermaphroditism, hypogonadism sexual infantilism, hypertension and hypokalemic alkalosis)
      - P-450scc (17,20-desmolase) deficiency
      - P-450c 17β-hydroxysteroid oxidoreductase (17 KS reductase) deficiency
    - Leydig cell hypoplasia
    - Testicular unresponsiveness (? luteinizing hormone receptor failure)
    - Androgen-resistant states and enzyme defects:
      - Testicular feminization (absence of androgen receptors)
      - Incomplete androgen insensitivity (Reiffenstein's syndrome)
      - 5α-reductase deficiency (pseudovaginal perineal scrotal hypospadius/familial incomplete male pseudohermaphroditism)

States causing hyperprolactinemia (incidence 1% to 5%)
- Hypothalamic disease
  - Tumors (craniopharyngioma), granulomas (sarcoidosis; histiocytosis X; tuberculoma)
- Pituitary disorders
  - Tumors
    - Functioning: microadenoma or macroadenoma, acromegaly
    - Nonfunctioning (pseudoprolactinoma]): stalk section (surgical, traumatic, meningioma)
- Drugs
  - Drugs may cause hyperprolactinemia secondary to either diminished synthesis or release of dopamine. In addition, certain drugs (α-methyldopamine and reserpine) are capable of depleting the central dopamine stores. Others block dopamine receptors, such as phenothiazine (*eg,* chlorpromazine), butyrophenones (haloperidol), and benzamide (metoclopramide, sulpiride, and domperidone). Metoclopramide, amoxapine, verapamil, cocaine, cimetidine, and opioids block the effect of endogenous dopamine and thus release lactotrophs from their hypothalamic inhibition.
- **Miscellaneous disorders**
  - Primary hypothyroidism
  - Diabetes
  - Chronic renal failure
  - Cirrhosis
  - Chest wall lesions (neurogenic mechanisms)
  - Stress
  - Idiopathic

Miscellaneous
- Systemic disease
  - Liver diseases (25% incidence of alcoholic cirrhosis with nonalcoholic liver cirrhosis and 75% incidence of erectile dysfunction with alcoholic cirrhosis)
  - Thyroid diseases (2% incidence of erectile dysfunction)
  - Chronic renal failure
  - Diabetes (60% incidence of erectile dysfunction)
  - Sickle disease
  - Sickle cell anemia (trait and disease)
  - Nutritional disorders (protein malnutrition, zinc deficiency)
  - Estrogen excess
- Autoimmune diseases
  - AIDS (autonomic neuropathy and hormonal)
  - Polyglandular autoimmune syndrome (multiple endocrine failure)

FIGURE 1-21. Endocrinologic erectile dysfunction (ED). The major endocrinologic disorders associated with impotence are hypogonadotropic hypogonadism, hypergonadotropic hypogonadism, and hyperprolactinemia [42]. In these disorders, the serum testosterone is abnormally low. Hyperprolactinemia is associated with low circulating testosterone levels, which appear to be secondary to the inhibition of normal gonadotropin-releasing hormone (GnRH) pulsation by elevated prolactin. Erectile complaints also may be associated with both the hyperthyroid and hypothyroid states. Hyperthyroid states commonly are associated with diminished libido and, less often, with ED. Impotence has been reported in hypothyroid states and may be secondary to associated low testosterone secretion and elevated prolactin levels.

ARTERIOGENIC ERECTILE DYSFUNCTION

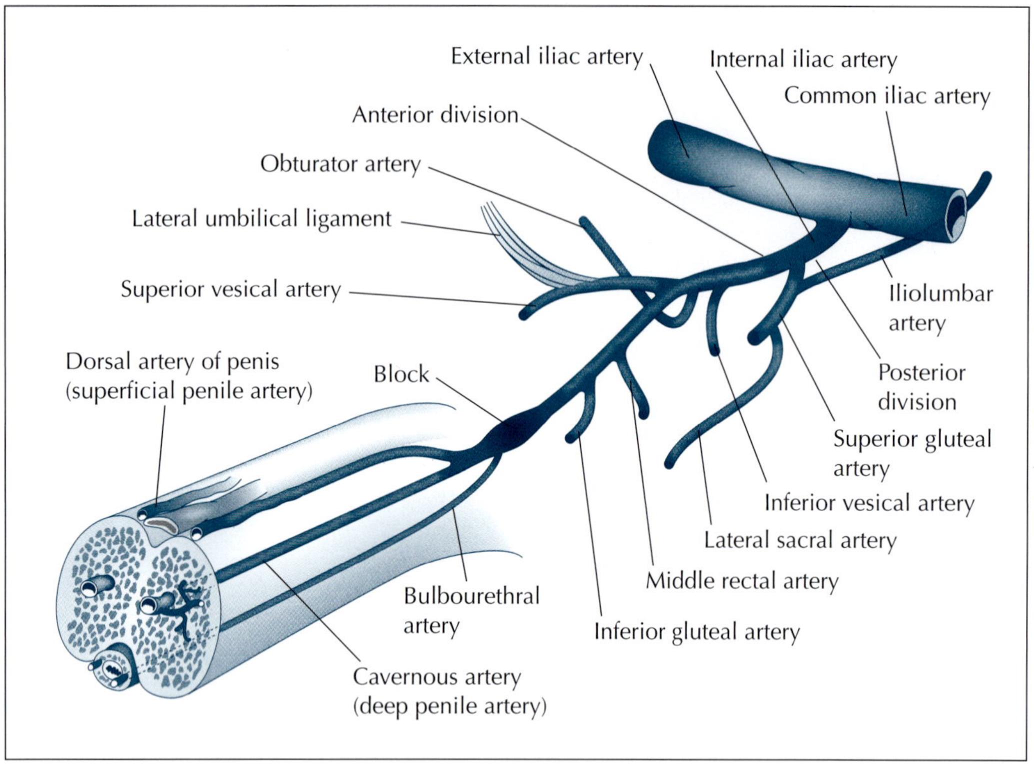

FIGURE 1-22. Arterial erectile dysfunction (ED). Atherosclerotic or traumatic arterial occlusive disease of the hypogastric-cavernous arterial bed can decrease the perfusion pressure and arterial flow to the lacunar spaces, thus decreasing the rigidity of the erect penis and the time to maximum erection, respectively. Common risk factors associated with arterial insufficiency include hypertension, hyperlipidemia, cigarette smoking, diabetes mellitus, blunt perineal or pelvic trauma and pelvic irradiation [39,43]. Arteriogenic ED can be suspected clinically by loss of spontaneity, constant diminished rigidity, difficulty maintaining erection, and morning erection often more rigid than erotic erection. Arteriographic signs of significant penile vascular occlusion include 1) delay in filling of cavernosal arteries compared to other penile vessels; 2) abrupt termination of arteries, particularly in the perineal segment of the penile artery; 3) late collateral filling; 4) retrograde filling of the cavernous artery from the dorsal artery; and 5) nicking, bending, or narrowing of the deep penile or cavernous artery and tributaries.

VENOGENIC ERECTILE DYSFUNCTION

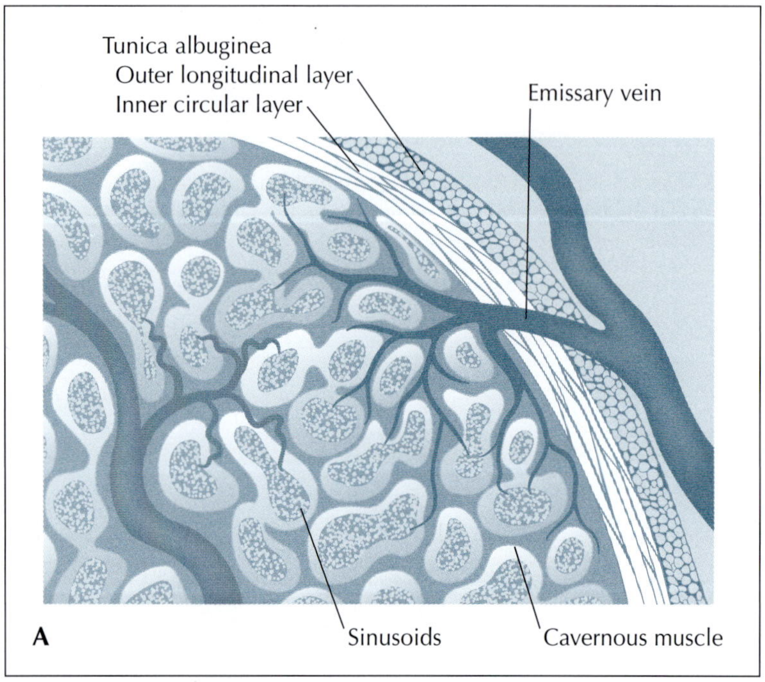

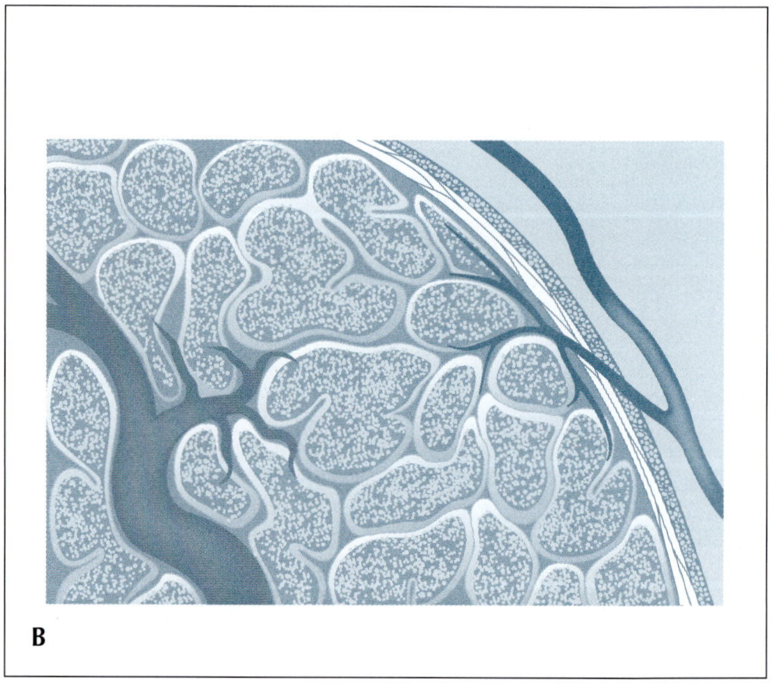

FIGURE 1-23. Venogenic erectile dysfunction. The erectile tissue of the corpus cavernosum is capable of considerable enlargement in both length and girth. Erection depends on the relaxing capabilities of the smooth muscle and on tissue expandability. **A,** Flaccid state. Impotent patients may have adequate arterial inflow to the penis but excessive outflow through the subtunical venules (*ie*, the corporal veno-occlusive mechanism is not functional). The perfusion pressure, although adequate, cannot compensate for the unrestricted outflow, so that adequate penile rigidity cannot be attained. **B,** Erection state. Veno-occlusive dysfunction may be primary or secondary, resulting from 1) large venous channels draining the corpora cavernosa; 2) degenerative changes in the tunica albuginea; 3) inadequate corporal smooth muscle relaxation; or 4) acquired venous shunts. (*Adapted from* Lue [44].)

Pharmacogenic Erectile Dysfunction

Medication	*Erectile Dysfunction*
Antidepressants	Decreased libido, ED, and ejaculatory inhibition The serotoninergic and anticholinergic properties of the heterocyclic antidepressant have been implicated. Serotonin antagonists (*eg,* cyproheptadine) and cholinergics (*eg,* bethanechol) have been reported to restore function.
Antipsychotics (neuroleptics)	Decreased libido, ED, and ejaculatory inhibition with or without priapism Neuroleptics decrease libido due to hyperprolactinemia resulting from dopamine receptor antagonism in the pituitary and hypothalamus, although other factors such as weight gain, central nervous system sedation, parkinsonism, and psychomotor retardation also may contribute. ED and ejaculatory impairment also are characteristic of those neuroleptics with high anticholinergic and α-adrenergic activity (lack of emission or erectile dysfunction, and they also may be associated with priapism).
Antihypertensives	These drugs induce impotence either by actions at the central level or peripheral level (α-adrenergic receptor agonists, *eg,* clonidine, have a 4% to 41% incidence of ED). Methyl-dopa (25% to 30% incidence of ED) acts by depleting neurotransmitters (plus increased prolactin, sedation, depression), by direct actions at the corporal level (intracellular calcium channel regulation), or by dropping the systemic blood pressure (reduced perfusion pressure) on which the patient has relied to maintain an intracorporal pressure sufficient for development of penile rigidity.
Diuretics	Diuretics alone rarely cause sexual disturbance. Spironolactone blocks testosterone synthesis and competitively binds to androgen receptor. Thiazide is a common cause of impotence. Hydrochlorothiazide (9%), bendrofluazide (36%), and spironolactone (4% to 30%) may cause decreased libido, gynecomastia, and mastodynia.
Cardiovascular drugs	The effect of digoxin is caused by elevated levels of estrogen and reduced levels of testosterone due to the similarity of chemical structure of digoxin and that of sex steroids. Digoxin induces erectile difficulties by blocking the Na-K-ATPase pump resulting in a net increase in intracellular calcium and subsequent increased tone in the corporal smooth muscle. Disopyramide: effect through potent anticholinergic activity Antihyperlipidemic drugs enhance hepatic metabolism of androgens Propranolol (at high doses) may impair libido and cause ED. The incidence is lower with atenolol. Note: ACE inhibitors (captopril, enalapril) and calcium channel blockers (verapamil) do not appear to cause significant erectile problems. Laboratory studies have demonstrated that α-blocking agents such as terazosin and doxazosin, ACE inhibitors such as enalapril, and calcium channel blockers such as nifedipine actually increase erectile function, both in vivo and in vitro.
Drugs of abuse	Alcohol: chronic use leads abnormal endocrine function due to increased aromatization of androgen, development of a peripheral autonomic neuropathy, and behavioral changes. Acute use leads to behavioral changes and temporary dysfunction that may be related to dopamine. Tobacco: causes vasoconstriction, endothelial damage, and reduced penile blood flow, and blocks corporal smooth muscle relaxation, thus preventing normal venous occlusion. Cocaine: causes diffuse arteriosclerotic changes in the arterial bed due to endothelial toxicity. Chronic use of cocaine and amphetamine indirectly increases α-adrenergic activity.
H_2 blockers	Cimetidine decreases libido and causes impotence in 50% of patients through antiandrogen activity, elevation of serum prolactin (gynecomastia), and blocking of androgen receptors. Peripheral H_2 receptor blockage acts at cavernosal smooth muscle level. Ranitidine causes prolactin secretion, loss of libido, and ED, but less commonly than cimetidine. Famotidine causes ED less than either cimetidine or ranitidine.
Antiandrogens	Antiandrogens block androgen synthesis. Finasteride has a 5% incidence of ED. Estrogen, spironolactone, ketoconazole, and digoxin lower serum testosterone.
Miscellaneous drugs	Metoclopramide affects the central nervous system dopamine receptor antagonist, which is similar to the way in which neuroleptics lead to hyperprolactinemia. Anticonvulsants increase hepatic enzyme induction, leading to increased androgen metabolism. Opioid effects are dose-related by alteration of testosterone level. Nonsteroidal anti-inflammatory agents (*eg,* indomethacin) inhibit prostaglandin formation. Barbiturates increase hepatic P-450 microsomal enzyme induction, increasing the metabolism of hormones.

FIGURE 1-24. Pharmacologic erectile dysfunction (ED). Drugs that interfere with hormonal, monoaminergic, adrenergic, and cholinergic mechanisms often are associated with impaired sexual desire, arousal, or ejaculation. In general, drugs that potentiate the action of dopamine or antagonize serotonin have stimulatory effects, whereas those that enhance serotoninergic activity or diminish dopaminergic activity interfere with sexual functions. Noradrenergic pathways in the brain may exert an inhibitory influence on penile erection. Inhibition of adrenergic activity in the central nervous system appears to depress male sexual behavior. Drug regimens that increase peripheral adrenergic tone have been reported to cause erectile failure, whereas those that decrease postsynaptic α1-adrenergic receptor activity are associated with reports of priapism. Drugs that have adrenergic or cholinergic actions commonly impair ejaculatory functions in older men. Some patients are more vulnerable because of contributing factors such as vascular or neurologic disease and hormonal disorders. ACE—angiotensin-converting enzyme; ATPase—adenosine triphosphatase; K—potassium; Na—sodium.

A. Iatrogenic Erectile Dysfunction

Trauma or surgery that interferes with the neurovascular supply to the penis
- Surgical procedures in proximity to the spinal cord
  - RPLND
  - Aortoiliac reconstruction
- Pelvic trauma
- Pelvic irradiation
- Radical or simple prostatectomies
- Transurethral procedures, *eg*, TURP

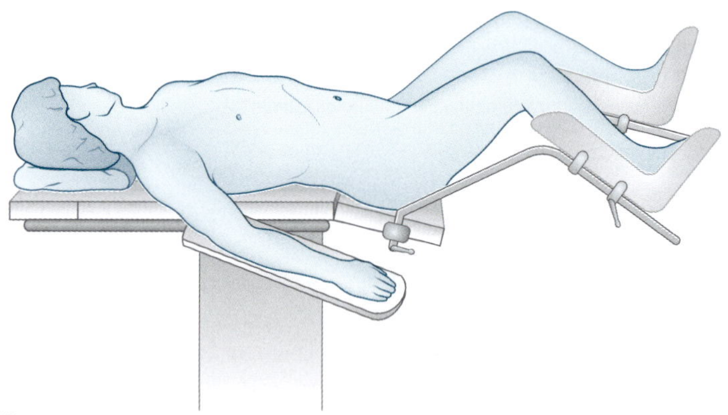

B

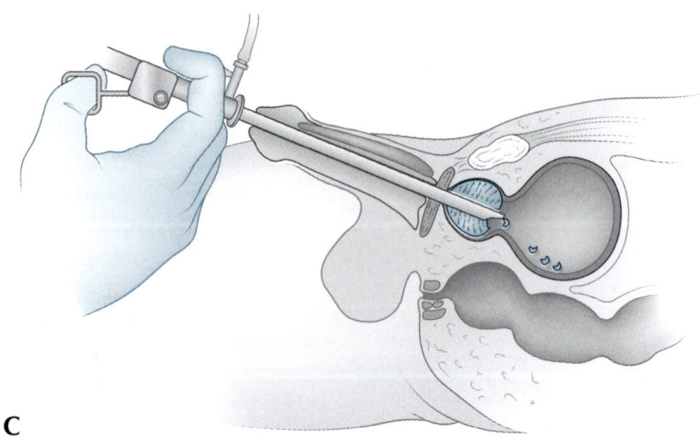

C

FIGURE 1-25. Iatrogenic erectile dysfunction (ED). Trauma or surgery that affects the neurovascular supply to the penis may result in ED (**A**). Surgical procedures in proximity to the spinal cord such as retroperitoneal lymph node dissection (RPLND) or aortoiliac reconstruction may also cause ED. Other iatrogenic etiologies of ED include pelvic trauma or irradiation and more commonly urologic surgery. Radical prostatectomy (**B**) may jeopardize the neurovascular bundle to the penis. The nerve-sparing procedure has been popularized to minimize inadvertent injury to the branches of the pelvic plexus innervating the corporal cavernosa. Transurethral procedures (**C**) are also associated with ED, because the nerves are located in the 5 and 7 o'clock positions in the prostatic urethra, 3 and 6 o'clock positions in the membranous urethra, and 11 and 1 o'clock positions in the penile urethra.

Specific Conditions Most Commonly Associated with Erectile Dysfunction

Condition	*Basis of Erectile Dysfunction*
Diabetes	Psychogenic
	Neurogenic (loss of fibers)
	Arterial (small vessel disease as well as atherosclerosis)
	Venous (myopathy leading to veno-occlusive dysfunction)
	Endothelial dysfunction
	Hormonal
Peyronie's disease	Loss of elastin
	Increased collagen formation
	Venocorporal dysfunction
Aging	Gradual decrease in desire and erectile response to penile sensitivity
	More dependent on direct physical stimulation
	Less responsive to visual psychologic stimulation
	Reduced duration and intensity of orgasm
	Prolonged refractory period
	Reduced force of emission and ejaculation
Uremia	Arterial (atherosclerosis)
	Neurologic (peripheral neuropathy)
	Psychologic (added stress and depression)
	Medication (hypertension medication)
	Endocrine (hyperprolactinemia, hypogonadism, hyperparathyroidism)
Alcoholism	Acute use: behavioral changes (central nervous system depression) and temporary ED possibly related to dopamine
	Chronic use: abnormal endocrine function as a result of increased androgen aromatization; development of peripheral neuropathy; behavioral and psychiatric changes
AIDS	Neuropathy (autonomic)
	Hormonal (hypogonadotropic hypogonadism, secondary defect in the hypothalamic-pituitary axis)

FIGURE 1-26. Conditions most commonly associated with erectile dysfunction (ED). This list of diseases associated with ED presents the physiologic or pathologic case of the erectile failure at the end organ.

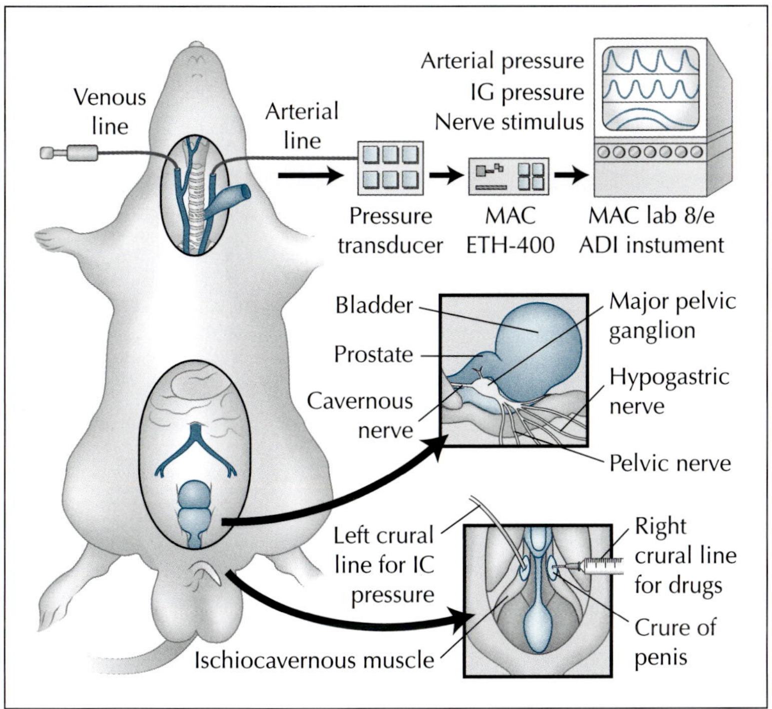

FIGURE 1-27. In vivo rat model. Diabetes has been the disease that is studied the most in animal models as a marker for erectile dysfunction (ED), and the classic method of inducing diabetes in an animal model is through the use of streptozotocin (STZ). This figure illustrates the experimental procedure. The rat is anesthesized and lying in supine position. An arterial line in the left carotid artery is connected to a data-acquisition board via a transducer and transducer amplifier for continuous monitoring of blood pressure. A right external jugular venous line is used for intravenous fluid administration and blood sampling. The prostate is exposed through a low midline incision. The *top inset* demonstrates the cavernous nerves that can be seen on the posterolateral surface of the prostate arising from the pelvic ganglion that is formed by joining of the hypogastric and pelvic nerves. The *bottom inset* shows the two corpora that have been exposed via inguinoscrotal incisions on both sides and degloving of the penis. A line is inserted into the right corpus for continuous monitoring of intracorporal pressure. Another line is placed in the left corpus for intravenous drug injection. Finally, current stimulation is delivered via a nerve stimulator probe placed around the cavernous nerve. (*Adapted from* Rehman *et al.* [45].)

A. Aging and Erectile Dysfunction

Aging-associated factors that can contribute to ED
- Decreased testosterone level
- Decreased elastin fiber concentration
- Decreased smooth muscle content
- Decreased corporal cavernosum compliance
- Decreased vibrotactile sensation
- Decreased cavernosal arterial inflow
- Decreased libido
- Increased medical comorbidities
  - Increased cardiovascular risk
  - Increased diabetes mellitus
  - Depression
  - Increased benign prostatic hyperplasia, prostate cancer
    - Increased urologic surgeries
- Possibly decreased nitric oxide and synthase activity
- Possibly partner availability

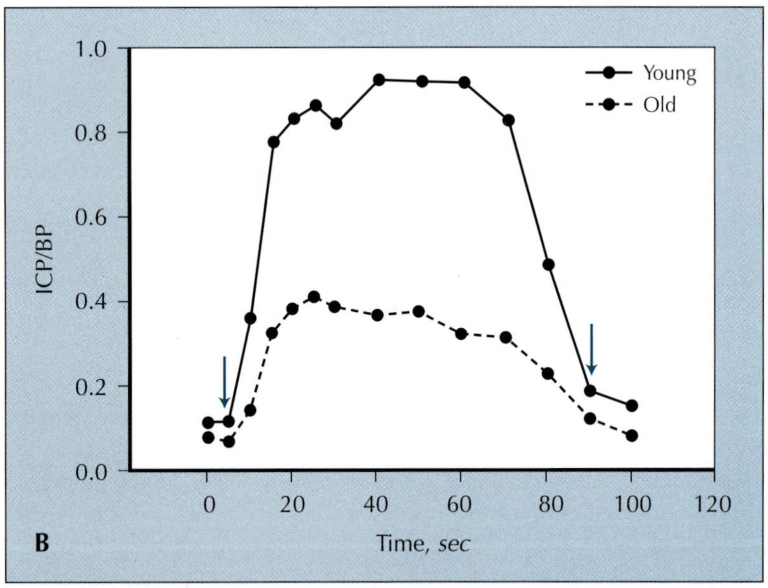

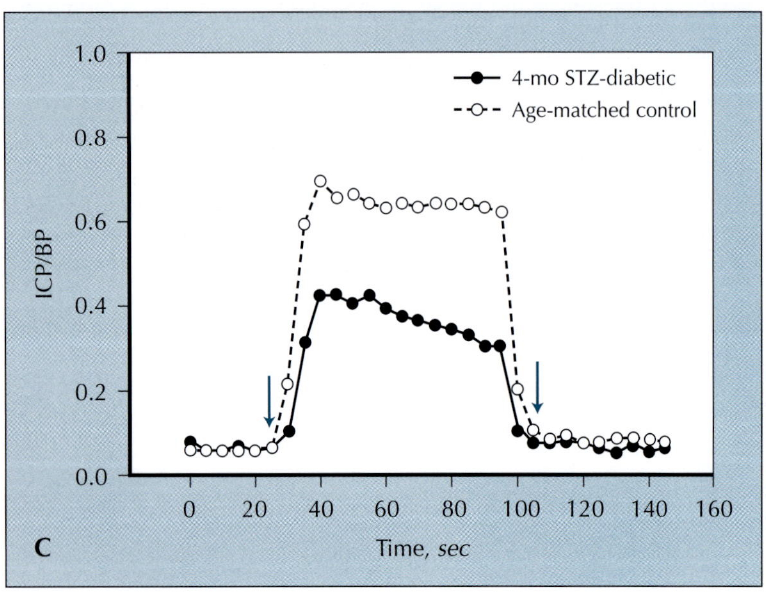

FIGURE 1-28. Aging and erectile dysfunction (ED). **A,** While men of any age may be afflicted with ED, the disease is more common in the elderly. A decrease in libido may contribute to ED in these men. Because the highest desired frequency of coitus is in the late teens, men in their 70s and 80s may only want to be sexually active once or twice per month. Elderly patients afflicted with chronic disease and depression may also have diminished libido. As men age, the hormonal milieu may be altered adversely, including a decrease in serum testosterone level. Significant structural changes also occur in the penis; for example, penile elastic fibers and smooth muscle content decrease with age along with alteration in the type I and III collagen ratio. The corporal bodies ultimately becomes less compliant and veno-occlusive dysfunction may also be encountered. Aging is also commonly associated with medical diseases such as renal disease and artherosclerosis, which can adversely affect blood flow to the penis [46].

B and **C,** Intracavernous pressure (ICP) changes during cavernous nerve stimulation. Representative examples of how both age and experimental diabetes mellitus are associated with a significant diminution in erectile function/capacity in vivo in the rat model. In both cases, experiments were conducted as described elsewhere [45,47,48]. These examples show the time course of the intracorporeal pressure (ICP) response to 2 (age diagram) or 4 mA (diabetes diagram) stimulation of the cavernous nerve. The *arrows* indicate when the neurostimulation was turned on and off. The old rat was a retired breeder that weighed more than 600 g and was approximately 15 months old. The young rat was approximately 12 weeks old. For the diabetes study, the rat shown was subjected to a single intraperitoneal injection of streptozotocin (35 mg/kg) and remained diabetic for 4 months prior to being studied. BP—blood pressure.

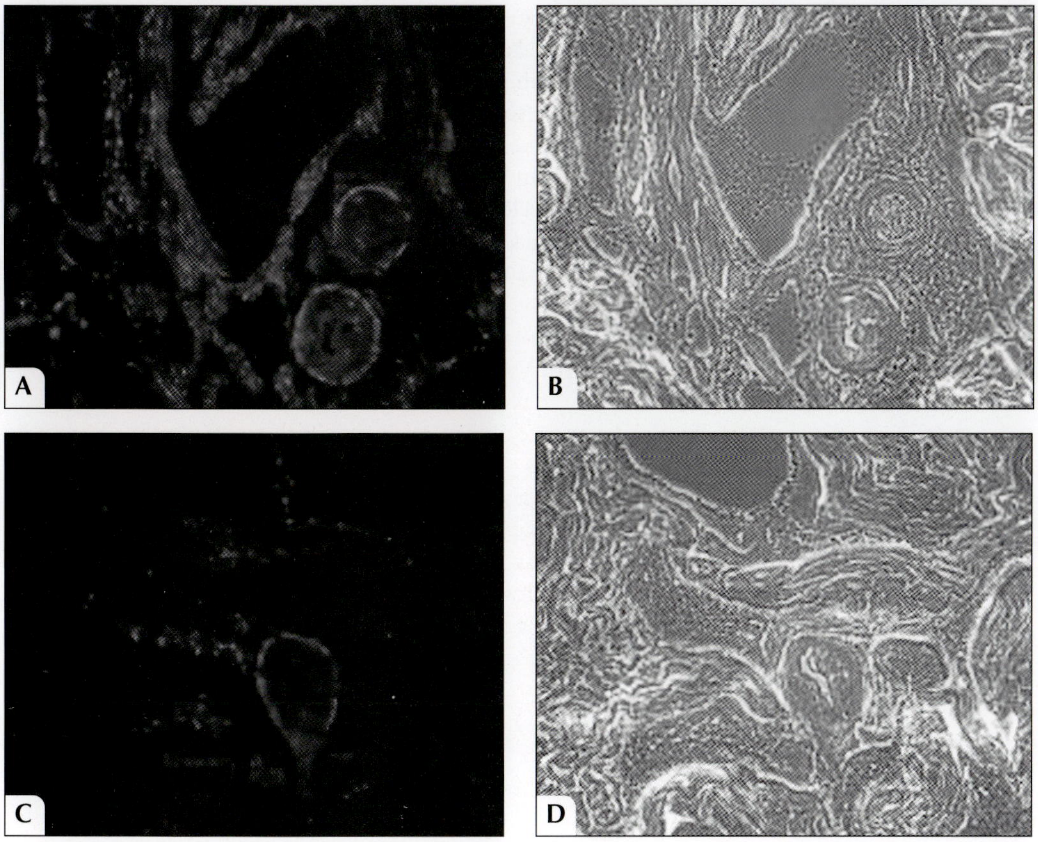

FIGURE 1-29. (*See Color Plate*) Streptozotocin (STZ)-diabetic corporal histology. Photomicrographs of immunohistochemical stain for synaptophysin (**A** and **C**) and phase-contrast images of the same sections of corporal tissue (**B** and **D**) from an age-matched control rat (**A** and **B**) and an 8-week STZ-diabetic rat (**C** and **D**). The sections were examined with a Nikon epifluorescence microscope with conventional optics. Images were stored on a pentium computer (200 × magnification). Note the obvious reduction in synaptophysin immunostaining in diabetic rat corpora, although not all rat corporal tissue at this time displayed such dramatic changes. These observations further emphasize the utility of the proposed integrative approach [45].

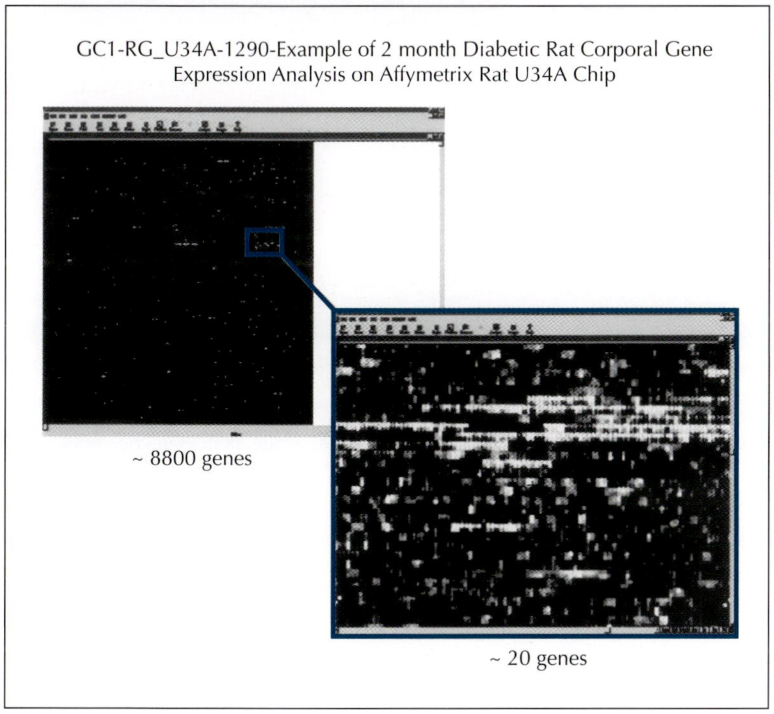

FIGURE 1-30. Microarrays. Representative gene expression analysis of diabetic rat corpora. The animals in this study were made diabetic for 2 months via a single intraperitoneal injection of streptozotocin [45]. As previously demonstrated, there is a significant decrease in the cavernous nerve stimulated intracavernous pressure response (ICP) in these animals, and not surprisingly, a host of gene alterations are observed. These data represent a work in progress, but it is clear that such analyses, when coupled with functional studies in vivo, will eventually permit a "molecular profile" of the diabetic state (or any other disease state for that matter) to be established. Such molecular profiles will be extremely useful for the improved pharmacotherapy of erectile dysfunction, as it will, at least in theory, permit the physician (urologist) to select a mechanism-based, patient-specific treatment modality. This particular Affymetrix (Affymetrix Inc., Santa Clara, CA) chip is capable of simultaneously evaluating the expression of more than 8000 genes. More robust chips are on the way, but this example clearly makes the point. Approximately 10% of these genes showed evidence of altered expression in this experiment. (The authors are grateful to Dr. Kelvin Davies for helping with the preparation of this figure.)

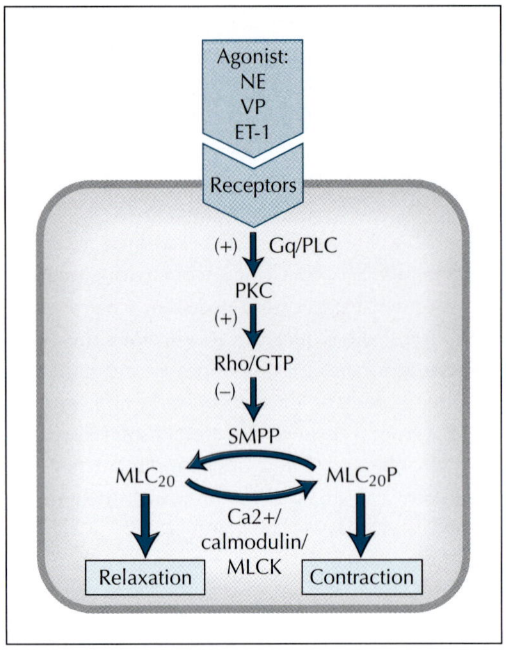

FIG 1-31. Rho-kinase.This diagram shows the calcium sensitization/Rho kinase pathway in corporal smooth muscle. Illustrated are the series of steps involved in myosin phosphorylation, as well as the subsequent regulation of myosin light chain phosphorylation by the Rho-kinase pathway. In this diagram, the *plus sign* denotes a stimulatory effect; the *minus sign* denotes an inhibitory effect. Note that inhibition of phosphatase by Rho-kinase is logically thought to be very high in the flaccid state. This scenario would be required to maintain the phosphorylated state of myosin, and thereby ensure tonic contraction of corporal smooth muscle in the presence of near-resting levels of intracellular calcium. G_q—subtype of the heteromeric G protein that couples receptor activation to Rho kinase activation; MLC20—myosin light chain; MLCK—myosin light chain kinase; SMPP—smooth muscle myosin phosphatase.

REFERENCES

1. Hinman F, Jr.: *Atlas of Urosurgical Anatomy*. Philadelphia: WB Saunders Co.; 1993.
2. Melman A, Gingell JC: The epidemiology and pathophysiology of erectile dysfunction. *J Urol* 1999, 161:5–11.
3. Melman A, Rehman J: Pathophysiology of erectile dysfunction. *Molecular Urology* 1999, 3:87–102.
4. Christ G J, Brink PR, Melman A, *et al.*: The role of gap junctions and ion channels in the modulation of electrical and chemical signals in human corpus cavernosum smooth muscle. *Int J Impot* 1993, 5:77–96.
5. Christ G J, Brink PR: An analysis of the presence and physiological relevance of subconducting states of connexin43-derived gap junction channels in cultured human corporal vascular smooth muscle cells. *Circ Res* 1999, 84:797–803.
6. Lagaud G, Davies KP, Venkateswarlu K, *et al.*: The physiology, pathophysiology and therapeutic potential of gap junctions in smooth muscle. *Current Drug Targets* 2002, 3:1–14.
7. Christ G J: Gap junctions and ion channels: relevance to erectile dysfunction. *Int J Impot* 2000, 12:S15–S25.
8. Venkateswarlu K, Giraldi A, Zhao W, *et al.*: Potassium channels and human corporeal smooth muscle cell tone: diabetes and relaxation of human corpus cavernosum smooth muscle by adenosine triphosphate sensitive potassium channel openers. *J Urol* 2002, 168:355–361.
9. Christ GJ: The penis as a vascular organ: the importance of corporal smooth muscle tone in the control of erection. *Urol Clin North Am* 1995, 22:727–745.
10. Palmer LS, Valcic M, Melman A, *et al.*: Characterization of cyclic AMP accumulation in cultured human corpus cavernosum smooth muscle cells. *J Urol* 1994, 152:1308–1314.
11. Trigo-Rocha F, Hsu GL, Donatucci CF, *et al.*: Intracellular mechanism of penile erection in monkeys. *Neurol Urodynamics* 1994, 13:71–80.
12. Miller MA, Morgan RJ: Eicosanoids, erections, and erectile dysfunction. *Prostaglandins Leukot Essent Fatty Acids* 1994, 51:1–9.
13. Pickard RS, Powell PH, Zar MA: Nitric oxide and cyclic GMP formation following relaxant nerve stimulation in isolated human corpus cavernosum. *Br J Urol* 1995, 75:516–522.
14. Cahn D, Melman A, Valcic M, Christ GJ: Forskolin: a promising new adjunct to intravenous pharmacotherapy. *J Urol* 1996, 155:1789–1794.
15. Christ GJ, Moreno AP, Melman AP, Spray DC: Gap junction-mediated intercellular diffusion of Ca^{2+} in cultured human corporal smooth muscle cells. *Am J Physiol* 1992, 263:C373–C383.
16. Giraldi A, Wen YP, Geliebter J, *et al.*: Differential gap junction mRNA expression in human corpus cavernosum: a significant regulatory in cell-to-cell communication? [abstract] *J Urol* 1995, 153:508A.
17. Autieri MV, Melman A, Christ GJ: Identification of a down-regulated mRNA transcript in corpus cavernosum from diabetic patients with erectile dysfunction. *Int J Impot Res* 1996, 8:69–73.
18. Anderson KE: Pharmacology of lower urinary tract smooth muscle cells and penile erectile tissues. *Pharmacol Rev* 1993, 45:253—309.
19. Fan SF, Brink PR, Melman A, Christ GJ: An analysis of the maxi-K^+ (KCa) channel in cultured human corporal smooth muscle cells. *J Urol* 1995, 153:818–825.
20. Kim N, Azadzoi KM, Goldstein I, Saenz de Tejada I: A nitric-oxidelike factor mediates nonadrenergic noncholinergic neurogenic relaxation of penile corpus cavernosum smooth muscle. *J Clin Invest* 1991, 88:112–118.
21. Ignarro LJ, Bush PA, Buga GM, *et al.*: Nitric oxide and cyclic GMP formation upon electric field stimulation cause relaxation of corpus cavernosum smooth muscle. *Biochem Biophys Res Commun* 1990, 170:843–850.
22. Rajfer J, Aronson WJ, Bush PA, *et al.*: Nitric oxide as a mediator of relaxation of the corpus cavernosum in response to nonadrenergic, noncholinergic neurotransmission. *N Engl J Med* 1992, 326:90–94.
23. Kirkeby HJ, Fahrenkrug J, Holmquist F, Ottesen B: Vasoactive intestinal polypeptide (VIP) and peptide histidine methionine (PHM) in human penile corpus cavernosum tissue and circumflex veins: localization and in vitro effects. *Eur J Clin Invest* 1992, 22:24–30.
24. Adaikan PG, Ratnam SS: Pharmacology of penile erection in humans. *Cardiovasc Intervent Radiol* 1988, 11:191–194.
25. Roy JB, Petrone RL, Said SI: A clinical trial of intracavernous vasoactive intestinal peptide to induce penile erection. *J Urol* 1990, 143:302–304.
26. Brindley GS: Pilot experiments on the actions of drugs injected into the human corpus cavernosum penis. *Br J Pharmacol* 1986, 87:495–500.
27. Loewy AD: Virus as transneuronal tracers for defining neural circuits. *Neurosci Biobehav Rev* 1998, 22:679–684.
28. Hosogai M, Matsuo S, Sibahara T, *et al.*: Projection of respiratory neurons in rat medullary raphe nuclei to the phrenic nuclei. *Respir Physiol* 1998, 112:37–50.
29. Rampin O, Giuliano F: Central control of the cardiovascular and erection systems: possible mechanisms and interactions. *Am J Cardiol* 2000, 86:19F–22F.
30. De Groat WC, Steers W: Neuroanatomy and neurophysiology of penile erection. In *Contemporary Management of Impotence and Infertility*. Edited by Tanagho E, Lue TF, McClure D. Baltimore: Williams & Wilkins; 1988.

31. De Groat WC, Booth AM: Neural control of penile erection. In *The Autonomic Nervous Control of the Urogenital System,* vol 3. Edited by Maggi CA. London: Harwood Academic Publishers; 1993:467–479.

32. Steers WD: Neural control of penile erection. *Semin Urol* 1990, 8:66–79.

33. MacLean PD, Ploog DW: Cerebral representation of penile erection. *J Neurophysiol* 1962, 25:29–55.

34. Wagner CK, Clemens LG: Projections of the paraventricular nucleus of the hypothalamus to the sexually dimorphic lumbosacral region of the spinal cord. *Brain Res* 1991, 539:254.

35. Chen K, Chan SHH, Chang CLS, Chan JYH: Participation of paraventricular nucleus of hypothalamus in central regulation of penile erection in rat. *J Urol* 1997, 158:238–244.

36. Murphy MR, Seckl JR, Burton S, *et al.*: Changes in oxytocin and vasopressin secretion during sexual activity in men. *J Clin Endocrinol Metab* 1987, 65:738–741.

37. Saenz de Tejada I, Ware JC, Blanco R, *et al.*: Pathophysiology of prolonged erection associated with trazodone use. *J Urol* 1991, 145:60–64.

38. van Ahlen H, Peichota HJ, Kias HJ, *et al.*: Opiate antagonists in erectile dysfunction: a possible new treatment option? Results of a pilot study with naltrexone. *Eur Urol* 1995, 28:246–250.

39. Feldman HA, Goldstein I, Hatzichristou D G, *et al.*: Impotence and its medical and psychosocial correlates: results of the Massachusetts Male Aging Study. *J Urol* 1994, 151:54–61.

40. Hartmann U: Psychological subtypes of erectile dysfunction: result of statistical analysis and clinical practice. *World J Urol* 1997, 15:56–64.

41. Comarr AE: Sexual function among patients with spinal cord injury. *Urol Int* 1970, 25:134–168.

42. Leonard MP, Nickel CJ, Morales A: Hyperprolactinemia and impotence: why, when, and how to investigate. *J Urol* 1989, 142:992–994.

43. Rehman J, Benet E, Melman A: *Arteriogenic Erectile Dysfunction: Evaluation and Treatment. Mediguide to Urology,* vol 8. Edited by Carson CC III. New York: Bayor Corp; 1996:1–7.

44. Lue TF: Male sexual dysfunction. In *Smith's General Urology,* edn 14. Edited by Tanagho EA, McAninch JW: Norwalk, CT:Appleton & Lange; 1994:776.

45. Rehman J, Chenven E, Brink PR, *et al.*: Diminished neurogenic but not pharmacological erections in the 2- to 3-month experimentally diabetic F-344 rat. *Am J Physiol* 1997, 272:H1960–H1971.

46. Seftel AD: Erectile dysfunction in the elderly: epidemiology, etiology and approaches to treatment. *J Urol* 2003, 169:1999–2007.

47. Christ G J, Rehman J, Day N, *et al.*: Intracorporal injection of hSlo cDNA in rats produces physiologically relevant alterations in penile function. *Am J Physiol* 1998, 275:H600–H608.

48. Melman A, Zhao W, Davies KP, *et al.*: The successful long-term treatment of age-related erectile dysfunction with hSlo cDNA in rats in vivo. *J Urol* 2003, 170:285–290.

Office Evaluation and Diagnostic Testing for Erectile Dysfunction

2

Drogo K. Montague
Milton M. Lakin

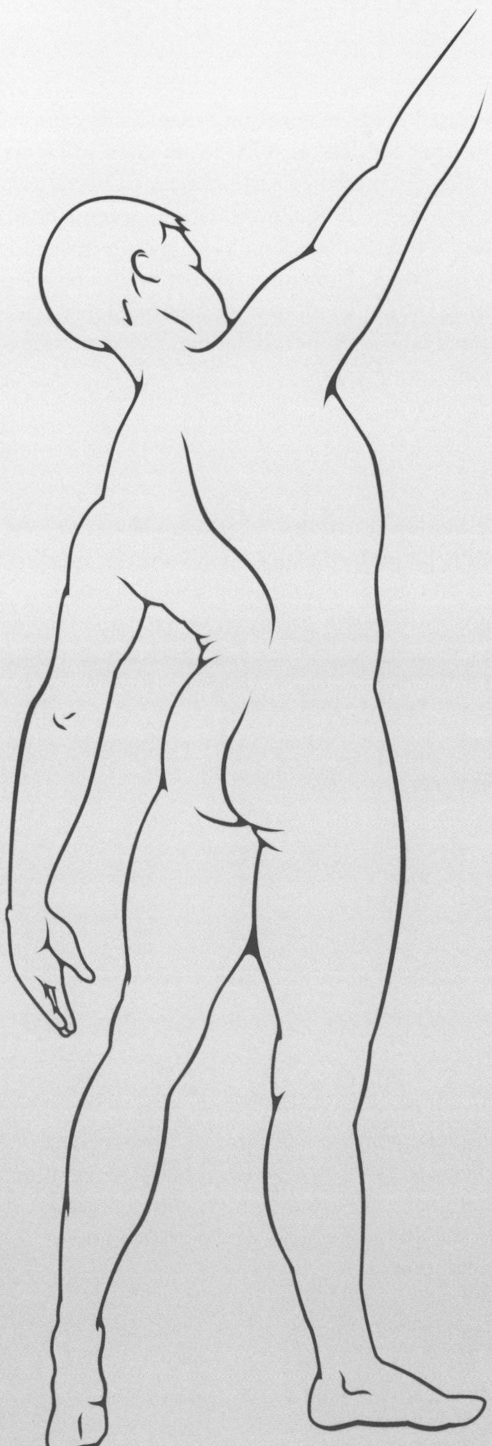

In the 1970s, treatment of erectile dysfunction (ED), the preferred term for impotence [1], was relatively simple. Sex therapy was the treatment of choice for psychogenic ED, and penile prosthesis implantation was the only reasonable treatment option for most men with organic ED. Clinical evaluation of ED was also relatively straightforward: differentiation between psychogenic and organic ED was usually made by taking a detailed sexual and medical history and by performing nocturnal penile tumescence testing.

A wide variety of treatment options are available today for ED including sex therapy, systemic therapy, vacuum constriction devices, intraurethral pharmacotherapy, penile injection therapy, penile prosthesis implantation, and penile vascular surgery. Numerous applicable diagnostic tests include nocturnal penile tumescence testing, intracavernosal test injections, duplex Doppler ultrasonography of the penile arteries, cavernosometry, and penile arteriography.

In 1990, Lue [2] introduced the concept of the "patient's goal-directed therapy" for ED. In this era of cost containment, Lue and many others have advocated an approach that provides the ED patient with a menu of treatment options. The patient selects the treatment option that appeals to him and his work-up is then tailored for that option. In the context of this goal-directed paradigm and in view of cost concerns, it is appropriate to ask the following questions: How much evaluation is necessary? Which tests, if any, should be performed? How valid are the current tests?

This chapter attempts to answer these questions and provides a guide for the rational use of office diagnostic testing.

RATIONALE FOR DIAGNOSTIC EVALUATION

Reasons for Diagnostic Assessment

To accurately identify the patient's complaint
To uncover significant systemic disease
To identify psychogenic ED in the patient considering surgery
The patient's need to know

FIGURE 2-1. Reasons for diagnostic assessment. In this era of specialized testing for erectile dysfunction (ED), history taking unfortunately is often abbreviated. Men presenting with an apparent chief complaint of ED actually may have premature ejaculation; because this is not correctly identified, they may undergo many unnecessary tests and treatments [3]. ED is often the presenting manifestation of a significant systemic disease, such as adult-onset diabetes mellitus [4] or atherosclerotic vascular disease. Much less often but still significantly, ED may be the first sign of a pituitary tumor [5,6]. Although differentiation between psychogenic and organic ED may not be of great importance for the patient considering nonsurgical therapy, it is paramount in one considering penile prosthesis implantation or any other form of surgical treatment. Finally, some patients want, if possible, to be given an explanation about why they have ED.

CLASSIFICATION OF MALE SEXUAL DYSFUNCTIONS

Male Sexual Dysfunctions

Decreased libido
Erectile dysfunction
  Primary
  Secondary
Ejaculatory disorders
  Premature ejaculation
  Retarded ejaculation

FIGURE 2-2. Male sexual dysfunctions. Decreased libido may be the patient's sole complaint or it may accompany erectile dysfunction (ED). Reasons for decreased libido are given in Figure 2-3. Primary ED has been lifelong (*ie,* present since first attempted coitus). Primary ED is relatively uncommon and often difficult to treat, especially if it is of long-term duration. Secondary ED presents after a well-established period of normal sexual functioning. Compared with primary ED, secondary ED is common and usually has a better prognosis. Premature ejaculation can be classified as ejaculation that occurs before intromission, during intromission, or after intromission. Men with retarded ejaculation usually have nocturnal seminal emissions and sometimes can masturbate to orgasm; however, they are unable to reach orgasm during coitus.

Reasons for Decreased Libido

Hypogonadism
Hyperprolactinemia
Depression
Relationship conflict
Secondary to erectile dysfunction
Systemic disease
Idiopathic
Medications and recreational drugs

FIGURE 2-3. Reasons for decreased libido. Libido or sexual desire has many determinants. Endocrine disorders, such as hypogonadism and hyperprolactinemia, are notable for causing decreased sexual desire [6]. Decreased libido is a prominent feature in men with depression [7]. In couples with a relationship conflict, an avoidance pattern with decreased sexual desire may develop [7]. Moreover, men who develop erectile dysfunction, for whatever reason, sometimes manifest decreased sexual desire as a result of repeated failures. Severe systemic diseases, such as chronic renal failure or hepatic failure, also are frequently associated with decreased libido. Various medications and recreational drugs have been associated with reduced sexual desire [8]. Finally, men may develop low libido for reasons that are not readily apparent.

HISTORY

Erectile Dysfunction: History Elements

Sexual history
Psychosocial assessment
Medical history

FIGURE 2-4. Elements required for a complete history of erectile dysfunction (ED). History taking should begin with the patient's chief complaint and proceed through a review of sexual systems (*see* Fig. 2-5). Figure 2-6 provides psychosocial assessment; referral for formal psychologic consultation by a sex therapist is based on the results of this assessment. Finally, a complete medical history completes this portion of the evaluation. Of all the elements in the evaluation for ED, it is our opinion that proper history taking is the most important.

Sexual History

Chief complaint and duration of problem
Onset (sudden versus gradual) and progression
Sexual review of systems
  Libido
  Erections
  Ejaculations
Previous tests and treatments
Frequency and results of current attempts

FIGURE 2-5. Elements of a complete sexual history. The patient who consults a physician for a sexual problem is invariably ill at ease. If the problem that concerns him is promptly addressed, in a straightforward manner, by a doctor who is familiar with sexual problems and their evaluation, the patient is usually reassured. The onset, progression, and duration of the patient's complaints are explored. If the chief complaint is erectile dysfunction, specific inquiry should also include questions relating to libido, orgasm, and ejaculation. Results of previous tests and treatment should be discussed and an assessment of current sexual functioning should be made.

Psychosocial Assessment

Formal psychologic consultation is usually indicated when any of the following exist:
  Relationship conflict
  Drug or alcohol abuse
  Psychiatric disorder
  Hypochondriasis
  Litigious personality
  Psychogenic dysfunction

FIGURE 2-6. Psychosocial assessment. It is our opinion that not every man with erectile dysfunction needs a formal psychologic evaluation. However, history taking should explore the elements listed in this figure; consultation with a sex therapist is often indicated when any of these elements are present.

Sexual History in Erectile Dysfunction

Onset and duration of problem
  Sudden
  Gradual
Erections
  Situationally present
    Morning
    Nocturnal
    With masturbation
    With different partners
  Globally decreased or absent
  Quality of best erection
    Duration
    Rigidity
    Self-rating on scale of 0 to 10

FIGURE 2-7. Sexual history in erectile dysfunction. In the absence of a known precipitating event, such as trauma or pelvic surgery, sudden onset of erectile dysfunction suggests a psychogenic etiology. Erections that are normal under some circumstances but not others generally indicate a psychogenic cause. Erectile rigidity and its duration should be recorded based on the patient's self-rating. Pain with erection or erectile deformity should, when present, be recorded.

Medical History

Medical illnesses
Operations
Trauma
Radiation therapy
Medications
Alcohol and illicit drugs
Smoking
Sleep disorders

FIGURE 2-8. Elements of a complete medical history. Because erectile dysfunction (ED) often results from many diverse disease processes and circumstances, obtaining a complete medical and surgical history including all major or chronic illnesses and operations is important. Surgical treatment for carcinoma of the bladder, prostate, and rectum frequently causes erectile and ejaculatory dysfunction. Trauma to the back, spinal cord, pelvis, genitalia, and perineum are all potentially important. Radiation therapy, especially to the pelvis, should be noted. Drugs, prescribed and illicit, may be associated with ED, as are alcohol and smoking. A sleep disorder, often associated with ED, may be present in the man who has a history of excessive daytime sleepiness, loud snoring, sleep apnea, obesity, or hypertension. Diseases associated with endothelial dysfunction such as hypertension, hypercholesterolemia, diabetes mellitus, peripheral vascular disease, and cigarette smoking should be noted. Neurologic disorders such as stroke, multiple sclerosis, and Parkinson's disease also may play a role in ED.

PHYSICAL EXAMINATION

General Physical Examination
General appearance, affect
Blood pressure
Secondary sex characteristics
Gynecomastia
Abdominal examination
Peripheral pulses

FIGURE 2-9. General physical examination. The general physical examination places special emphasis on the items listed in this table. How does the patient look? Is he apparently healthy or does he appear chronically ill? Does he appear anxious or depressed? Hypertension is a significant risk factor in the development of vascular disease; any examination for erectile dysfunction should include blood pressure determination. Long-standing hypogonadism may produce abnormal secondary sex characteristics, such as diminished axillary and pubic hair or gynecomastia. Abdominal examination should look for, among other things, hepatomegaly, abdominal aortic bruit or aneurysm, and masses. Carotid, femoral, and lower extremity peripheral pulses should be examined.

Genital and Rectal Examinations
Circumcision status
Penile plaques
Corporeal induration
Penile stretch
Testicular size and consistency
Rectal sphincter tone
Prostatic examination

FIGURE 2-10. Genital and rectal examinations. Note whether the patient is circumcised. If not, the presence of phimosis or balanitis should be noted. The surface of the corporeal bodies should be examined for plaque; occasionally we find this even in men who are not complaining of erectile deformity. Both corpora should be compressed from a dorsal to ventral direction to identify induration that suggests the presence of corporeal fibrosis. The amount of stretch in the flaccid penis should be noted; this correlates best with erect length after intracavernosal injection [9] and after penile prosthesis implantation. Decreased testicular size and consistency may indicate hypogonadism. On rectal examination, anal sphincter tone and size and consistency of the prostate must be noted.

Neurologic Examination
Gait
Motor and sensory examinations
Deep tendon reflexes
Lower back, gluteal cleft examination
Bulbocavernosus reflex
Saddle sensation

FIGURE 2-11. Neurologic examination. The patient's gait should be examined; a foot drop or duck waddling gait suggests motor impairment to lower extremity muscles. Motor and sensory examinations of the lower extremities are performed; knee and ankle deep-tendon reflexes are also examined. An abnormal gluteal cleft or the presence of a dimple or nevus at the top of the gluteal cleft may suggest the presence of spinal dysraphism. Perineal (saddle) sensation should be determined. Normal sphincter tone detected during the rectal examination alerts the examiner to the presence of the bulbocavernosus reflex.

LABORATORY (BLOOD AND URINE) TESTS

Laboratory Tests
CBC
Kidney/liver profile
Lipid profile
Hemoglobin A1C
PSA
Testosterone
Prolactin
Urinalysis

FIGURE 2-12. Laboratory tests for erectile dysfunction (ED). A complete blood count (CBC), kidney/liver profile, and urinalysis are ordered to help detect occult systemic disease. Because atherosclerotic vascular disease is a leading cause of ED, obtaining a lipid profile may also be in order. ED may be the presenting manifestation of adult onset diabetes mellitus; hemoglobin A1C determination helps evaluate this possibility. A serum prostate specific antigen (PSA) should be drawn if the man is in the appropriate age range for prostate carcinoma screening. Serum testosterone should be determined because hypogonadism can be detected by physical examination only when it is long-standing. Serum prolactin should also be determined because hyperprolactinemia may also be associated with ED.

Intracavernosal Drugs Used for Erectile Dysfunction Testing

Papaverine
Papaverine and phentolamine
Prostaglandin E_1
Prostaglandin E_1 and phentolamine
Papaverine, phentolamine, and prostaglandin E_1

FIGURE 2-13. Intracavernosal drugs used for erectile dysfunction testing. The drugs listed here are injected intracavernosally either singly or in combination and used diagnostically alone or together with other procedures, such as duplex ultrasonography or cavernosometry.

Diagnostic Intracavernous Injection

Diagnostic injection alone
- Plus manual stimulation [10]
- Plus visual sexual stimulation [11]
- Plus visual sexual and manual stimulation

FIGURE 2-14. Diagnostic intracavernous injection. A diagnostic intracavernous injection is probably the most frequently performed test for erectile dysfunction (ED) and is also useful in assessing the degree of curvature in men with congenital curvature or acquired curvature due to Peyronie's disease. If a man obtains a full, well-sustained erection in response to the injection of a vasoactive drug or drug mixture (*see* Fig. 2-13) alone or in combination with manual or visual sexual stimulation, his ED may be psychogenic, neurogenic, or mildly vasculogenic. However, if he fails to respond with a normal erection, nothing at all can be said about his ED. Anxiety mediated through the sympathetic nervous system may prevent complete cavernosal smooth muscle relaxation, thus causing a falsely abnormal test [3,12].

Duplex Doppler Ultrasonography of Penile Arteries

Intracavernosal injection of vasoactive drug(s)
Ultrasonic imaging of penile arteries
Doppler determination of:
- Arterial wave forms
- Peak systolic velocities
- End diastolic velocities

FIGURE 2-15. Duplex Doppler ultrasonography of penile arteries. This test not only images the penile arteries but does so during the development of an erection. It also determines the velocity of blood flow through these vessels. Thus, it is a dynamic study and the most useful test to evaluate penile arterial status. Peak systolic velocities in men with normal erections range from 32.9 cm/s in men 70 to 79 years of age to 53.7 cm/s in men 20 to 29 years of age [13]. Peak systolic velocities are used as an indirect measurement of arterial function and need to be reported with time after injection. With development of an adequate erection, peak systolic velocity decreases. The degree of erection produced by the injection must be recorded. It has been suggested that high-end diastolic velocities indicate corporovenous occlusive dysfunction [14]. However, the failure to achieve complete cavernous smooth muscle relaxation after vasoactive drug injection, which often results from anxiety, makes this portion of the examination much less certain.

Dynamic Infusion Cavernosometry and Cavernosography

Intracavernosal injection of vasoactive drugs
Infusion of normal saline to obtain a full erection
Determination of maintenance flow rate
Infusion is stopped and pressure fall over 30 seconds is determined
Infusion cavernosography is performed using contrast material

FIGURE 2-16. Dynamic infusion cavernosometry and cavernosography (DICC). This test determines the presence or absence of corporovenous occlusive dysfunction (CVOD) [15]. If CVOD is identified during the examination, is it because the man has organic CVOD due, for example, to cavernosal smooth muscle disease, or is it because he failed to achieve complete smooth muscle relaxation following the injection of the vasoactive drug(s)? We found a poor correlation between nocturnal penile tumescence and rigidity (NPTR) and DICC results in two groups of men, one with psychogenic and one with organic erectile dysfunction [12]. It is likely that anxiety mediated through the sympathetic nervous system or other factors not yet identified can prevent complete smooth muscle relaxation during this test in some men who clearly have psychogenic and normal NPTR. Results of DICC should therefore be interpreted with caution.

Penile Arteriography

Intracavernosal injection of vasoactive drugs
Flush pelvic arteriogram
Bilateral selective internal pudendal arteriography

FIGURE 2-17. Penile arteriography. During penile flaccidity, the penile arteries have a small diameter and relatively low blood flow. Visualization of the vessels is improved if arteriography is performed following intracavernosal vasoactive drug injection [16]. Penile arteriography provides a "road map" of the vasculature, which is necessary if penile arterial revascularization is being considered. However, this examination, which is relatively expensive and entails some risks, does not supply the functional information concerning penile arterial status afforded by cheaper and safer duplex Doppler ultrasonography. Penile arteriography should therefore only be done in men who are candidates for penile arterial revascularization. For the most part arterial surgery is limited to young men with arterial occlusion following pelvic or perineal trauma.

NOCTURNAL PENILE TUMESCENCE TESTING

Basis for Nocturnal Penile Tumescence Testing

Normal males of all ages have sleep erections
These erections are usually associated with REM stage of sleep
NPT usually implies a psychogenic etiology*
Abnormal NPT usually implies an organic etiology*

** In men with erectile dysfunction.*

FIGURE 2-18. Basis for nocturnal penile tumescence (NPT) testing. The pioneering work of Fisher *et al.* [17] and Karacan [18] led to work demonstrating that normal men of all ages have erections during sleep. Most sleep erections occur during the rapid eye movement (REM) stage of sleep. Men typically have three to five sleep erections per night with many episodes lasting 30 to 60 minutes. In men with erectile dysfunction (ED), NPT testing has been used to help differentiate psychogenic from organic ED. NPT testing may be falsely positive (normal) in men with neurogenic ED and in men with vasculogenic pelvic steal syndrome. NPT may be falsely negative (abnormal) in men with hypogonadism, sleep disorders, or a major depressive episode. For these reasons, NPT results need to be correlated with all other parts of the ED evaluation [19].

Methods for Measuring Nocturnal Penile Tumescence

Stamp test
Snap Gauge
Strain gauge
RigiScan
Sleep laboratory

FIGURE 2-19. Methods for measuring nocturnal penile tumescence (NPT). Stamps (*eg,* Christmas Seals, Easter Seals; not postal stamps) applied to the flaccid penis at bedtime have been used to record the presence of sleep erections [20]. If the perforations between the stamps are broken, it is presumed that a sleep erection has occurred. This simple test has many obvious limitations. It does not record the number or duration of episodes of NPT. It does not record the degree of tumescence, and it records rigidity in a very simple fashion. Snap Gauges (Imagyn Medical Technologies, Augusta, GA) wrap around the penis and function much like the stamp test except that rigidity is recorded at three different levels [21]. Strain gauges record the number and duration of NPT episodes; they also record the amount of tumescence. However, tumescence and rigidity do not always correlate directly; rigidity is more important for coitus than tumescence [22]. NPT testing can be done with a strain gauge in a sleep laboratory, which has the advantage of recording NPT in real-time while an electroencephalogram is being recorded to document the presence and stages of sleep. The attendant who is present for this test can measure penile axial rigidity by employing a buckling meter. Sleep laboratory testing has many advantages; its principal disadvantage is its expense. The RigiScan device records both tumescence and radial rigidity in real-time [23]. It can be used by the patient in the privacy of his home.

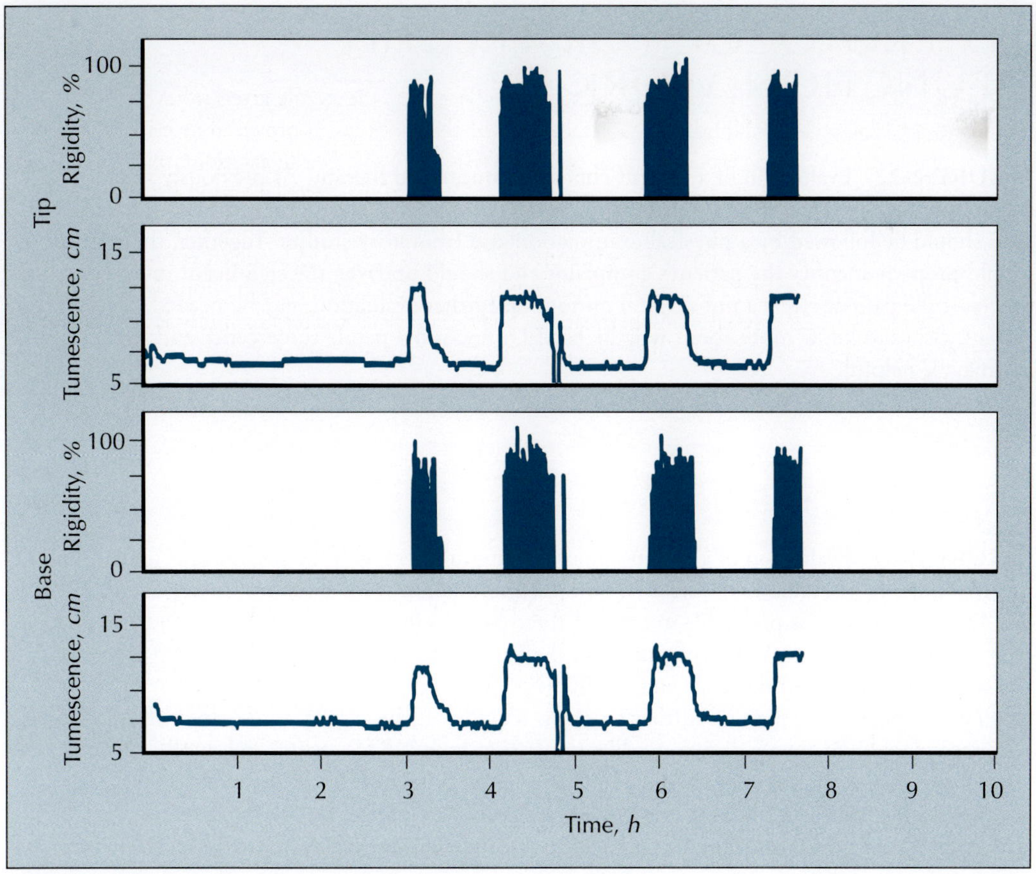

FIGURE 2-20. Normal RigiScan (Timm Medical Technologies, Eden Prairie, MN) nocturnal penile tumescence (NPT) reading in a patient with psychogenic erectile dysfunction. Marks along the horizontal axis represent time in hours. Shown along the vertical axis are base and tip tumescence in centimeters and base and tip radial rigidity on a percentage scale. This patient had four episodes of NPT ranging from approximately 15 to 45 minutes. Tumescence was normal with an average increase in penile circumference of 5 cm at the base and 4 cm at the tip. Radial rigidity is approximately 70% to 80% at both the base and the tip. The lower limits of normal for NPT testing with the RigiScan device is rigidity of 70% lasting 10 minutes [23].

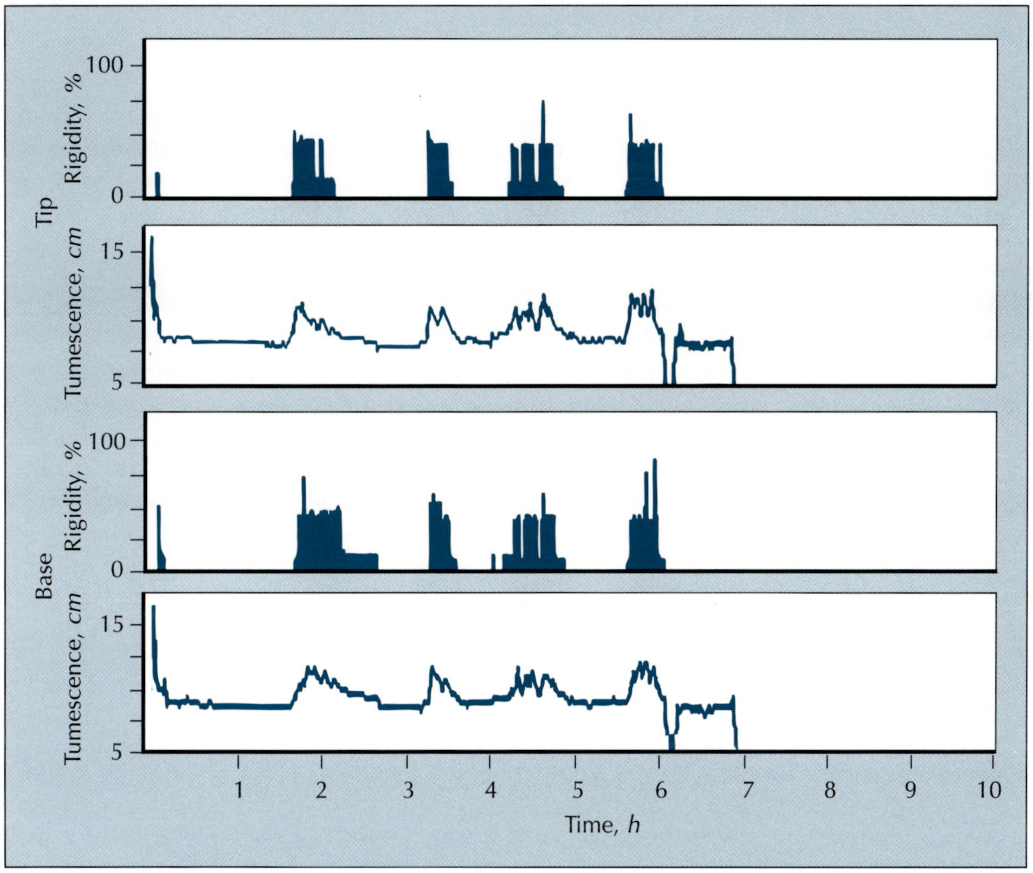

FIGURE 2-21. Abnormal RigiScan (Timm Medical Technologies, Eden Prairie, MN) nocturnal penile tumescence and rigidity (NPTR) test in a man with vasculogenic erectile dysfunction (ED). This man clearly has sleep erections; four episodes were recorded. However, both tumescence and rigidity are impaired and poorly sustained. Base and tip tumescence average 2 cm and the tumescence waves are peaked, indicating poorly sustained sleep erections. Base and tip rigidity average 40%. These findings are common in men with vasculogenic ED.

SUGGESTED PROTOCOL FOR ERECTILE DYSFUNCTION WORK-UP

Evaluation of Patient Choosing Nonsurgical Therapy

History
Physical examination
Laboratory studies
Nocturnal penile tumescence and rigidity studies (optional)

FIGURE 2-22. Evaluation of a patient choosing nonsurgical therapy. As previously stated, a thorough history is the most important single item in the evaluation of erectile dysfunction (ED). This should be followed by a physical examination and laboratory studies. Together, these items should properly identify the patient's complaint and should uncover any significant underlying disorders. If the patient elects a nonsurgical option, no further evaluation may be needed. If the patient wishes to know more about why he has ED, nocturnal penile tumescence and rigidity testing may be helpful.

Evaluation of Patient Choosing Surgical Therapy

History
Physical examination
Laboratory studies
Nocturnal penile tumescence and rigidity testing
Optional studies
- Duplex Doppler ultrasound
- Cavernosometry/cavernosography
- Penile arteriography

FIGURE 2-23. Evaluation of a patient choosing surgical therapy. If the patient opts for surgical treatment, the basic evaluation of history, physical examination, and laboratory studies is still carried out. In our opinion, it is preferable in most of these patients to have some objective evidence that their erectile dysfunction (ED) is organic, and the best test to differentiate organic from psychogenic ED is nocturnal penile tumescence and rigidity (NPTR) testing. If the intended surgery is penile prosthesis implantation, then no further testing is required. If the surgery is to correct erectile deformity secondary to Peyronie's disease, we like to perform both NPTR testing and duplex Doppler ultrasonography preoperatively. We do this in an attempt to identify those men who are likely to develop erectile failure following surgery to correct Peyronie's disease. As previously mentioned, penile arteriography is reserved for those few men who are candidates for penile arterial surgery.

OVERVIEW OF TREATMENT OPTIONS FOLLOWING DIAGNOSIS

Treatment Options for Erectile Dysfunction

First-line options
- Systemic therapy
- Hormonal

Second-line options
- Vacuum erection device therapy
- Intraurethral pharmacotherapy
- Penile injection therapy

Third-line options
- Penile prosthesis implantation

FIGURE 2-24. Treatment options for erectile dysfunction (ED). For most patients, the first line of treatment for ED will be systemic therapy. Currently, the most effective agents available are sildenafil citrate [24] and vardenafil hydrochloride [25] type 5 phosphodiesterase inhibitors (*see* Figs. 2-25 to 2-28). A third type 5 phosphodiesterase inhibitor, tadalafil [26], is expected to receive US Food and Drug Administration approval and will be available in the near future (*see* Figures 2-25 to 2-28). For a minority of men in whom hypogonadism or hyperprolactinemia is present, systemic therapy for these disorders is indicated. If the first-line treatments either fail or are not indicated, the patient and his partner should consider other nonsurgical methods of treatment, including vacuum erection device therapy, penile injection pharmacotherapy, and intraurethral pharmacotherapy. If these methods fail, the patient and his partner may wish to consider penile prosthesis implantation.

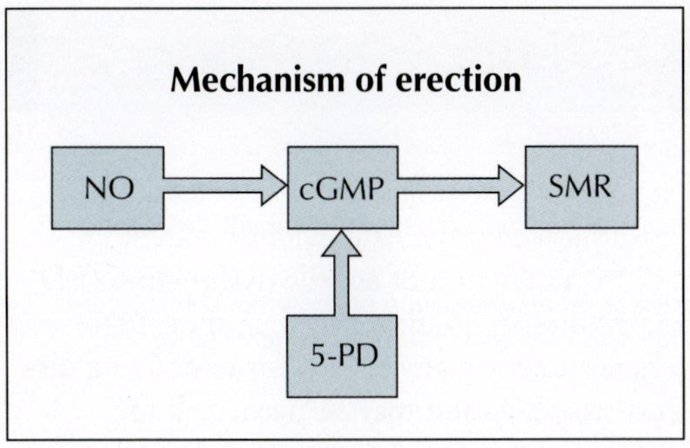

FIGURE 2-25. Mechanism of erection. Sexual stimulation results in the release of nitric oxide (NO) in the corpus cavernosum. NO activates the enzyme guanylate cyclase, which results in the formation of cyclic guanosine monophosphate (cGMP). Increased levels of cGMP promote cavernosal smooth muscle relaxation (SMR) and increase blood flow to the penis, resulting in erection. Type 5 phosphodiesterase (5-PD) breaks down cGMP, helping to prevent prolonged erections.

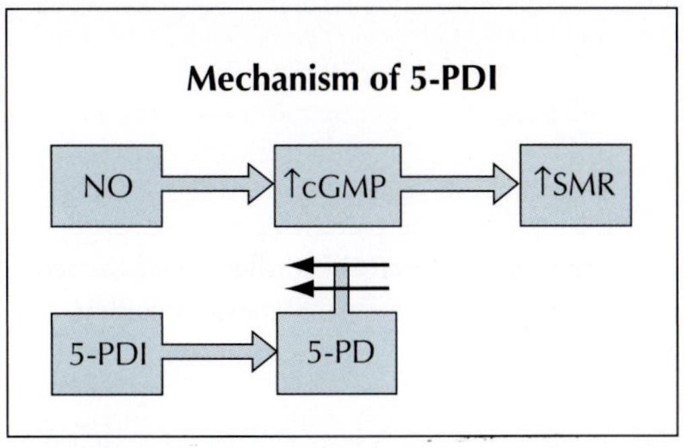

FIGURE 2-26. Sildenafil, vardenafil, and tadalafil are selective competitive inhibitors of type 5 phosphodiesterase (5-PDI). This results in less 5-PD activity, with resulting increased levels of cGMP. In many men with erectile dysfunction, administration of these agents results in increased levels of cGMP, leading to firmer and better maintained erections in response to sexual stimulation.

Phosphodiesterase Inhibitors

Oral, 1 hour before coitus
Does not produce an erection
Enhances erections
Requires sexual stimulation

FIGURE 2-27. Phosphodiesterase inhibitors. Peak blood levels of sildenafil and vardenafil are reached approximately 1 hour after ingestion. The half-life of sildenafil and vardenafil is about 4 hours. Tadalafil has a half-life of 17.5 hours and peak blood levels are obtained in about 2 hours. These agents do not affect libido, sensation, orgasm, or ejaculation. These three drugs do enhance sexually induced erections in many men with erectile dysfunction of various causes.

Side Effects of Phospodiesterase Inhibitors

Headaches
Flushing
Dyspepsia
Nasal congestion
Color vision (100 mg)

FIGURE 2-28. Side effects of type 5 phosphodiesterase inhibitors. Type 5 phosphodiesterase inhibitors potentiate the hypotensive effects of nitrates (coronary vasodilators), and their use in men taking organic nitrates in any form is strictly contraindicated. Side effects of these agents are generally mild and include, in decreasing frequency, headaches, flushing, dyspepsia, and nasal congestion. Some men taking higher doses of sildenafil and rarely vardenafil experience mild, temporary visual side effects. With tadalafil, additional adverse events include myalgia and back pain.

REFERENCES

1. NIH Consensus Panel on Impotence: Impotence. *JAMA* 1993, 270:83–90.
2. Lue TF: Impotence: a patient's goal-directed approach to treatment. *World J Urol* 1990, 8:67–74.
3. Montague DK, Lakin MM: False diagnoses of venous leak impotence. *J Urol* 1992, 148:148–149.
4. Deutsch S, Sherman L: Previously unrecognized diabetes mellitus in sexually impotent men. *JAMA* 1980, 244:2430–2432.
5. Leonard MP, Nickel CJ, Morales A: Hyperprolactinemia and impotence: why, when, and how to investigate. *J Urol* 1989, 142:992–994.
6. Zonszein J: Diagnosis and management of endocrine disorders of erectile dysfunction. *Urol Clin North Am* 1995, 22:789–802.
7. Hartmann U: Psychological subtypes of erectile dysfunction: results of statistical analyses and clinical practice. *World J Urol* 1997, 15:56–64.
8. Lakin MM: Diagnostic assessment of disorders of male sexual function. In *Disorders of Male Sexual Function.* Edited by Montague DK. Chicago: Year Book Medical Publishers; 1988:26–43.
9. Wessells H, Lue TF, McAninch JW: Penile length in the flaccid and erect states: guidelines for penile augmentation. *J Urol* 1996, 156:995–997.
10. Lue TF, Donatucci CF: The combined intracavernous injection and stimulation test: diagnostic accuracy. *J Urol* 1992, 184:61–62.
11. Martins FE, Reis JP: Visual erotic stimulation test for initial screening of psychogenic erectile dysfunction: a reliable noninvasive alternative? *J Urol* 1997, 157:134–139.
12. Montague DK, Lakin MM, Medendorp SV, Tesar LJ: Infusion pharmacocavernosometry and nocturnal penile tumescence findings in men with erectile dysfunction. *J Urol* 1991, 145:768–771.
13. Broderick GA, Arger PA: Penile blood flow study: age specific reference ranges. *J Urol* 1994, 151:A371.
14. Broderick GA: Noninvasive arterial evaluation of the patient complaining of erectile dysfunction with color duplex Doppler ultrasound. In *Diagnosis and Management of Male Sexual Dysfunction.* Edited by Mulcahy JJ. New York, Tokyo: Igaku-Shoin; 1997:89–126.
15. Padma-Nathan H, Gasior B, Roddy T, *et al.*: Dynamic infusion cavernosometry and cavernosography (DICC): the interaction of arterial and veno-occlusive function [abstract]. *J Urol* 1989, 141:221A.
16. Benet AE, Rehman J, Melman A: Penile revascularization. In *Diagnosis and Management of Male Sexual Dysfunction.* Edited by Mulcahy JJ. New York, Tokyo: Igaku–Shoin; 1997:127–147.
17. Fisher C, Schiavi RC, Edwards A, *et al.*: Evaluation of nocturnal penile tumescence in the differential diagnosis of sexual impotence: a quantitative study. *Arch Gen Psychiatry* 1979, 36:431–437.
18. Karacan I: *The Developmental Aspect and the Effect of Certain Clinical Conditions upon Penile Erection during Sleep: International Congress Series.* Princeton, NJ: Excerpta Medica; 1966.
19. Daitch JA, Lakin MM, Montague DK: Nocturnal penile tumescence monitoring. In *Diagnosis and Management of Male Sexual Dysfunction (Topics in Clinical Urology).* Edited by Mulcahy JJ. Tokyo: Igaku-Shoin; 1997:55–73.
20. Barry JM, Blank B, Boileau M: Nocturnal penile tumescence monitoring with stamps. *Urology* 1980, 15:171–172.
21. Ek A, Bradley WE, Krane RJ: Nocturnal penile rigidity measured by the Snap-Gauge band. *J Urol* 1983, 129:964–966.
22. Wein AJ, Fishkin R, Carpiniello VL, Malloy TR: Expansion without significant rigidity during nocturnal penile tumescence testing: a potential source of misinterpretation. *J Urol* 1981, 126:343–344.
23. Bradley WE, Timm GW, Gallagher JM, *et al.*: New method for continuous measurement of nocturnal penile tumescence and rigidity. *Urology* 1985, 26:4–9.
24. Goldstein I, Lue TF, Padma-Nathan H, *et al.*: Oral sildenafil in the treatment of erectile dysfunction: Sildenafil Study Group. *N Engl J Med* 1998, 339:1397–1404.
25. Hellstrom WJ, Gittleman M, Karlin G, *et al.*: Sustained efficacy and tolerability of vardenafil, a highly potent selective phosphodiesterase type 5 inhibitor, in men with erectile dysfunction: results of a randomized, double-blind, 26-week placebo-controlled pivotal trial. *Urology* 2003, 61 (suppl 1):8–14.
26. Porst H, Padma-Nathan H, Giuliano F, *et al.*: Efficacy of tadalafil for the treatment of erectile dysfunction at 24 and 36 hours after dosing: a randomized controlled trial. *Urology* 2003, 62:121–125.

Vascular Assessment of Erectile Dysfunction

3

Gregory A. Broderick

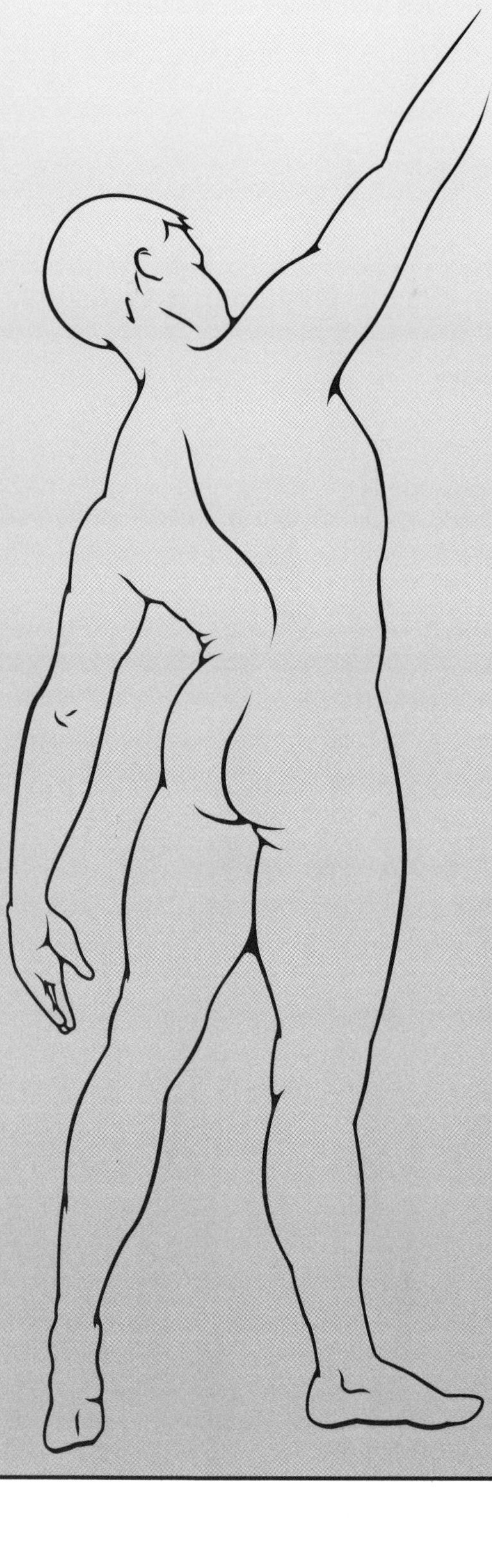

The discovery that penile erection is a vascular phenomenon the quality of which is adversely affected by identifiable clinical factors coincided with the advent of multiple technologies for penile imaging. The 1980s and 1990s saw the development of many penile diagnostics; of these technologies, color duplex Doppler ultrasound is the least invasive and most informative. Before the wide availability of Doppler technology, a vasoactive penile injection administered in the office permitted the physician to roughly distinguish between severe arterial disease and psychogenic erectile dysfunction (ED). Whether the agent is papaverine, prostaglandin E_1, or a combination of vasoactive medications, the addition of duplex Doppler ultrasound provides greater objective criteria for evaluating penile responses.

All vascular evaluations are aimed at identifying and quantifying arterial and veno-occlusive erectile function. The primary causes of arteriogenic ED are atherosclerotic vascular disease and traumatic arterial occlusion (following pelvic or perineal trauma). The quality of penile inflow has been directly related to common vascular comorbidities of age, diabetes mellitus, hypertension, atherosclerotic coronary/peripheral vascular disease, hyperlipidemia, and cigarette smoking. Veno-occlusion is a no less essential hydraulic phenomenon regulating intrapenile pressure changes by penile outflow. The quality of veno-occlusion depends on the tone of cavernous smooth muscle. Clinically imaging and quantifying veno-occlusion is more difficult than documenting penile arterial inflows. Regulation of cavernosal smooth muscle (CSM) tone is complex; specific clinical risk factors for veno-occlusive ED have not yet been identified. The forces at play include neuropharmacologically mediated adrenergic tone, smooth muscle versus extracellular matrix composition, molecular mediators of contraction, and cell-to-cell communication.

In practice, vascular ED is subclassified as arterial, veno-occlusive, or mixed vascular insufficiency. These clinical distinctions correspond with our appreciation of the mechanisms of erection. Color duplex Doppler has enhanced penile diagnostics by speeding the acquisition of data especially in low-flow states associated with arterial disease, providing the only noninvasive imaging of intrapenile circulation, and lending itself easily to sexual stimulation protocols (visual, audiovisual, self-erotic).

The introduction of sildenafil in 1998 dramatically changed practice patterns in ED—increasing the number of patients acknowledging the complaint, and shifting the burden of evaluation and management away from the urologist and toward the family practitioner. Currently both the American Urological Association and the First International Consultation on ED recommend sildenafil for patients based on good sexual history, assessment of medical risks, and physical examination. The primary purpose of establishing a specific diagnosis is to formulate a treatment plan; in most cases of ED this can be done without extensive testing. Conversely, without diagnostic testing, efficacy and satisfaction with pharmacotherapies becomes a matter of chance. Effectiveness of sildenafil in the average ED patient ranges from 60% to 80%, and declines as the number of risk factors the patient has increases. The next decade will see the development of multiple oral agents for the management of vascular ED. Currently with only one class of agents widely available (phosphodiesterase type-5 [PDE-5] inhibitors), clinicians categorize patients as PDE-5 inhibitor successes or PDE-5 inhibitor failures. Patients failing first-line therapy by primary caregivers or confused by the variety of options should be encouraged to seek the expertise of specialists. They may simply want to know what is wrong with them, or which specific agent is best for them, or why a PDE-5 inhibitor has failed to reverse their ED. Optimally, ED testing needs to create vascular profiles to predict which drug or combination of drugs (oral, cutaneous, urethral, intracavenosal) will effectively restore erection, spare patients the frustration and the potential side effects of multiple empiric trials, and determine whether patients would best be served by a mechanical or surgical solution.

This chapter visually highlights a variety of vascular imaging modalities for the patient with ED, Peyronie's disease, and penile implant problems. When diagnostics are indicated, the penile blood flow study, which typically uses intracavernous injection and assessment by color duplex Doppler ultrasound, is the most informative and least invasive means of evaluating vasculogenic ED. This testing may be all that is needed to define and determine severity. Pharmacotesting with duplex Doppler certainly should be used before more invasive technology is considered.

THE INITIAL EVALUATION

Characteristics of the Average Erectile Dysfunction Patient

Age ≥ 50 y
Stable relationship
Gradually progressive ED
ED for more than 1 y
One or more vascular risk factors for ED
- Diabetes mellitus
- Hypertension
- Atherosclerotic coronary and/or peripheral vascular disease
- Hyperlipidemia
- Cigarette smoking

Good mental health

FIGURE 3-1. The average erectile dysfunction (ED) patient. Vascular, neurologic, and psychologic testing are not mandatory for the average ED patient.

The Initial Erectile Dysfunction Evaluation

Comprehensive history
- Medical
- Sexual
- Psychosocial

Focused physical examination
- Male secondary sexual characteristics
- Genitalia, prostate
- Lower extremity vascular integrity
- Lower extremity neurologic integrity

Recommended testing
- Testosterone assay
- Fasting glucose
- HbA1c
- Lipid profile
- *PSA (for all men ≥ 50 y old, for African American men ≥ 40 y old, for all men ≥ 40 y old with strong family history of prostate cancer); for all when considering testosterone treatment

Interventions
- Trial of oral therapy
- Modify risk factors
- Basic counseling

**Modified from the Recommendations of the First International Consultation on ED, Paris, 1999.*

FIGURE 3-2. The initial erectile dysfunction (ED) evaluation. Physician–patient dialogue is the cornerstone in the clinical assessment of ED.

SPECIALIZED EVALUATIONS

Indications for Specialized Referral and/or Diagnostics

Patient request
Treatment failure
Primary ED (poorly sustained erections, life-long)
Anatomic penile deformities
- Peyronie's disease
- Congenital: hypospadius, chordee
- Trauma
- Phimosis
- Short penis, buried penis

Pelvic/perineal trauma
Endocrinopathy
Psychiatric or psychosexual disorder
Relationship problems
Complex vascular problems
Complex neurologic problems

FIGURE 3-3. Indications for specialized referral and/or diagnostics. ED—erectile dysfunction.

Erectile Dysfunction Diagnostics

Self-report measures
- Self-administered questionnaires
- Structured interviews
- Event logs/diaries

Evidence-based assessments
- Vascular
  - ICI
  - Penile blood flow study: ICI and color duplex Doppler
  - Arteriography
  - CT angiography
  - MRI
  - Infrared spectrophotometry
  - Radioisotope penography
  - DICC
- AVSS
  - Independent or jointly with vascular testing
  - With or without pharmacologic stimulation (oral, ICI)
- Neurologic
  - NPTR
  - Erectiometer/rigidometer
  - Biothesiometry (vibratory thresholds)
  - Dorsal nerve conduction velocity
  - Bulbocavernosus reflex latency
  - Plethysmography/electrobioimpedence
  - CC-EMG
  - MRI, PET scanning of brain (response to sexual stimulation)

FIGURE 3-4. Erectile dysfunction (ED) diagnostics. Self-report measures have the advantage of providing a broader assessment of sexual function, including erection, orgasm, desire, and satisfaction. They are very cost-effective for clinical trials and may serve as an adjunct to the clinical interview. There has been poor correlation when self-report measures are compared with evidence-based assessments, most likely because the potential for patient bias is greater with the former. Many evidence-based assessments require a high degree of technical expertise and are typically performed by centers of excellence. ED diagnostics most commonly performed by the specialist include intracavernous injection pharmacotesting (ICI), color duplex Doppler, audiovisual sexual stimulation (AVSS), nocturnal penile tumescence and rigidity (NPTR), and dynamic cavernosometry and cavernosonography (DICC) [1]. CC-EMG—corpus cavernosum electromyography.

A. Erection Hemodynamics and Doppler Waveforms

Flaccid phase, minimal peak systolic cavernous flows
Latent phase
Tumescence phase, maximal peak systolic and diastolic waveforms
Full erection, narrowing and some reduction in peak systolic flows
Rigid erection, with reversal of cavernous flow during diastole
Rigid erection, with suppression of cavernous flow during diastole
Detumescence begins with significant decrease in peak systolic cavernous flows and reappearance of antegrade diastolic flows

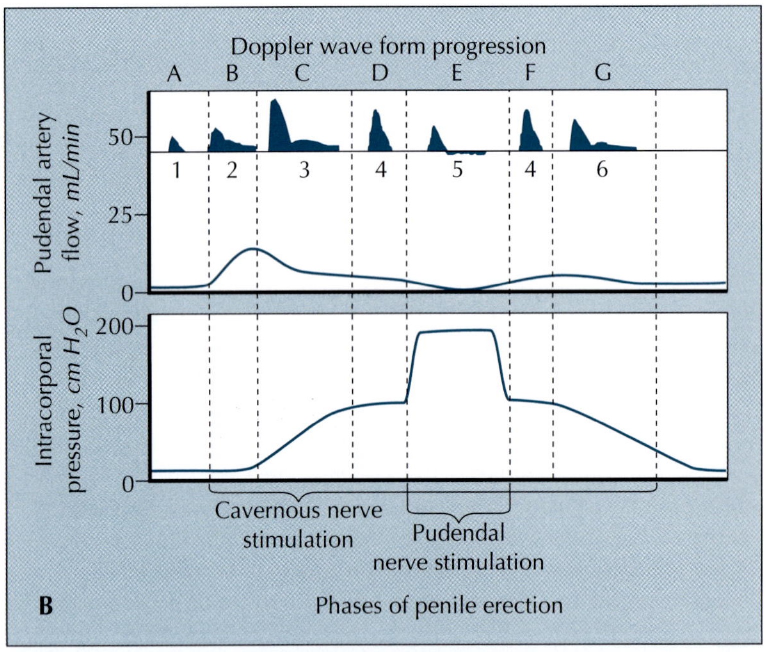

FIGURE 3-5. Erection hemodynamics and Doppler waveforms. Lue and others have studied the hemodynamics of erection in mammals, using cavernous and pudendal nerve stimulation techniques. **A,** Outline of phases. **B,** A summary of events from flaccidity to erection in the monkey. In the flaccid penis, arterioles and smooth muscle sinusoids are contracted. During the filling phase, penile vascular resistance decreases; there is increasing blood flow through the pudendal and cavernous arteries. In clinical testing there are many variables that may alter the normal progression of erection: pharmacokinetics, anxiety, and patient pathology. In a normal man, a pattern of spectral wave form progression during Doppler ultrasound is evident and reproducible. In the filling phase, sinusoidal and arterial resistance is low and the Doppler waveform is characterized by high forward flows during systole and diastole. As intrapenile pressures rise diastolic antegrade flows diminish, with full erection systolic waveforms peak, and diastolic flow is either suppressed or reversed [2–4].

Pharmacotesting

Pharmacotesting includes:
- ICI
- Visual rating of erection
  - Compared to best home erection
  - Inadequate, adequate, unbending rigidity
- Simple, minimally invasive, office test
- A positive response in a neurologically intact patient implies psychogenic impotence
- A normal injection test indicates normal veno-occlusion (normal DICC)
- Despite pharmacologic erection, there may be borderline arterial function

FIGURE 3-6. Pharmacotesting. This is the most common in office diagnostic for vascular erectile dysfunction (ED). In most cases it is performed without monitoring equipment. Comparison to other hemodynamic tests suggests that a normal pharmacotest result is associated with normal veno-occlusion (flow to maintain rigidity values of 0.5 to 3 mL/min). Pharmacotesting may be normal (false-negative) in as many as 20% of patients with borderline arterial inflow (when normal is defined as > 35 cm/sec peak systolic flow on Doppler, and borderline is defined as 25 to 35 cm/sec). False-positives occur most commonly because of patient anxiety or inadequate pharmacologic stimulation. Many vasoactive agents have been described for pharmacotesting, the most commonly used agent being prostaglandin E1 at a dosage from 10 to 20 μg for initial injection [4–9]. DICC—dynamic cavernosometry and cavernosonography; ICI—intracavernous injection.

A. Penile Arteriography: Advantages, Disadvantages, Indications

Advantages
- Best anatomic information about pelvic inflows
- Road map for paired penile vessels:
  - Pudendal artery
  - Common penile artery trifurcates
    - Cavernous artery
    - Bulbourethral artery
    - Dorsal artery
- Set the initial standards for the diagnosis of vascular ED

Disadvantages
- Requires: intracavernous and intra-arterial vasodilators
- Exposure to ionizing radiation
- Painful
- Differentiating congenital variations from acquired abnormalities
- Correlating complaints and hemo dynamics with vascular patterns of penile inflow

Indications: prior to vascular bypass procedures
- Pelvic trauma
- Posterior urethral disruptions
- Penile trauma
  - Fracture
  - Straddle injury

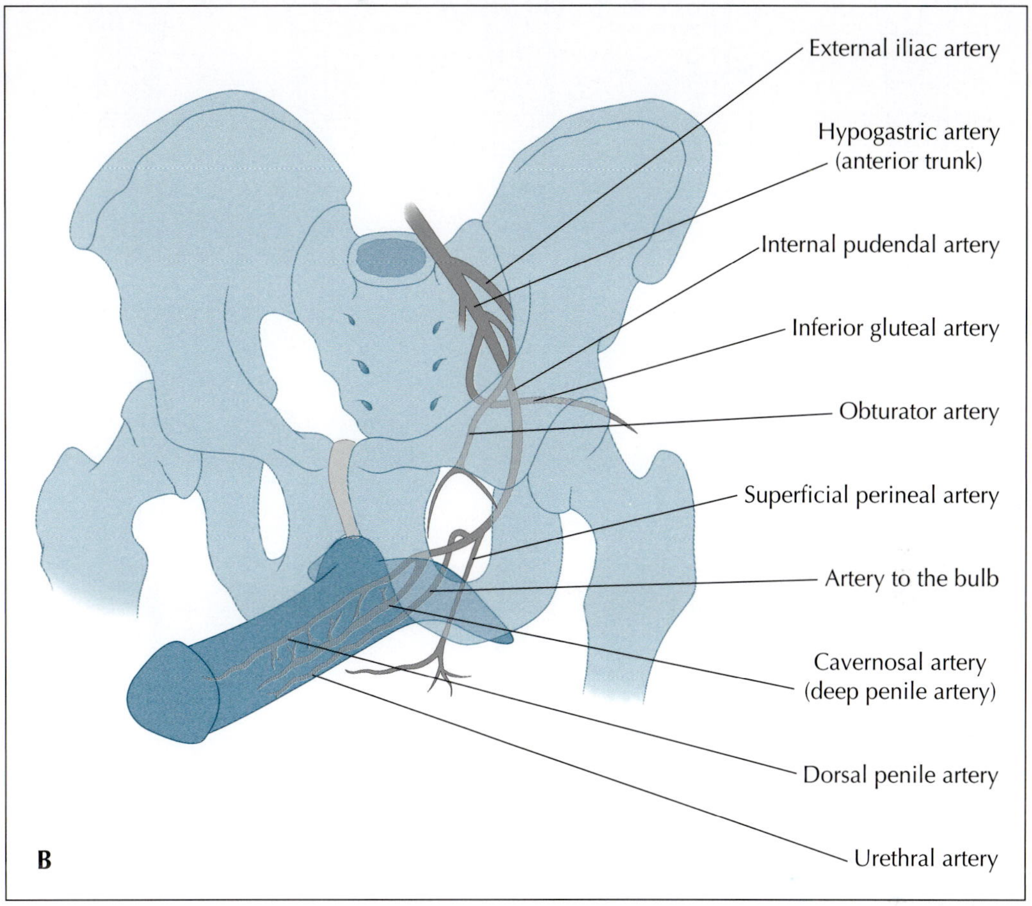

FIGURE 3-7. Aspects of penile arteriography. **A,** Outline of advantages and disadvantages. Infusion of intra-arterial contrast agents is painful and may cause vasospasm. Penile arteriograms require both intra-arterial and intrapenile injections of vasodilators, and use of low-osmolality nonionic contrast agents. Digital subtraction techniques and selective catheterization of internal pudendal artery, accessory pudendal and inferior epigastric arteries provide the vascular "roadmap" needed to plan penile arterial bypass operations. **B,** Schematic of left penile inflow. The common penile artery trifurcates, giving origin to the bulbourethral, cavernous, and dorsal arteries.

(*Continued on next page*)

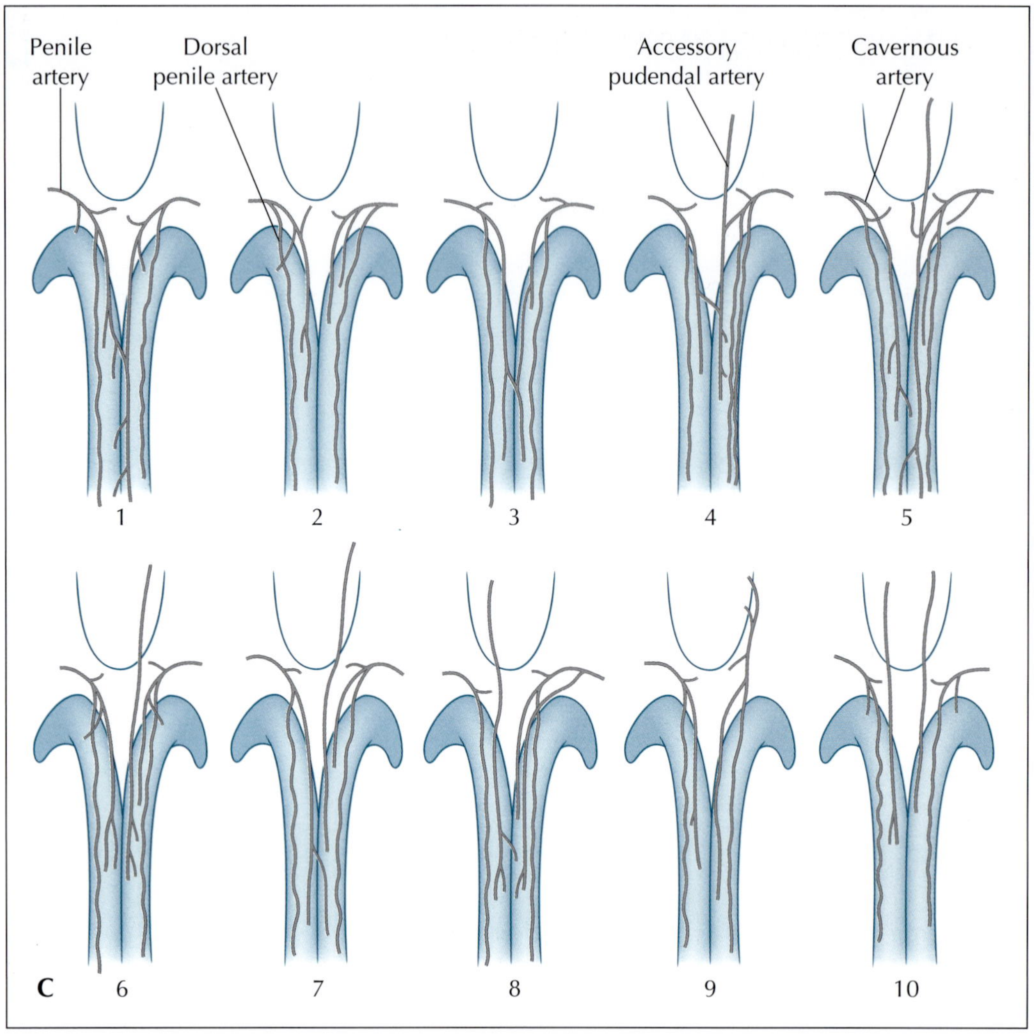

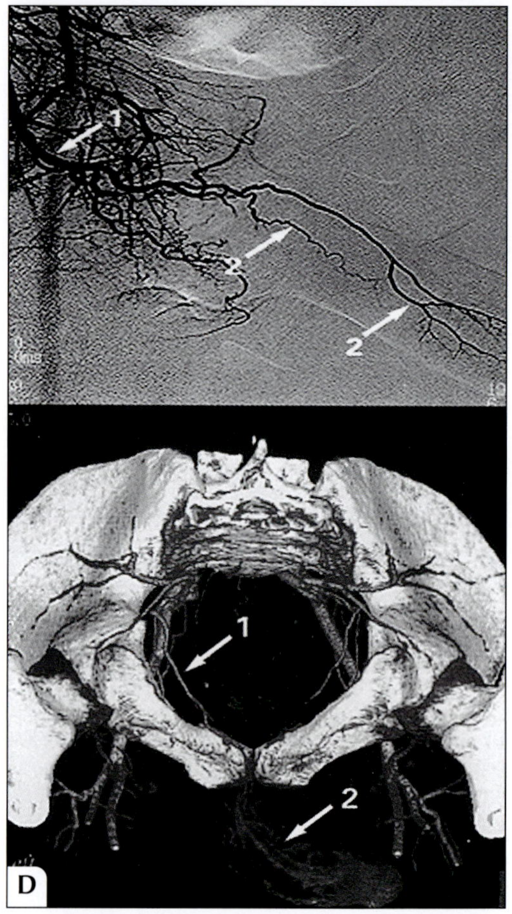

FIGURE 3-7. *(Continued)* **C,** Congenital deviations among the paired penile arteries have been documented in 50% of healthy volunteers. When planning a bypass operation, the most important of these variations to identify are unilateral hypoplasia of a dorsal artery and dorsal to cavernous collaterals. **D,** Magnetic resonance and CT angiography. Traditional digital subtraction angiography (DSA) is being replaced by more advanced techniques not requiring selective catheterization or intra-arterial dilators: magnetic resonance angiography and CT angiography, which in one study had a 79% accuracy compared with DSA [10–12].

PENILE BLOOD FLOW STUDY

Role of Penile Blood Flow Study in 2003

Advantages
- Minimally invasive
- Pairs two methods: ICI and Doppler sonography
- Power Doppler visualizes small vessel anatomy

Evidence-based assessments of
- Organic vs psychogenic
  - Arterial insufficiency
  - Venous insufficiency
  - Mixed vascular disease
- Trauma
- High-flow priapism
- Drug therapy failures
- Peyronie's disease

Qualify the severity of ED
- Intracavernous pharmacotesting
- PDE-5 inhibitor testing
- Visual erotic stimulation testing

Plan the surgery
- Peyronie's disease
- Microvascular arterial bypass
- Venous ligations

FIGURE 3-8. Role of penile blood flow study (PBFS) in 2003. PBFS is the least invasive technology for evaluating vascular erectile dysfunction (ED), distinguishing high-flow from low-flow priapism, and Peyronie's disease.

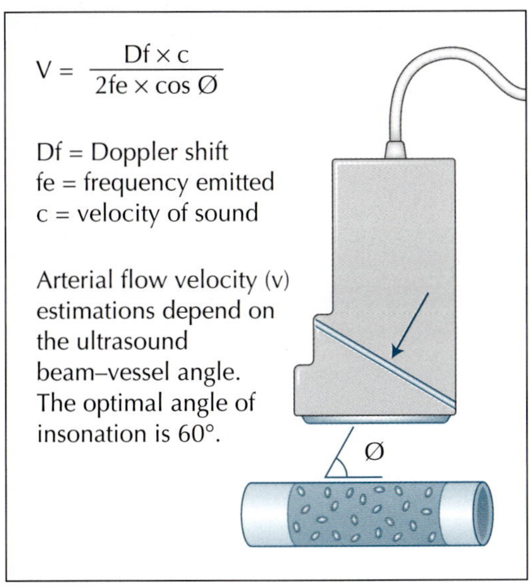

FIGURE 3-9. Schematic representation of the penile blood flow study. Gray scale, color flow, and power Doppler utilize the principles of pulsed Doppler: a pulse of ultrasound is emitted from the transducer, reflected back, and recorded. The returning echo in penile ultrasound is the signal blood moving in the penile vessel; this returning echo has a different frequency from the emitted signal—a Doppler shift. This Doppler shift depends on several physical factors: frequency of the transducer, velocity of the moving object (blood flow), speed of sound through the medium (penile tissues), and angle between the Doppler beam and direction of blood flow [13].

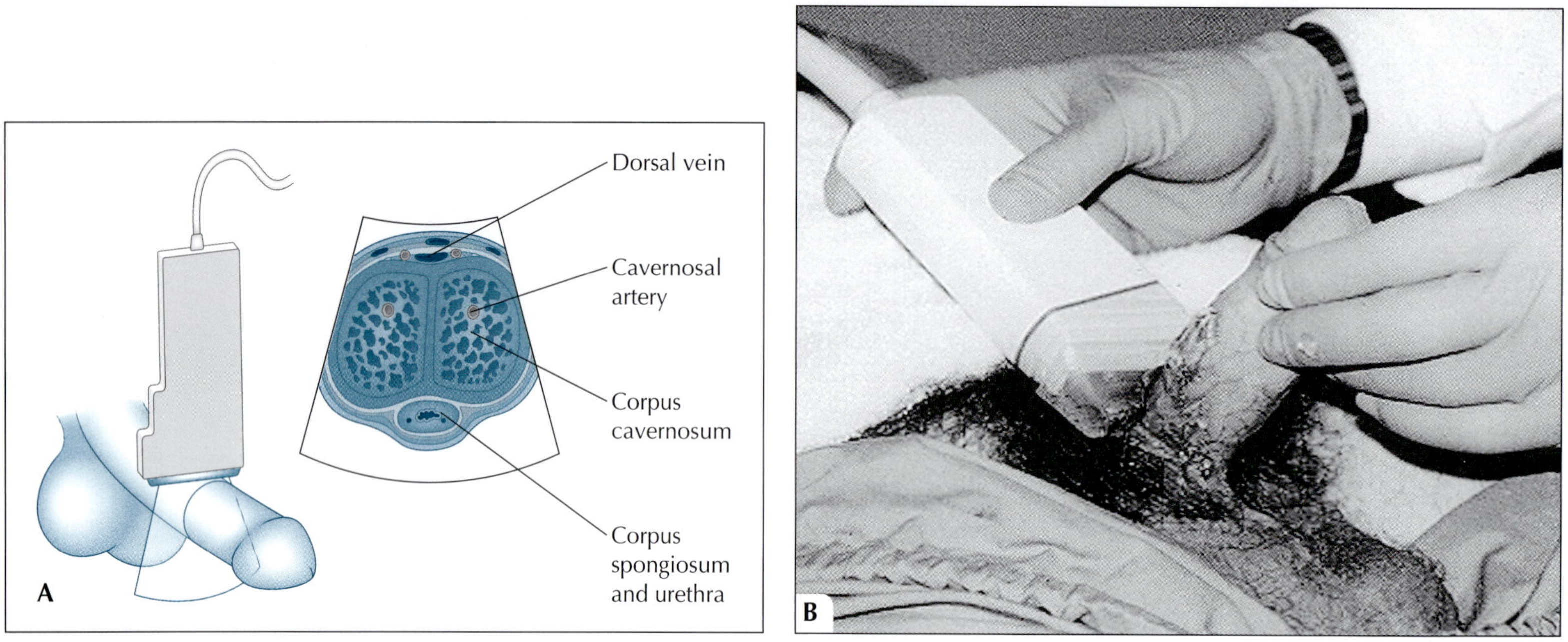

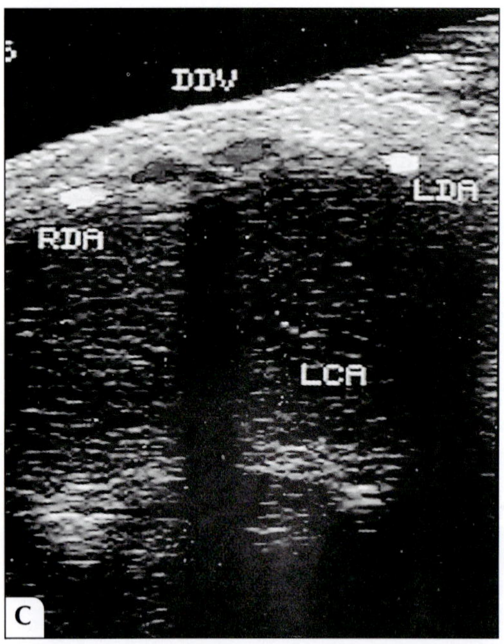

FIGURE 3-10. (*See Color Plate*) Penile blood flow study (PBFS) procedure. The examination requires a warm, secure examination room to reduce patient anxiety and facilitate relaxation of cavernous smooth muscle by intracavernous injection pharmacotesting. More recent investigations use visual sexual stimulation through headsets or monitors. The penis should first be examined in the early phase of erection (latent, tumescence), typically 5 to 10 minutes following injection. **A**, The corporal bodies are scanned from base to tip in the transverse plane. **B**, With color flow all intrapenile vessels can be identified in their anatomic locations: paired dorsal arteries (right dorsal artery, left dorsal artery), deep dorsal vein complex, and paired cavernous arteries (right cavernous arteries, left cavernous arteries). **C**, The echotexture of the corporal tissue should be homogeneously hypoechoic. Fibrosis is relatively hyperechoic in comparison.

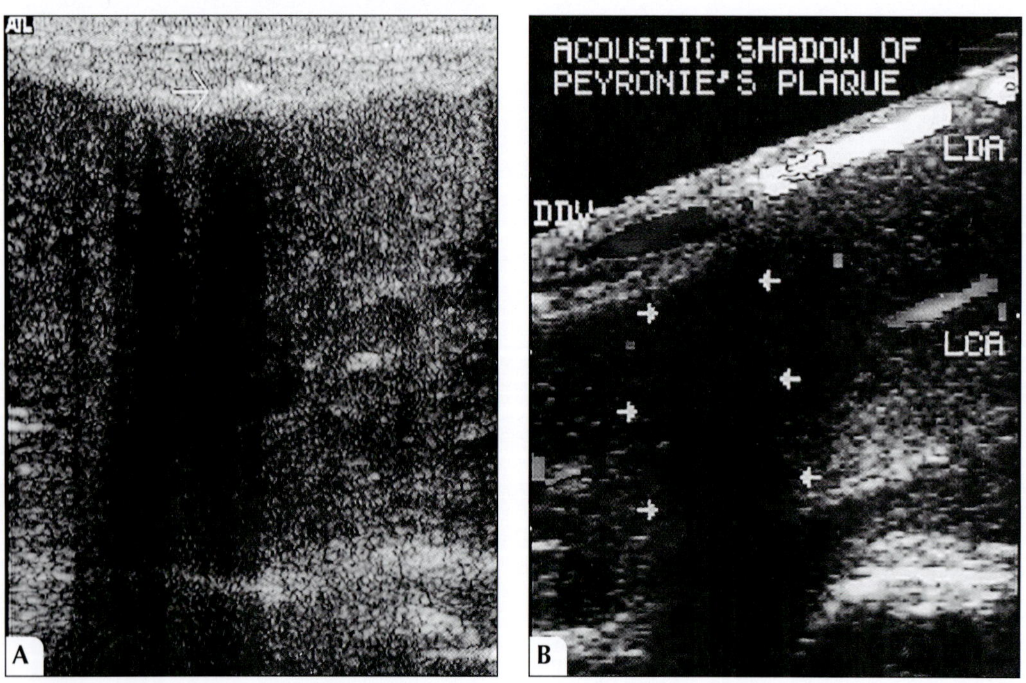

FIGURE 3-11. (*See Color Plate*) Acoustic shadows of Peyronie's plaques. Peyronie's plaques are denser than the normal tunica albuginea and will be relatively hyperechoic and thick compared with normal surrounding tunica; calcified plaques will cast an acoustic shadow, such as a renal stone. Gray-scale imaging (**A**) and color Doppler (**B**), both reveal focal Peyronie's plaque with acoustic shadowing below (*arrows in* **B**).

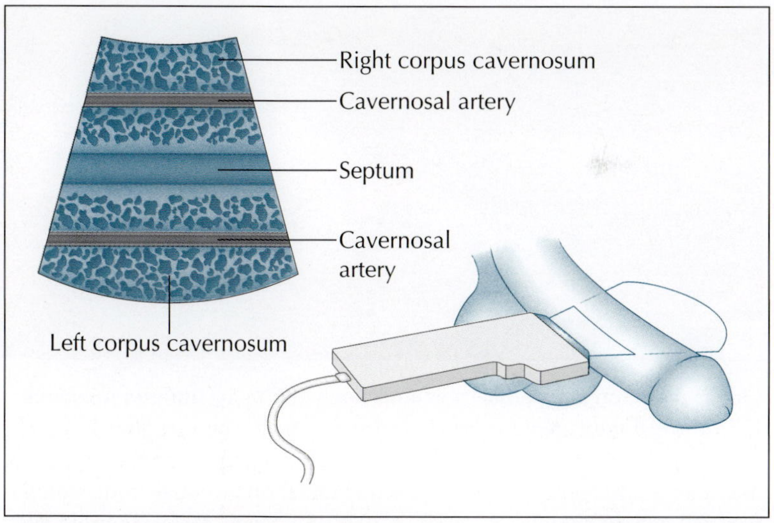

FIGURE 3-12. Assessing the sagittal planes. The penile vessels and flow velocities are assessed in the sagittal planes (parallel to the long axis of the penis). Lateral scanning (from 3 or 9 o'clock) will reveal both cavernous vessels in the same image, separated by the hyperechoic septum.

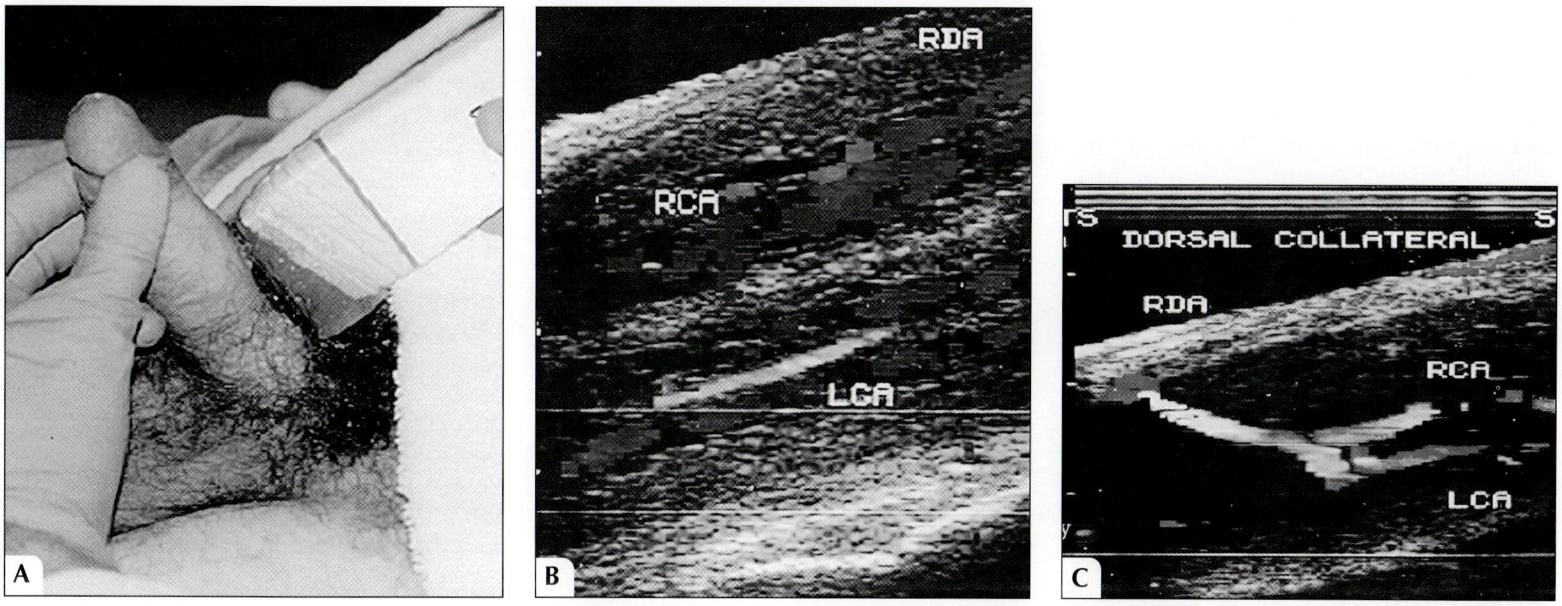

FIGURE 3-13. (*See Color Plate*) Dorsal scanning. **A,** Dorsal scanning will image the dorsal artery (DA) and underlying cavernous artery (CA). **B** and **C,** Dorsal to cavernous collaterals have been demonstrated in normal men and are congenital. They assume unique importance in the aging patient and should especially be documented if Peyronie's reconstruction is planned. Dorsal to cavernous collaterals may be an important source of inflow in the aging patient, with cavernous arterial insufficiency. Mobilization of the neurovascular bundle to resect a Peyronie's plaque will sacrifice dorsal to cavernous arterial collaterals, and could result in postoperative erectile dysfunction. LCA—left cavernous artery; RCA—right cavernous artery; RDA—right dorsal artery.

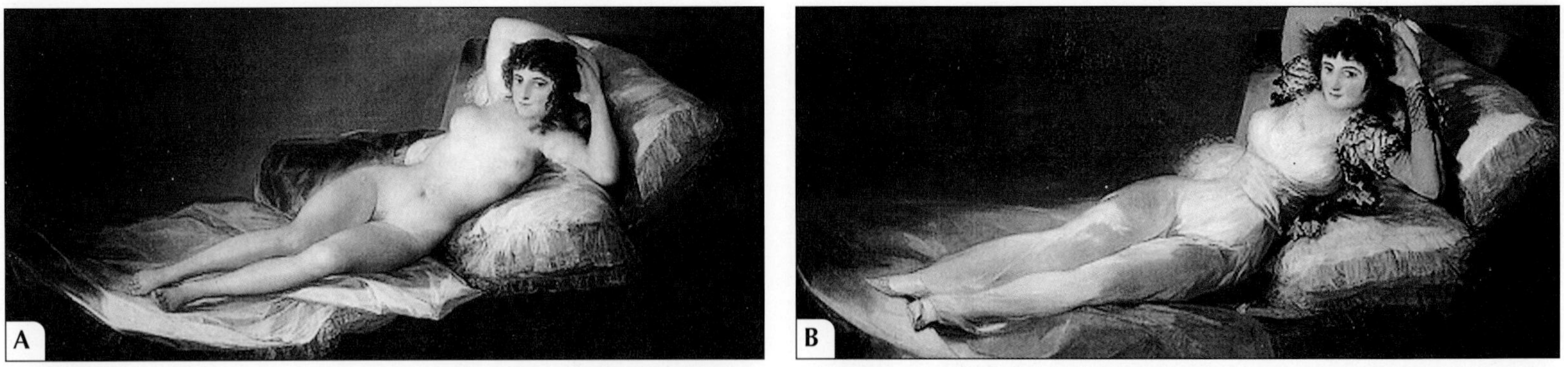

FIGURE 3-14. *La Maja Desnuda* and *La Maja Vestida* by Francisco Goya. These famous paintings by Francisco Goya are of the same model. Goya was compelled by the punative morality of the Spanish Inquisition to hide his original nude portrait (**A**) of the female figure and painted the same model dressed (**B**). In many ways the contemporary urologist faces a similar dilemma: sexual testing is optimized by sexual stimulation, but sexual stimulation is perceived as incongruous if not forbidden in the practice of clinical medicine. Timing is important in the penile blood flow study (PBFS) protocol. Arterial diameters and cavernous flows will maximize before rigid erection. Some investigators have recommended periodic measurements up to 30 minutes following intracavernous injection (ICI). Others have noted maximal cavernous flows at 5 to 10 minutes following ICI. If initial measurements are recorded at 5 to 10 minutes after ICI and full or rigid erection waveforms have not occurred, repeating the measurements after a period of privacy and self-stimulation or visual erotic stimulation will enhance penile responses in 70% of patients. Redosing protocols have also been used, if erectile response is not equal to that achieved at home. In one study, initial dosing of 10 µg of prostaglandin E_1 was followed at 10 minutes by repeat dosing or genital plus audiovisual sexual stimulation. Erections following audiovisual sexual stimulation were significantly better than after redosing [14–17].

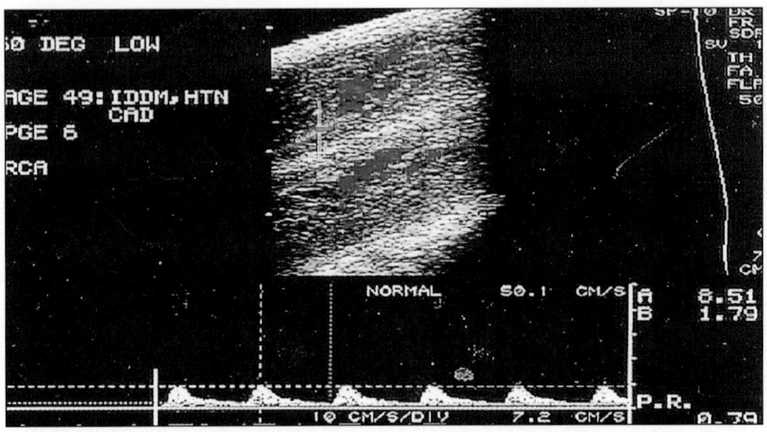

FIGURE 3-15. (*See Color Plate*) Parameters measured by the penile blood flow study (PBFS). These parameters include cavernous arterial diameters; peak systolic arterial velocity (PSV), which is the maximum of the systolic waveform; end diastolic arterial velocity (EDV); systolic rise time (measured in milliseconds from the start of systole to maximum value); cavernous artery acceleration time (AT, which is PSV divided by systolic rise time), and index of vascular resistance (RI, which is PSV minus EDV divided by PSV).

Peak systolic arterial velocity less than 25 cm/sec following intracavernous injection and sexual stimulation has a 100% sensitivity and 95% specificity in selecting patients with abnormal penile arteriography. PSV less than 25 cm/sec reflects severe cavernous arterial insufficiency; however, a PSV greater than 35 cm/sec consistently is associated with normal arteriography and defines normal cavernous artery inflow.

In this image, PSV is 8.5 cm/sec, and the patient did not improve with redosing of prostaglandin E_1 to 20 µg; the diagnosis is severe arterial insufficiency in a 49-year-old insulin-dependent diabetic, with coronary artery disease and hypertension [18–21].

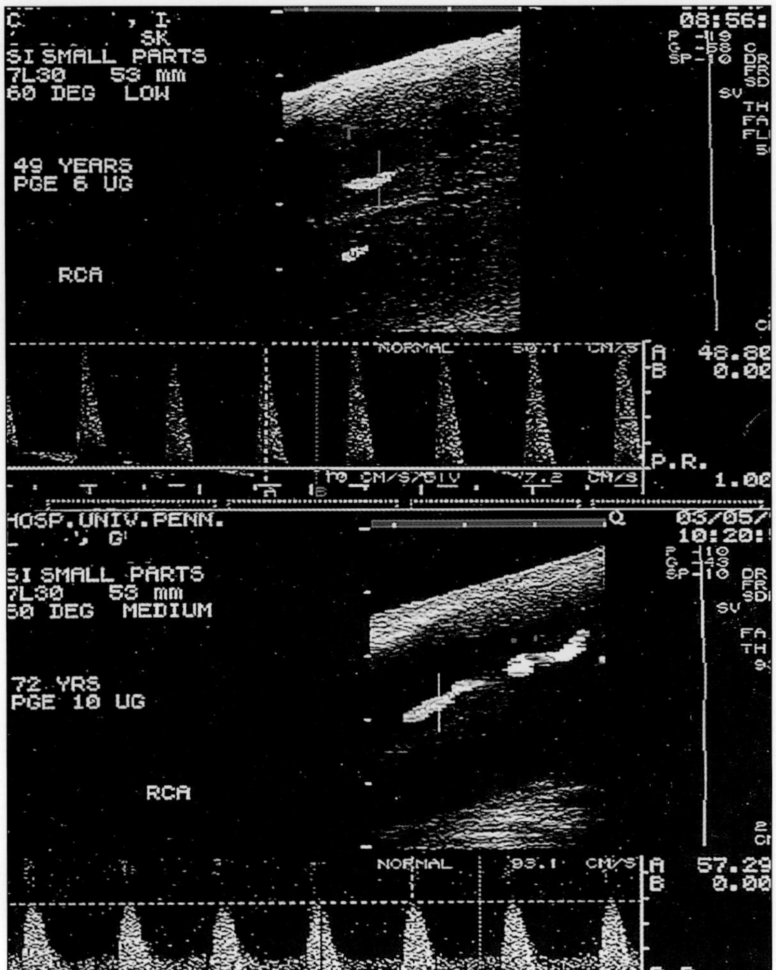

FIGURE 3-16. (*See Color Plate*) The normal study. Unbending rigidity of at least 20 minutes is a "normal" response in pharmacotesting. The observer should record the quality of erection any time Doppler parameters are recorded: inadequate, adequate, normal unbending rigidity. Correlation of the visual erection rating and Doppler parameters is an essential element in the diagnostic protocol. Excellent rigidity is associated with peak systolic velocities in the cavernous arteries at 35 cm/sec or higher. When intracorporal pressure exceeds 80 to 90 mm Hg, cavernous flow transiently reverses during diastole. Reversal of diastolic flow is another Doppler waveform parameter of excellent rigidity.

In this image, two different patients are tested. On the *top* is a 49-year-old man who received 6 μg of prostaglandin E_1 and developed a rigid erection (PSV 48.8 cm/sec). On the *bottom* is a 72-year-old man who was dosed with 10 μg of prostaglandin E_1 and achieved a rigid erection with PSV 57 cm/sec and reversal of diastolic flows.

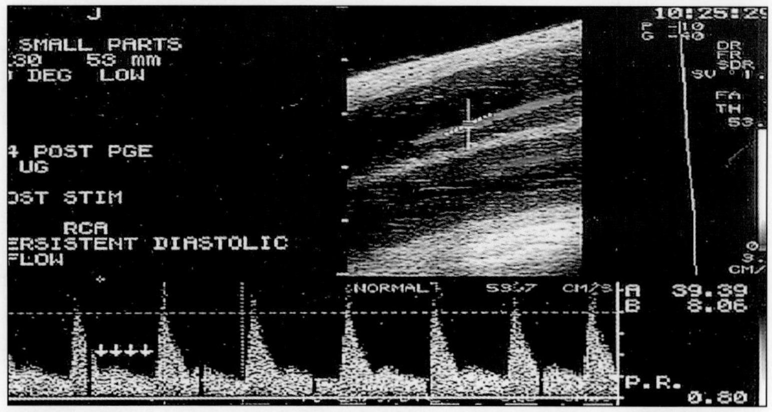

FIGURE 3-17. (*See Color Plate*) Venous leakage. The suspicion of venous leakage is raised when the older patient complains of easily initiated put poorly sustained erections. In the young patient who complains of never having sustained rigidity to climax, primary erectile dysfunction secondary to veno-occlusive disease should also be suspected.

Failure of the veno-occlusive mechanism is reflected in the Doppler spectral waveform of the cavernous arteries: a partial erection associated with PSV greater than 35 cm/sec, end-diastolic arterial velocity (EDV) greater than 3 to 5 cm/sec, and index of vascular resistance (RI) less than 0.9. When the spectral waveform shows elevated diastolic flows despite peak systolic arterial velocity (PSV) greater than 35 cm/sec, a low resistance state persists in the sinusoids. The examiner may also note that quality of rigidity is improved in the standing position and lessened by recumbency [22–25].

In this image, a 34-year-old patient who complained of lifelong erectile dysfunction (primary ED), was dosed with 4 μg of prostaglandin E_1. He achieved a partial erection (following self-stimulation) that was similar to his erection at home; PSV is 39 cm/sec, EDV is 8 cm/sec, and RI is 0.80. *Arrows* indicate that the diastolic waveform persists.

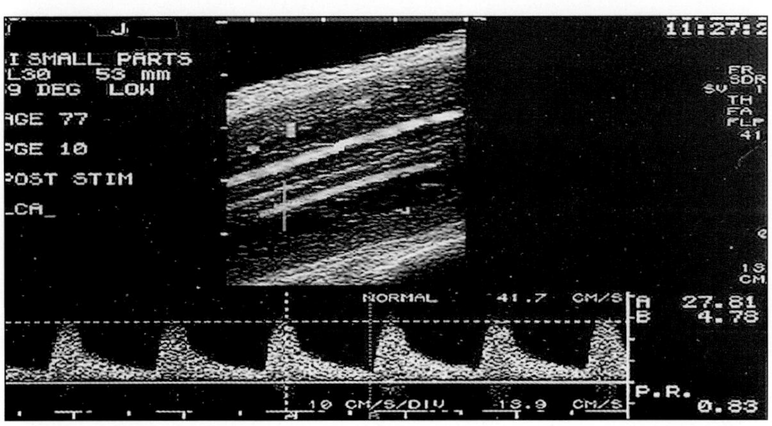

FIGURE 3-18. (*See Color Plate*) Erectile dysfunction due to mixed vascular insufficiency. This diagnosis is made when Doppler parameters reveal a peak systolic arterial velocity (PSV) less than 35 cm/sec and greater than 25 cm/sec, and index of vascular resistance (RI) less than 0.9.

A recent study characterized sildenafil failures by Doppler diagnostics [18]. The cavernous flow parameters suggested that 40% had severe arterial insufficiency (PSV < 25 cm/sec), 28% had cavernous venous occlusive disease (PSV > 35 cm/sec and RI < 0.9), and 21% had mixed vascular disease. Interestingly, 10% of sildenafil failures had normal erections and Doppler parameters.

In this image, PSV is 27.8 cm/sec, end-diastolic arterial velocity is 4.7 cm/sec, and RI is 0.83.

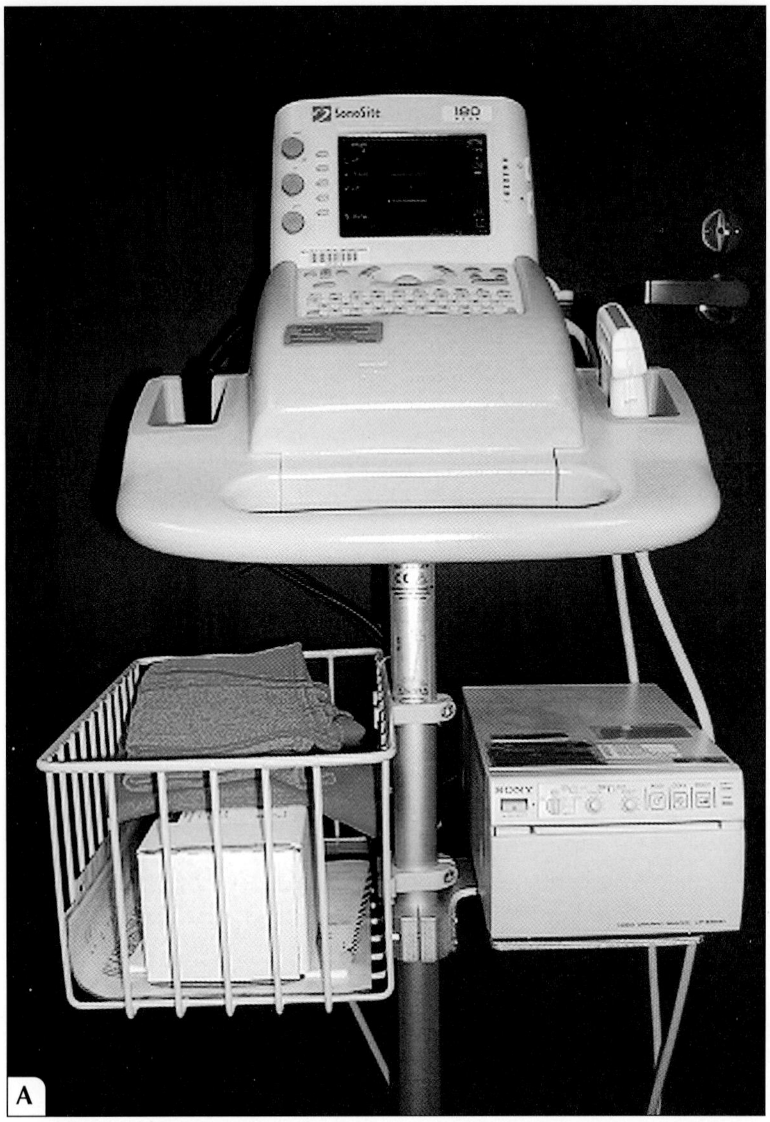

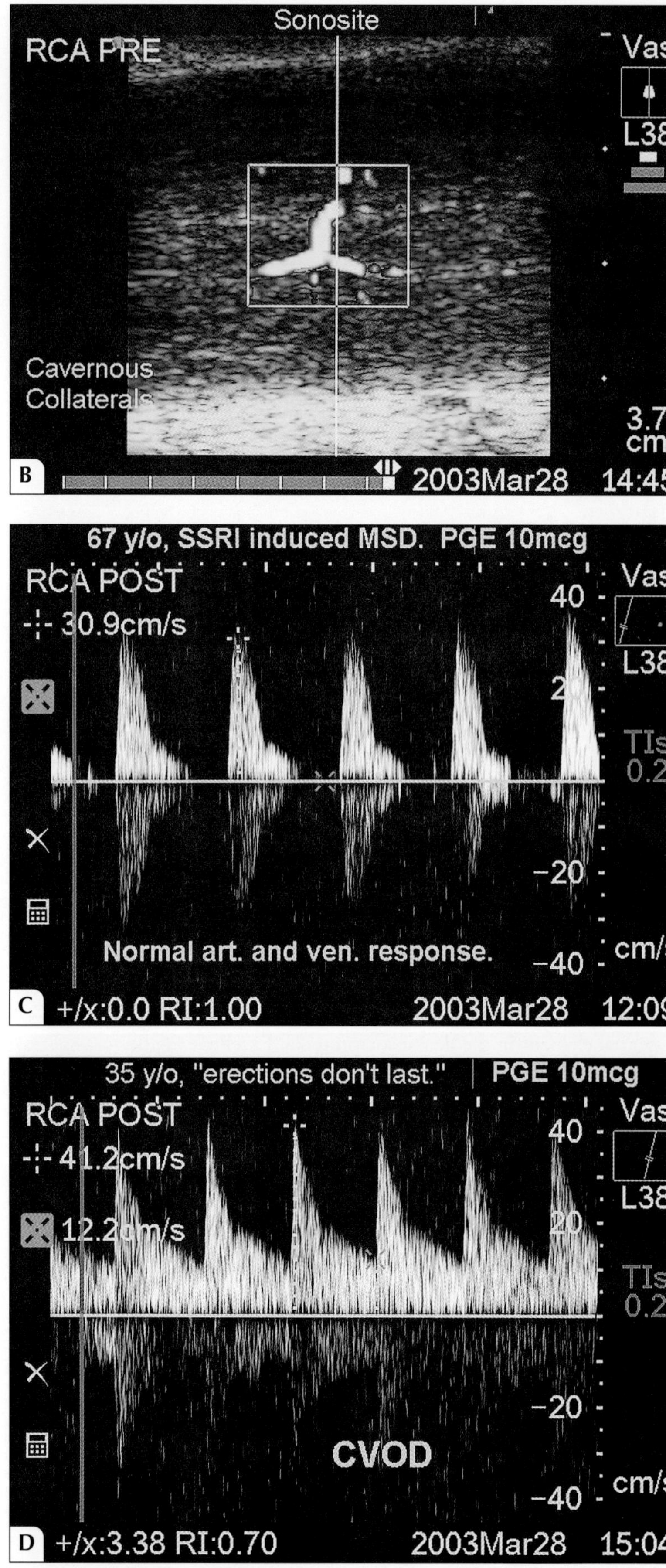

FIGURE 3-19. (*See Color Plate*) Power Doppler imaging. Recent advances in Doppler technology have increased resolution, reduced size of hardware, and dramatically reduced costs. Power Doppler imaging visualizes three orders of branching distal to the main cavernous artery; the hue and brightness of the signal is a function of the number of flowing red blood cells causing the Doppler shift. The dynamic range of imaging is increased, yielding higher resolution of small vessels and low flows. **A,** One such machine is highly portable and lends itself easily to a specialty urology practice: the SonoSite 180 Plus (SonoSite, Inc., Bothell,WA). The device has a linear array 10.5-mHz probe, a color plasma screen monitor, and entire studies can be downloaded to a computer.

B, Power Doppler image of cavernous to cavernous collateral. **C,** Power Doppler spectral waveform on a normal arterial and venous response in a 67-year-old patient complaining of drug-induced erectile dysfunction: peak systolic arterial velocity (PSV) is 30.9 cm/sec, and index of vascular resistance (RI) is 1.0. **D,** Power Doppler spectral waveform of cavernous venous occlusive disease (CVOD). The patient is a 35-year-old man with a lifelong complaint of short-lived erections. Note that PSV is 41 cm/sec and is RI 0.70, after prostaglandin E_1 10 μg administration and visual sexual stimulation.

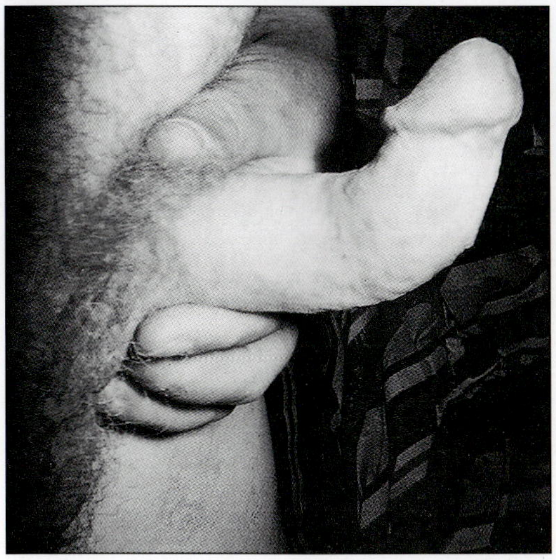

FIGURE 3-20. Preoperative assessment of Peyronie's disease. Preoperative assessment should include a photograph of the best home erection and in-office penile blood flow study (PBFS) to define relationship of plaques to dorsal arteries and collaterals. Erectile quality may be altered secondary to vascular insufficiency as well as penile deformity. PBFS permits the surgeon to confirm the presence and extent of curvature, and determine whether the area of greatest curvature localizes to the palpable plaque. Patients need to be counseled as to the likelihood of normal erections following correction of penile deviation, the need for postoperative pharmacotherapy, or the advisability of simultaneous placement of penile prosthesis.

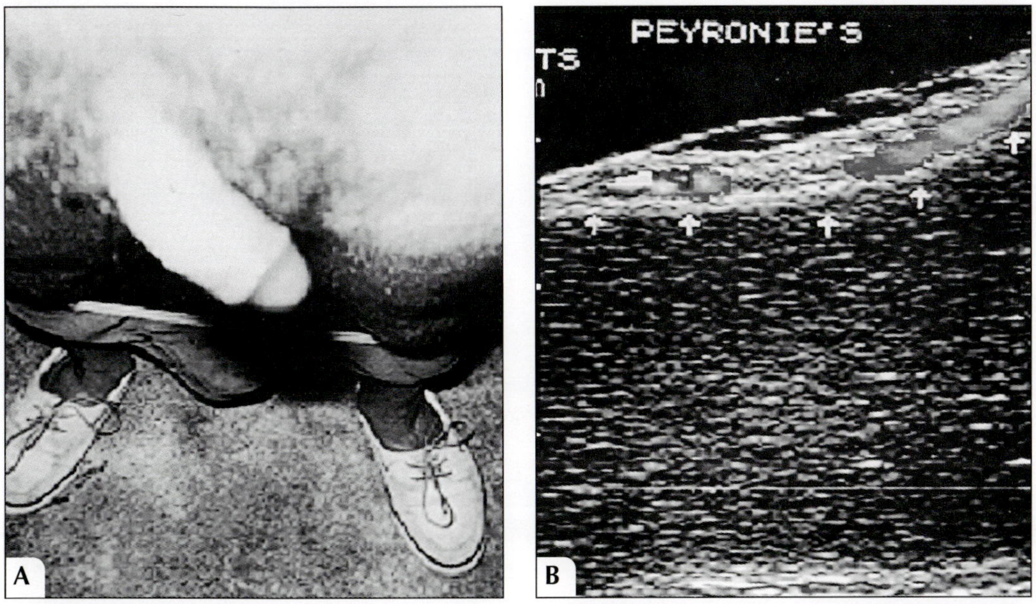

FIGURE 3-21. (*See Color Plate*) Penile plaques are hyperechoic thickenings of the tunica albuginea; typically they underlie the dorsal neurovascular bundle. Imaging of the plaque should be attempted prior to the rigid phase of erection; while the penis may still be flattened against the transducer, a cushion of ultrasound gel is helpful to keep contact with the bending surface. **A,** Home photograph of "best" erection, showing dorsolateral curvature. **B,** Color duplex Doppler of same patient. *Arrows* show Peyronie's curvature in relation to dorsal artery.

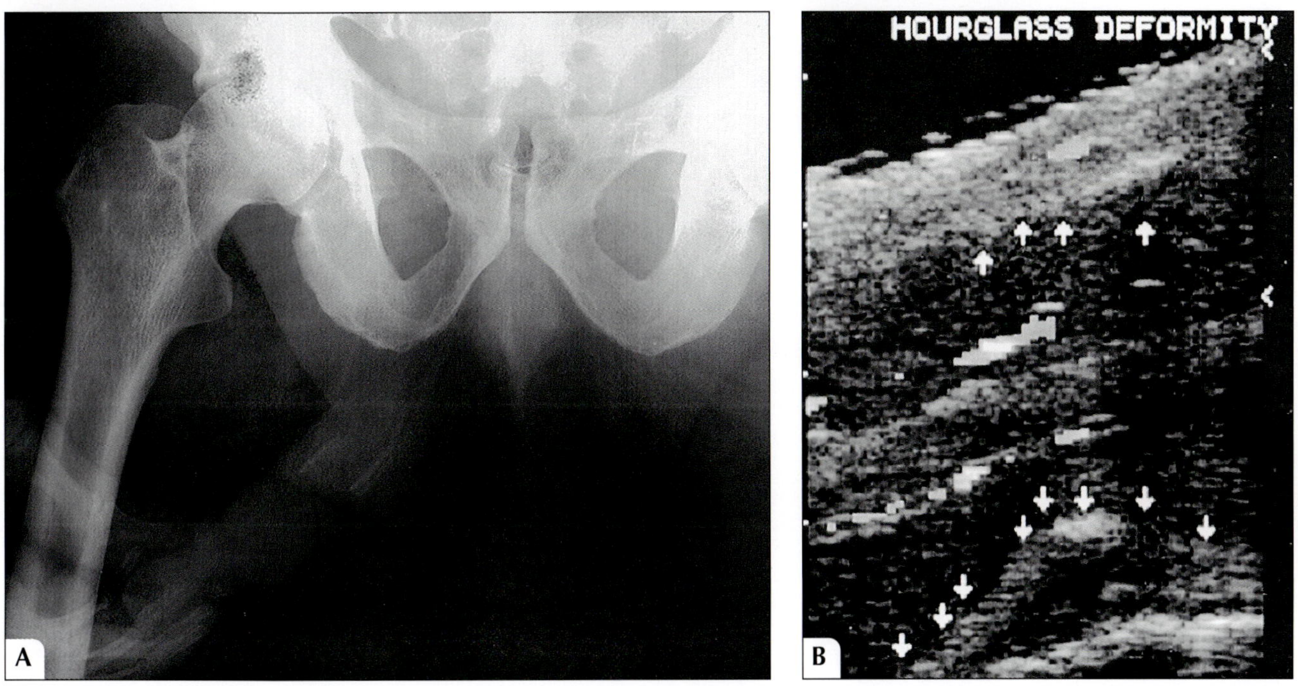

FIGURE 3-22. (*See Color Plate*) Visualizing of plaque using radiography and penile blood flow study (PBFS). **A,** Calcified plaques may be visualized on plain radiographs. **B,** Circumferential narrowing caused by a plaque may be identified during PBFS as a ring of thickened tunica, resulting in an hourglass deformity of the cavernous bodies.

High-flow Priapism

Definition:
- Arterial priapism (nonischemic) is a nonsexual persistent erection caused by unregulated cavernous arterial inflow
- Typically the penis is neither fully rigid nor painful
- Antecedent trauma either acute or remote is the commonly described etiology

Pathophysiology
- Dysregulation of cavernous arterial inflow
- Fistula forms between the cavernous arterioles and lacunar sinusoids
- Cavernous blood gases are normal, nonhypoxic, nonacidotic

Etiologies
- Straddle injury
- Coital trauma
- Needle laceration
- Complication of penile revascularization

Workup
- Penile blood–gas
- Color duplex Doppler sonography
- Pudendal arteriogram

Interventions
- Watchful waiting and periodic reimaging
- Selective pudendal arteriography and embolization
- Surgery
  - Intraoperative Doppler sonography
  - Site-specific ligation

FIGURE 3-23. High-flow priapism.

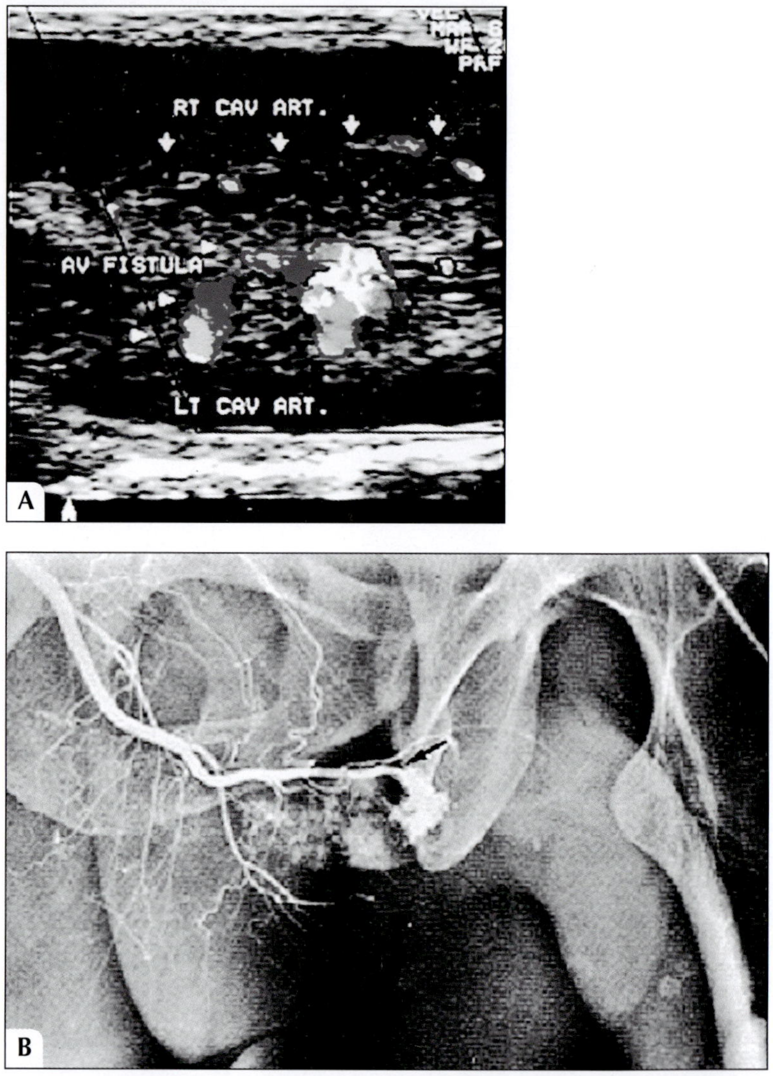

FIGURE 3-24. (*See Color Plate*) High-flow priapism caused by a straddle injury. **A,** Color duplex Doppler image done without intracavernous injection pharmacotesting. The penis was full but not rigid. Right cavernous artery (RT CAV ART) is intact and contracted. The left cavernous artery is disrupted; arterial sinusoidal fistula cause the high-flow priapism.

B, Selective internal pudendal arteriogram. The arrow shows a "blush" of fistula arising from cavernous artery. Phalloarteriography is invasive and should be reserved for therapeutic embolization.

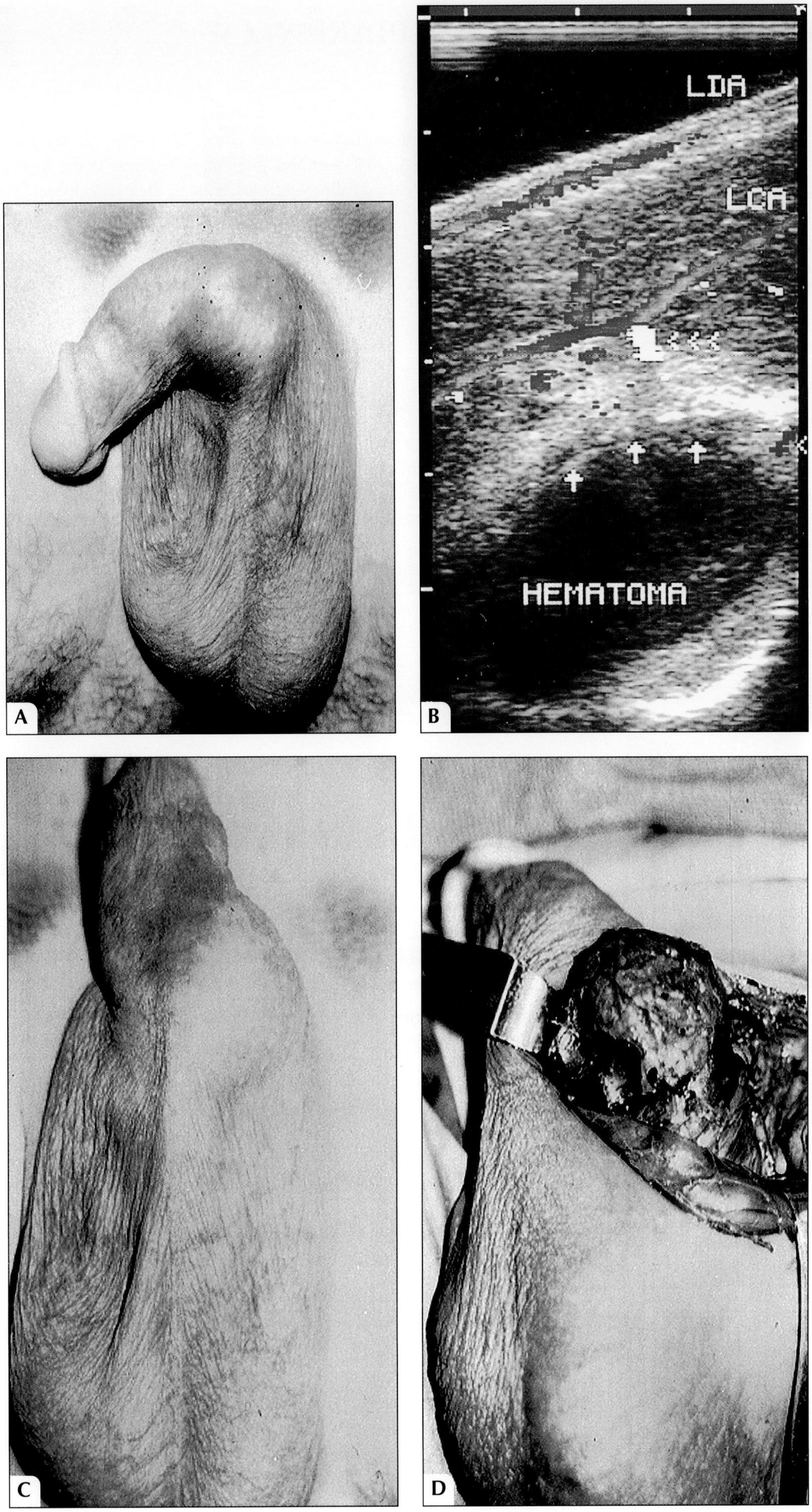

FIGURE 3-25. (*See Color Plate*) Pseudoaneurysm. **A,** Residual ecchymosis from penile trauma suffered weeks before this photograph was taken. The patient heard "a pop" during coital thrusting associated with sharp deflection of the penis against partner's perineum and prompt detumescence. In the weeks following he noted that a lump would develop on the left of the shaft only during nocturnal erections.

B, Penile blood flow study performed following 2 μg of prostaglandin E_1. The left dorsal artery (LDA) and left cavernous artery (LCA) are visualized. The tunica on the left is disrupted (*arrows*) and a pseudoaneurysm has formed, with flow arising from the LCA.

C and **D,** At time of operation, the pseudoaneurysm is identified.

DYNAMIC TESTING AND RADIOGRAPHY OF PENILE VENOUS OUTFLOW

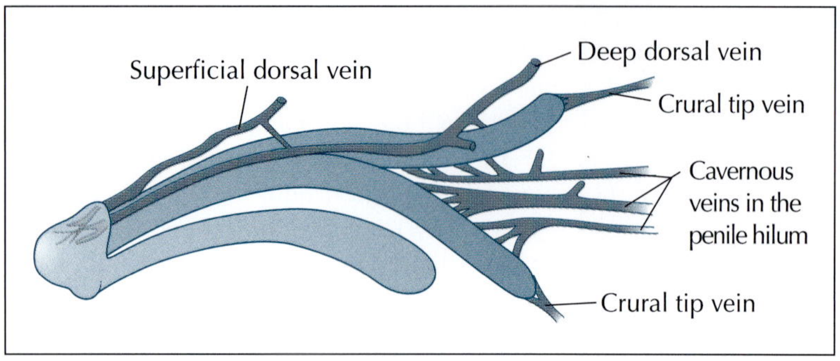

FIGURE 3-26. Venous outflow anatomy of the penis. The venous outflow anatomy of the penis demonstrates three main systems: 1) the superficial and deep dorsal veins, 2) the cavernous veins in the penile hilum, and 3) the crural tip veins.

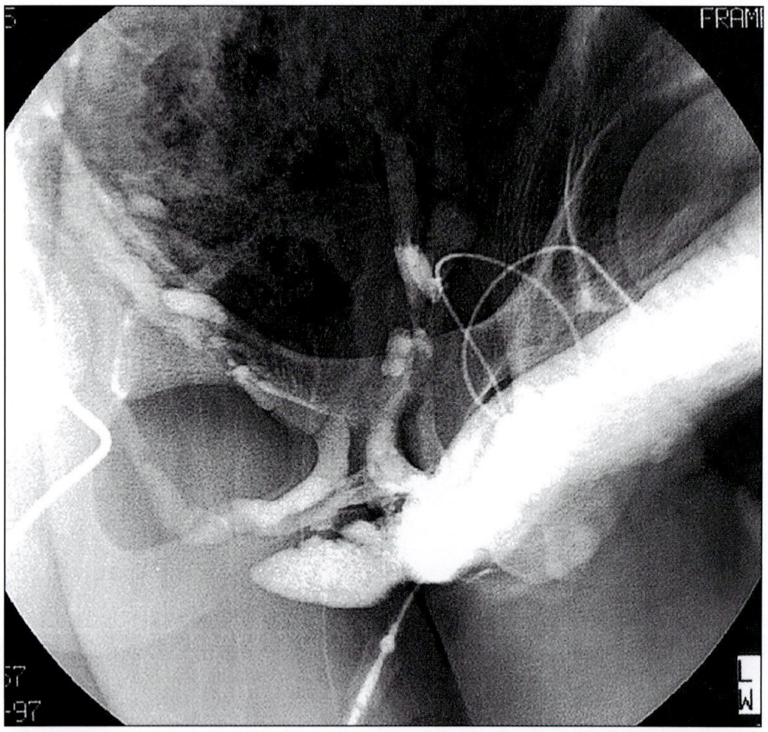

FIGURE 3-27. Dynamic infusion cavernosometry and cavernosography (DICC). DICC is an invasive evaluation of erection hemodynamics, requiring a needle in each corporal body (one infusing, one recording). It is reserved for young men who might be candidates for penile vascular operations, specifically those with a history of pelvic trauma or lifelong erectile dysfunction (primary ED).

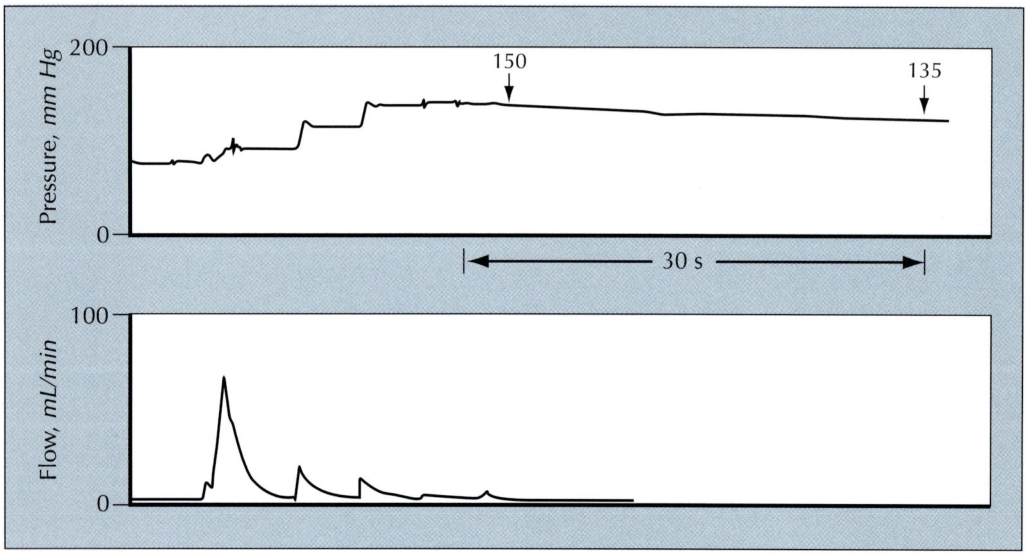

FIGURE 3-28. Normal cavernosometry study. The flow rates (*bottom*) required to maintain three corporeal pressures (*top*) are low (< 10 mL/min) and, following termination of flow at a corporeal pressure of 150 mm Hg, the ensuing drop in pressure from this suprasystolic pressure is low (< 45 mm Hg) over the subsequent 30-sec observation period. (*Courtesy of* Irwin Goldstein, MD, Boston, MA.)

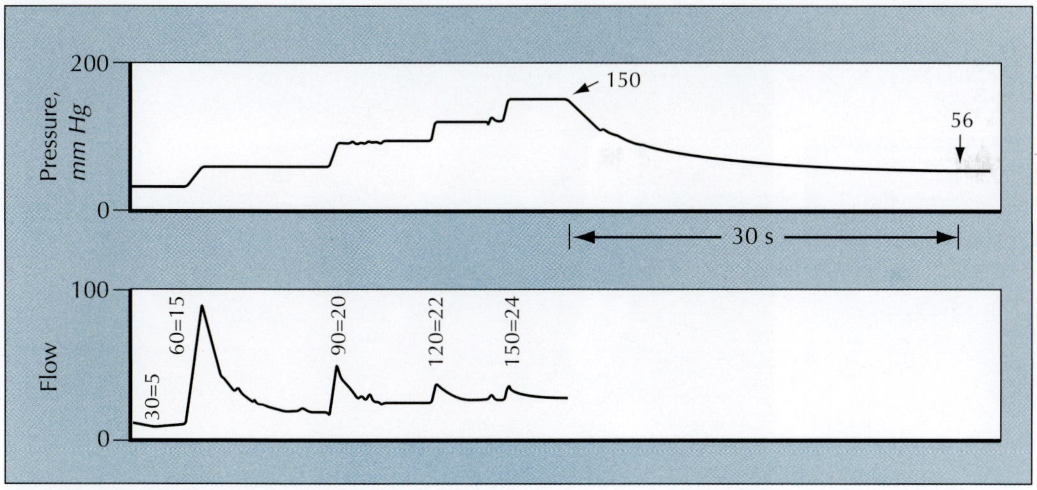

FIGURE 3-29. An abnormal cavernosometry study. In this case, the flow rates are high (> 10 mm Hg) and the pressure decay from 150 mm Hg is also abnormally increased. (*Courtesy of* Irwin Goldstein, MD, Boston, MA.)

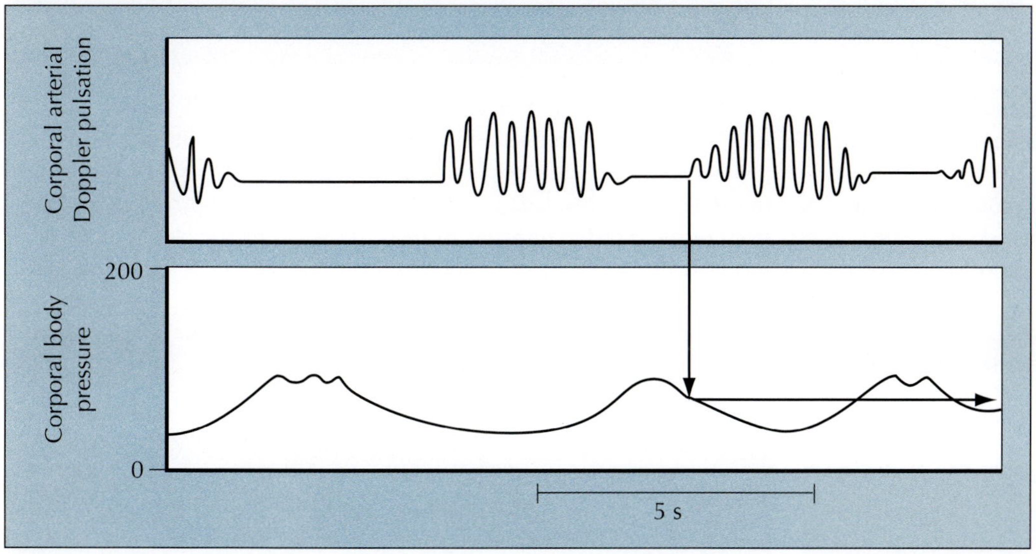

FIGURE 3-30. The cavernosal artery opening pressure. This is defined as the intracavernosal pressure at which the cavernosal artery flow returns following occlusion of the pulsatile flow by suprasystolic elevation of the intracavernosal pressure by saline infusions at cavernosometry. A brachial (systemic) cavernosal artery pressure gradient greater than 35 mm Hg has been correlated with arteriography to demonstrate a hemodynamically significant occlusive lesion [26]. (*Adapted from* Padma-Nathan [28].)

MAGNETIC RESONANCE IMAGING

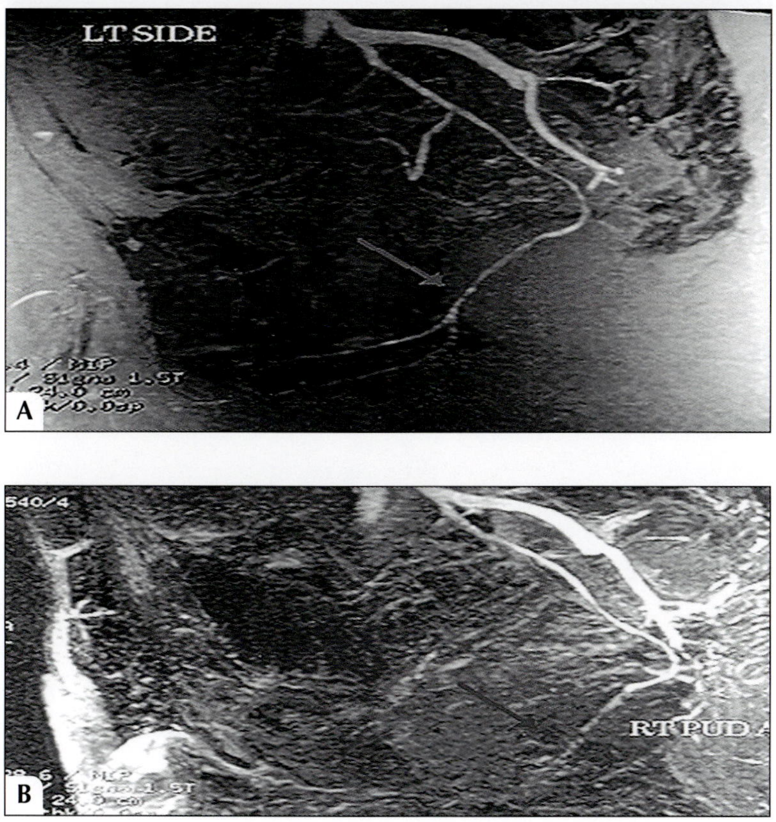

FIGURE 3-31. Noninvasive magnetic resonance angiography (MRA). MRA may have a role in screening men with erectile dysfunction (ED) following severe pelvic trauma (fractures). This is true especially if these men are undergoing MRI to evaluate pelvic fractures. MRA can localize vascular disruptions from the level of the iliac arteries down to the internal pudendal vessels.

A, The left iliac, internal pudendal, and common penile arteries (*arrow*) are normal. **B**, MRA demonstrates no flow distal to the right internal pudendal artery; the patient had suffered pelvic crush injury and subsequent ED.

A. Long-term Complications with Inflatable Implants

- Device failure, leak
- Pain
- Infection
- Pump erosion
- Glans erosion
- Proximal perforation
- Suboptimal placement, sizing
- Aneurysmal dilation
- Pump migration
- Corporal rupture

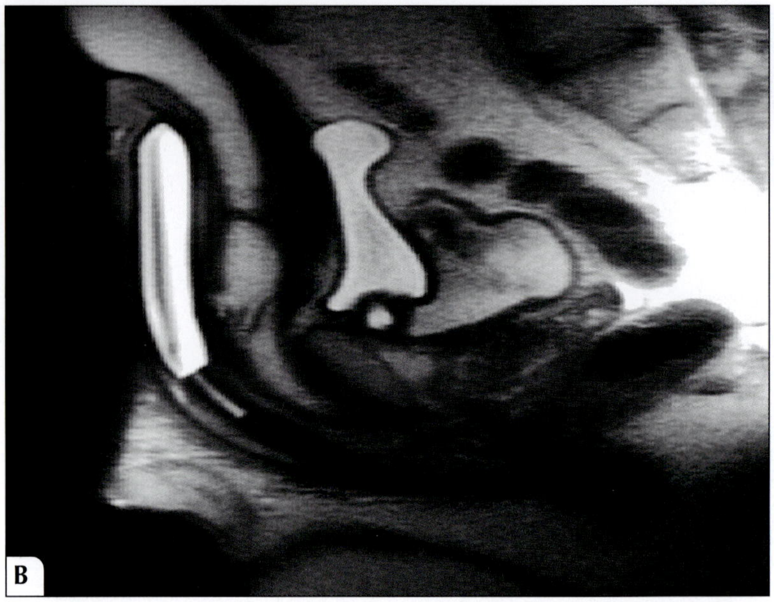

FIGURE 3-32. Long-term complications with inflatable implants. Revision of penile prosthesis has always been challenging, and despite device modifications, revision rates vary from 1% to 20%. MRI may be helpful preoperatively in select patients. MRI may be contraindicated with ferromagnetic implants primarily because of the risks associated with movement or dislodgment: induction of electrical current, excessive heating, and misinterpretation of artifact.

Many types of penile implants have been characterized for safety by MRI, including all currently used inflatable devices by American Medical Systems and Mentor Corporation.

A, Listing of long-term complications. **B,** Sagittal MRI of a fully functional inflatable implant in a patient complaining of chronic penile pain. The penile implant is inflated and slightly compressed against the abdomen by blanket. The reservoir is partially collapsed and sits in front of the bladder. Implants made of silicon or plastic elastomer are relatively devoid of signal; fluid-filled cylinders have high signal intensity (TSE T_2 with fat suppression). MRI revealed good sizing, no buckling, no crossovers, no corporal rupture. The patient, a diabetic who also had lower extremity dysesthesias, responded to neurontin.

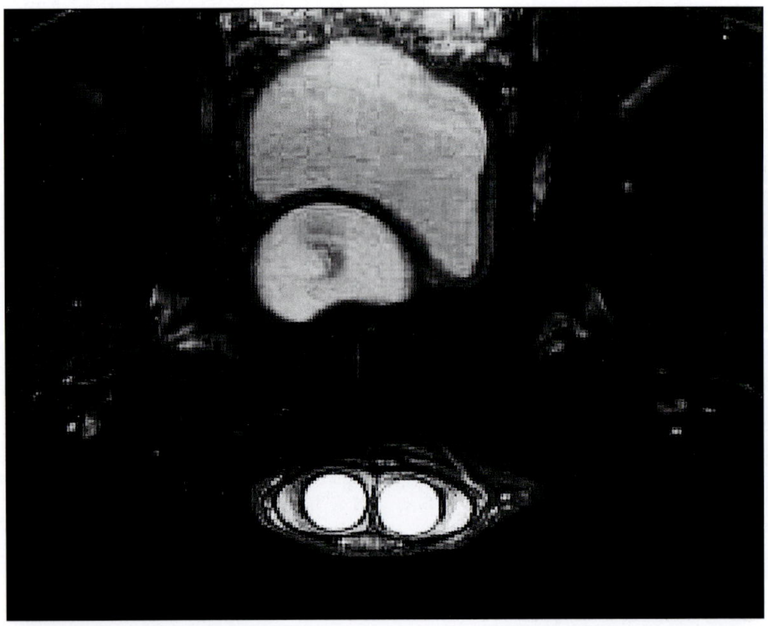

FIGURE 3-33. Magnetic resonance image (T_2-weighted with fat suppression). This transverse image demonstrates medium signal intensity of both the corpus spongiosum and residual corpus cavernosum tissues surrounding the high-signal fluid-filled cylinders. The tunica is a thin homogenous layer of low signal intensity.

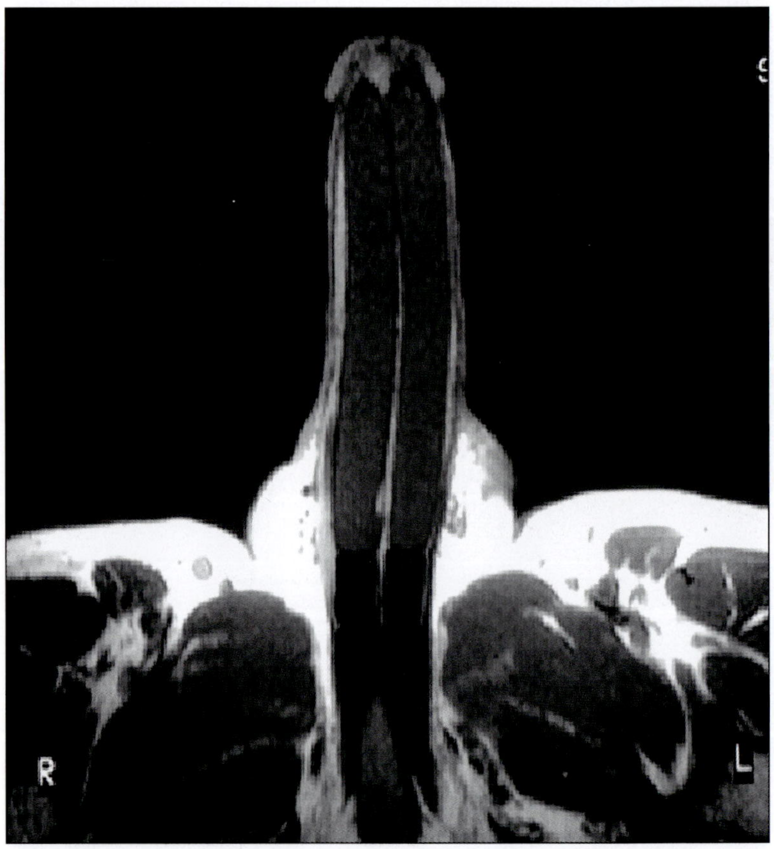

FIGURE 3-34. T_1-weighted MRI transverse image of inflated cylinders. Note symmetry of length and rear tip positioning.

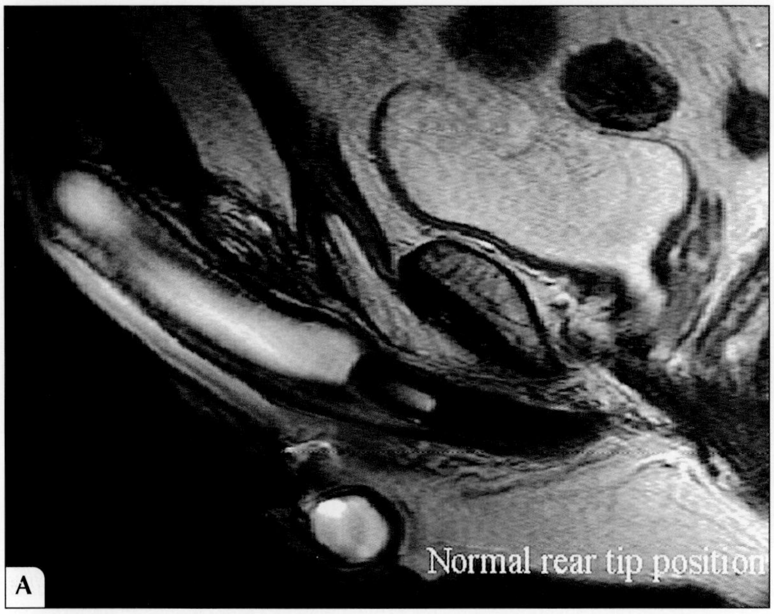

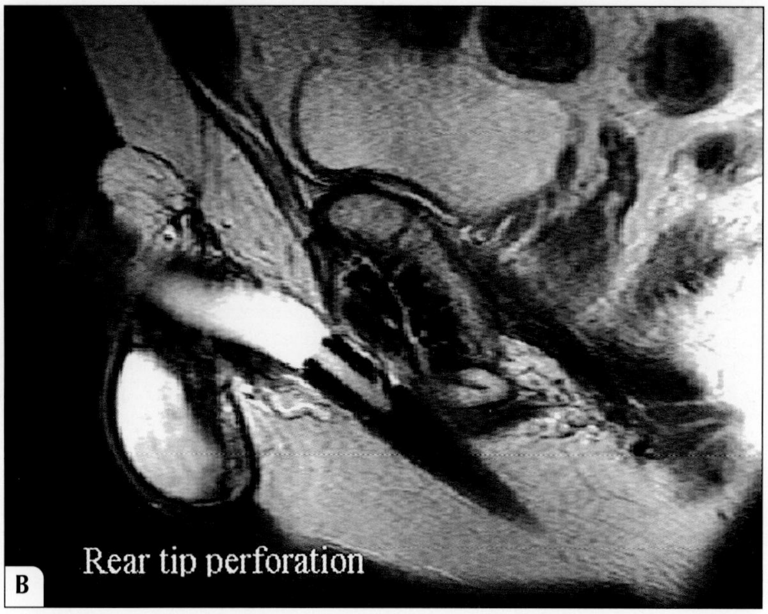

FIGURE 3-35. Normal rear tip position and rear tip perforation. **A,** Sagittal image of rear tip extender and scrotal pump in normal position (TSE T_2 with fat suppression). **B,** Sagittal image of rear tip extender perforated through proximal crura into perirectal fat. (TSE T_2 with fat suppression).

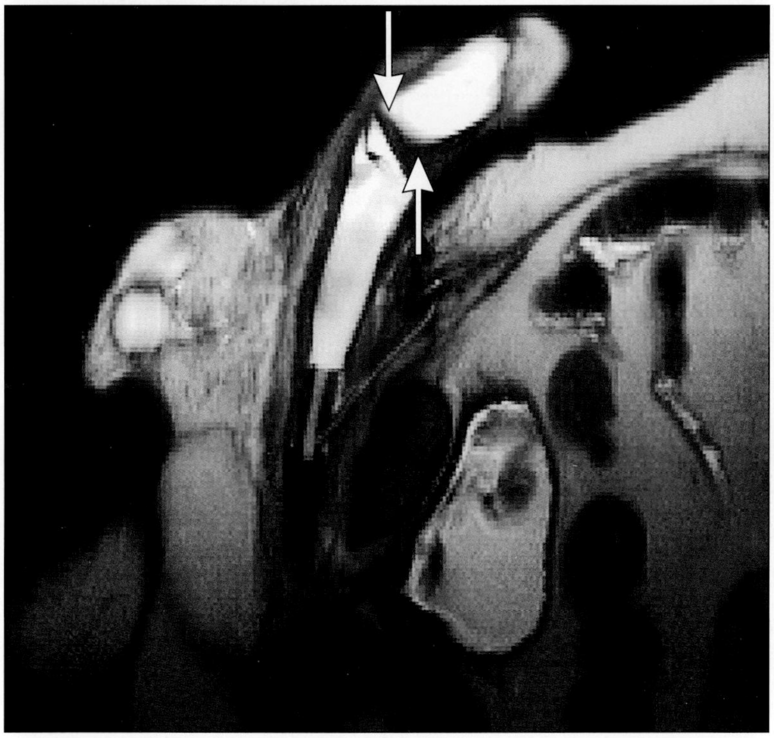

FIGURE 3-36. Sagittal image showing normal position of rear tip extender with tubing exiting at good angle (TSE T_2 with fat suppression). This patient could not fully inflate the device. Note circumferential thickening of tunica (*arrows*). Patient had severe Peyronie's hourglass deformity not addressed at the time of implantation.

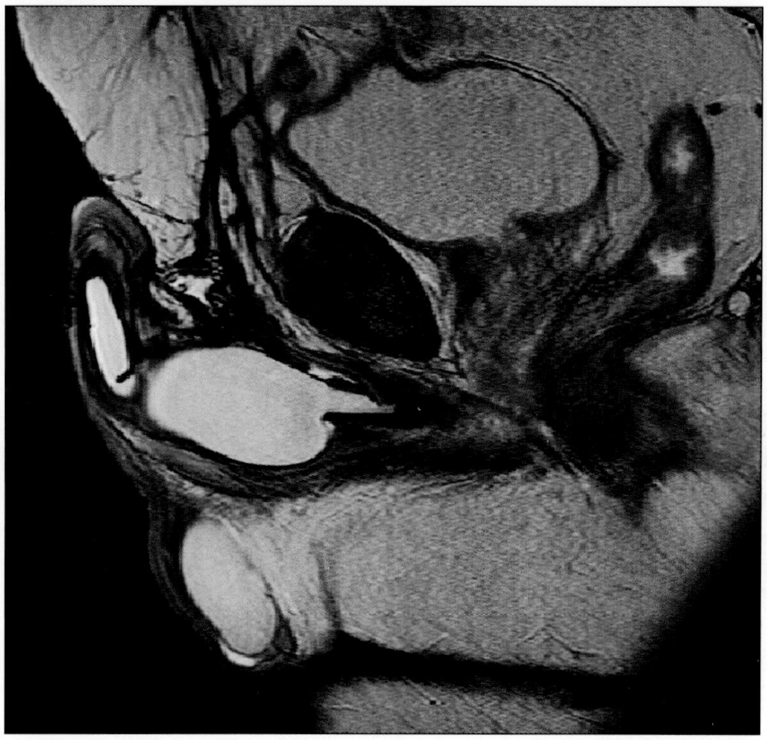

FIGURE 3-37. Sagittal image showing aneurysmal dilation of penile cylinder causing proximal filling and distortion, but little filling distal.

REFERENCES

1. Blander DS, Sanchez-Ortiz RF, Broderick GA: Sex questionnaires: can they replace etiology specific testing? *Urology* 1999, 54:719–723.
2. Aboseif SR, Lue TF. Hemodynamics of penile erection. *Urol Clin N Am* 1988, 15:1–7.
3. Andersson K-E, Wagner G: Physiology of penile erection. *Physiol Rev* 1995, 75:191–236.
4. Sanchez-Ortiz R, Broderick GA: Vascular Evaluation of ED. In *Male Sexual Function: A Guide to Clinical Management.* Edited by Mulcahy JJ. Totowa, NJ: Humana Press; 2001: 167–199.
5. Virag R, Frydman D, Legman M, Virag H: Intracavernous injection of papaverine as a diagnostic and therapeutic method in erectile failure. *Angiology* 1984, 35:79–87.
6. Pescatori ED, Hatzichristou DG, Namburi S, Goldstein I: A positive intracavernous injection test implies normal veno-occlusive but not necessarily normal arterial function: a hemodynamic study. *J Urol* 1994, 151:1209–1216.
7. Cormio L, Nisen H, Selvaggi FP, Ruutu M: A positive pharmacological erection test does not rule out arteriogenic erectile dysfunction. *J Urol* 1996, 156:1628–1630.
8. Elhanbly S, Schoor R, Elmogy M, *et al.*: What nonresponse to intracavernous injection really indicates: a determination by quantitative analysis. *J Urol* 2002, 167:192–196.
9. Aversa A, Isidori AM, Caprio M, *et al.*: Penile pharmacotesting in diagnosing male erectile dysfunction: evidence for lack of accuracy and specificity. *Int J Androl* 2002, 25:6–10.
10. Curet P, Grellet J, Perrin D, *et al.*: Technical and anatomic factors in filling of distal portion of internal pudendal artery during arteriography. *Urology* 1987, 29:333–338.
11. Bahren W, Gall H, Scherb W, *et al.*: Arterial anatomy and arteriographic diagnosis of arteriogenic impotence. *Cardiovasc Intervent Radiol* 1988, 11:195–210.
12. Kawanishi Y, Lee KD, Kimura K, Kojima A, *et al.*: Feasibility of multi-slice computed tomography in the diagnosis of arteriogenic erectile dysfunction. *BJU Int* 2001, 88:390–395.
13. Sanchez-Ortiz R, Broderick GA: Vascular Evaluation of ED. In *Male Sexual Function: A Guide to Clinical Management.* Edited by Mulcahy JJ. Totowa, NJ: Humana Press; 2001:167–199.
14. Govier FE, Asase D, Hefty TR, *et al.*: Timing of penile color flow duplex ultrasonography using a triple drug mixture. *J Urol* 1995, 153:1472–1475.
15. Meuleman EJ, Bemelmans BLH, van Asten W, *et al.*: Assessment of penile blood flow by duplex ultrasonography in 44 men with normal erectile potency in different phases of erection. *J Urol* 1992, 147:51–56.
16. Lue TF, Donatuci CF: The combined intracavernous injection and stimulation test: diagnostic accuracy. *J Urol* 1992, 148:61–62.
17. Montorsi F, Guazzoni G, Barbieri L, *et al.*: The effect of intracorporal injection plus genital and audiovisual sexual stimulation versus second injection on penile color doppler sonography parameters. *J Urol* 1996, 155:536–540.
18. Pinkstuff DM, Broderick GA: Contemporary management of erectile dysfunction: the challenge for second-generation PDE inhibitors. 3rd Fall Meeting of the Sexual Medicine Society of North America, December 2001. *Int J Impot Res* 2001, 13:S63.
19. McMahon CG, Daley J: Correlation of duplex ultrasonography, PBI, DICC and angiography in the diagnosis of impotence. *Int J Impot Res* 1994, 6:A32.
20. Sasteschi LM, Montorsi F, Fabris FM, *et al.*: Cavernous arterial and arteriolar circulation in patients with erectile dysfunction: power doppler study. *J Urol* 1998, 159:428–432.
21. Speel TG, van Langen H, Wijkstra H, Meuleman EJ: Penile duplex pharmacoultrasonography revisited: revalidation of the parameters of the cavernous arterial response. *J Urol* 2003, 169:216–220.
22. Schwartz AN, Lowe MA, Berger RE, *et al.*: Assessment of normal and abnormal erectile function; color doppler sonography versus conventional techniques. *Radiol Sci North Am* 1991, 180:105–109.
23. Merckx LA, De Bruyne RG, Goes E, *et al.*: The value of dynamic color duplex scanning in the diagnosis of venogenic impotence. *J Urol* 1992, 148:318–320.
24. Teh HS, Lin MB Tsou IY, *et al.*: Penile color duplex ultrasonography as a screening tool for venogenic erectile dysfunction. *Ann Acad Med Singapore* 2002, 31:165–169.
25. Kayigil O, Metin A: Relaxation degree: a new concept in erectile dysfunction. *Int Urol Nephrol* 2001, 32:391–394.
26. Broderick GA: Contemporary management of erectile dysfunction: the challenge for 2nd generation PDE inhibitors. *Int J Impot Res* 2001, 13:S45.
27 Lue TF, Hricak H, Marich KW, *et al.*: Vasculogenic impotence evaluated by high-resolution ultrasonography and pulsed Doppler spectrum analysis. *Radiology* 1985, 155:777.
28. Padma-Nathan H: My approach to evaluating erectile dysfunction. *Contemp Urol* 1995, 7:53–63.

4

Hormones and Male Sexual Dysfunction

Alvaro Morales
Jeremy Heaton

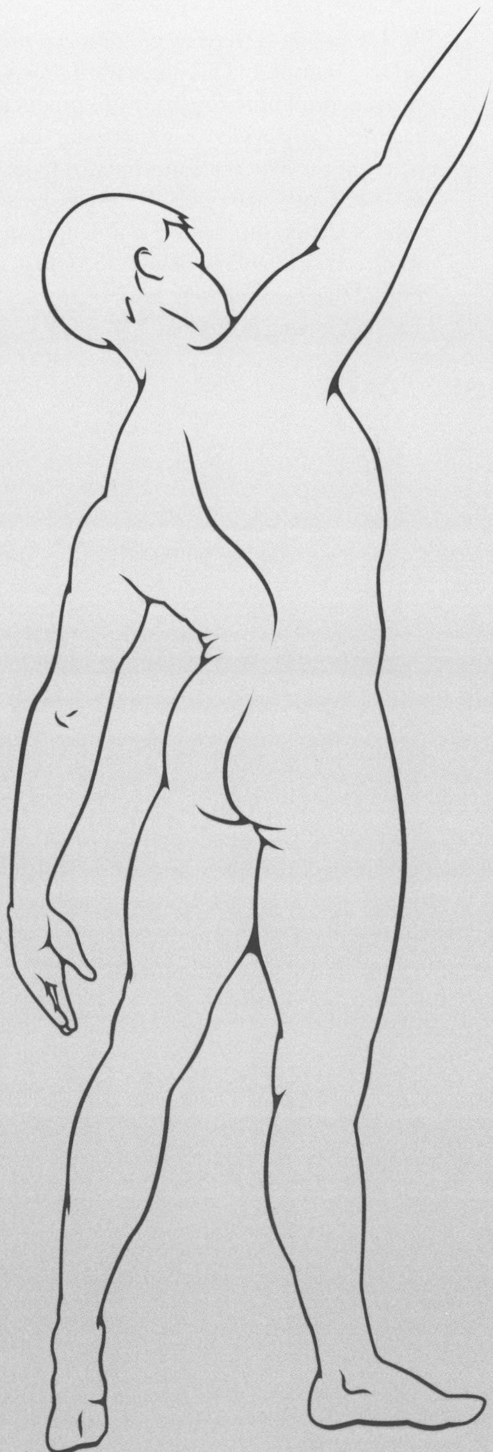

Androgens support the growth and function of all tissues related to erectile function. At any time in life, profound disturbances of the androgen milieu may have a corresponding impact on erections. The minor fluctuations of aging and disease may, in certain individuals, also have effects that necessitate therapy. Yet androgens per se are not a treatment for general erectile disorders. Modern therapy incorporates several different forms of administration and the need for caution especially directed at prostate health and red cell mass.

ENDOCRINE FACTORS

Endocrine Factors in Sexual Function

- Sex steroids
- Prolactin
- Insulin
- Others
  - Thyroxine
  - Growth hormone
  - Melatonin
  - Leptin

FIGURE 4-1. Endocrine factors in sexual function. Sex steroids are the most influential hormones affecting the human sexual response, although other hormones play, directly or indirectly, a pivotal role. Details of their function are beyond the scope of this chapter, but we wish to point out that diabetes mellitus is the most common endocrinopathy associated with erectile dysfunction and one of the most difficult to treat.

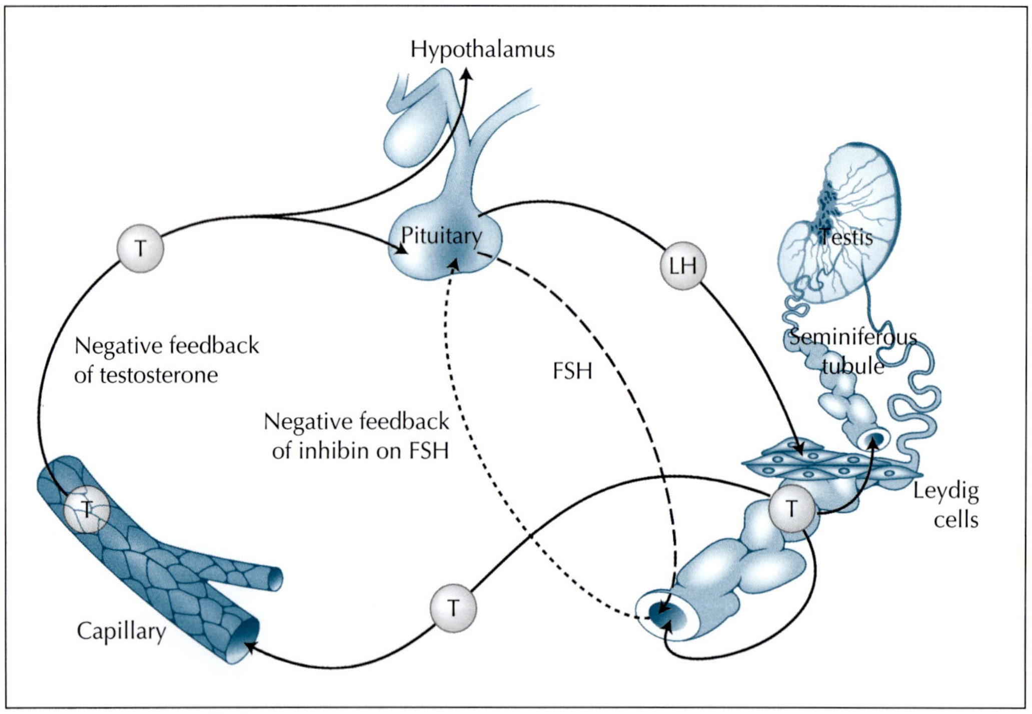

FIGURE 4-2. Overview of androgen production and transport. This illustration shows the central control of testosterone (T) production by the testis. Early evidence is appearing that centers in the hypothalamus (medial preoptic area, paraventricular nucleus) have influence on both sex steroid production and neurotransmitters directly controlling penile erection. FSH—follicle-stimulating hormone; LH—luteinizing hormone.

Overall Sites of Androgen Action

- Sexual system (brain to penis)
- Muscle
- Bone
- Central nervous system
- Prostate
- Bone marrow

FIGURE 4-3. Proerectile signals are sent from the brain through the spinal cord to the genitals, where peripheral penile nerves produce nitric oxide (NO). NO promotes penile smooth muscle relaxation, which allows the corpora cavernosa to engorge with blood and leads to erection of the penis. Suppression of circulating androgens promptly results in a marked decrease in central sexual function (sexual interest) and peripheral performance (erectile dysfunction). Essentially all of this pathway is subject to testosterone modulation.

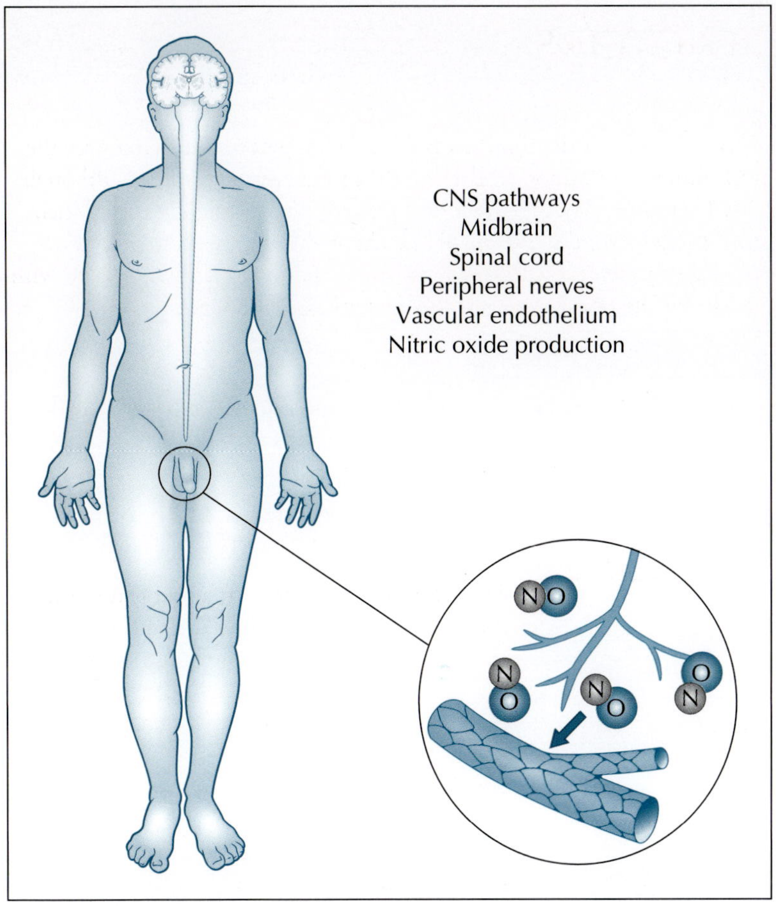

FIGURE 4-4. Androgens exert influence in many organ systems. Hypogonadism frequently exhibits marked changes in the items listed in this table. Urologists are familiar with the profound hypogonadism occurring during treatment for metastatic prostate cancer. In adult hypogonadism associated with aging, the changes are more subtle and are frequently missed. CNS—central nervous system.

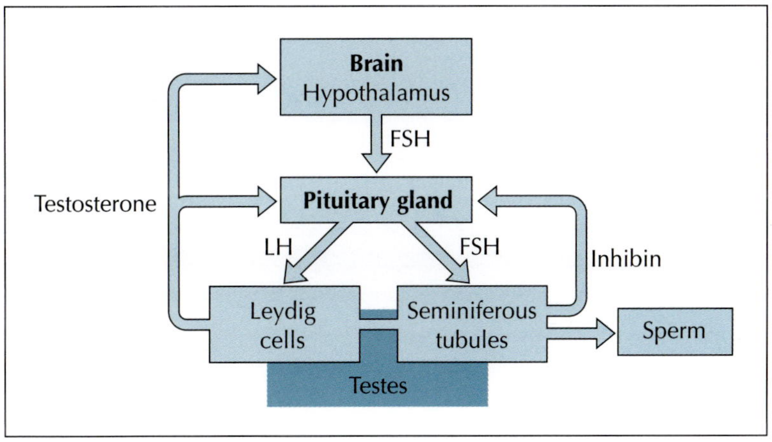

FIGURE 4-5. Basic male reproductive physiology. This image shows the closed loop and feedback mechanisms of testosterone production. Note should be made of the fact that the secretion of control hormones is pulsatile, not constant. FSH—follicle-stimulating hormone; LH—luteinizing hormone.

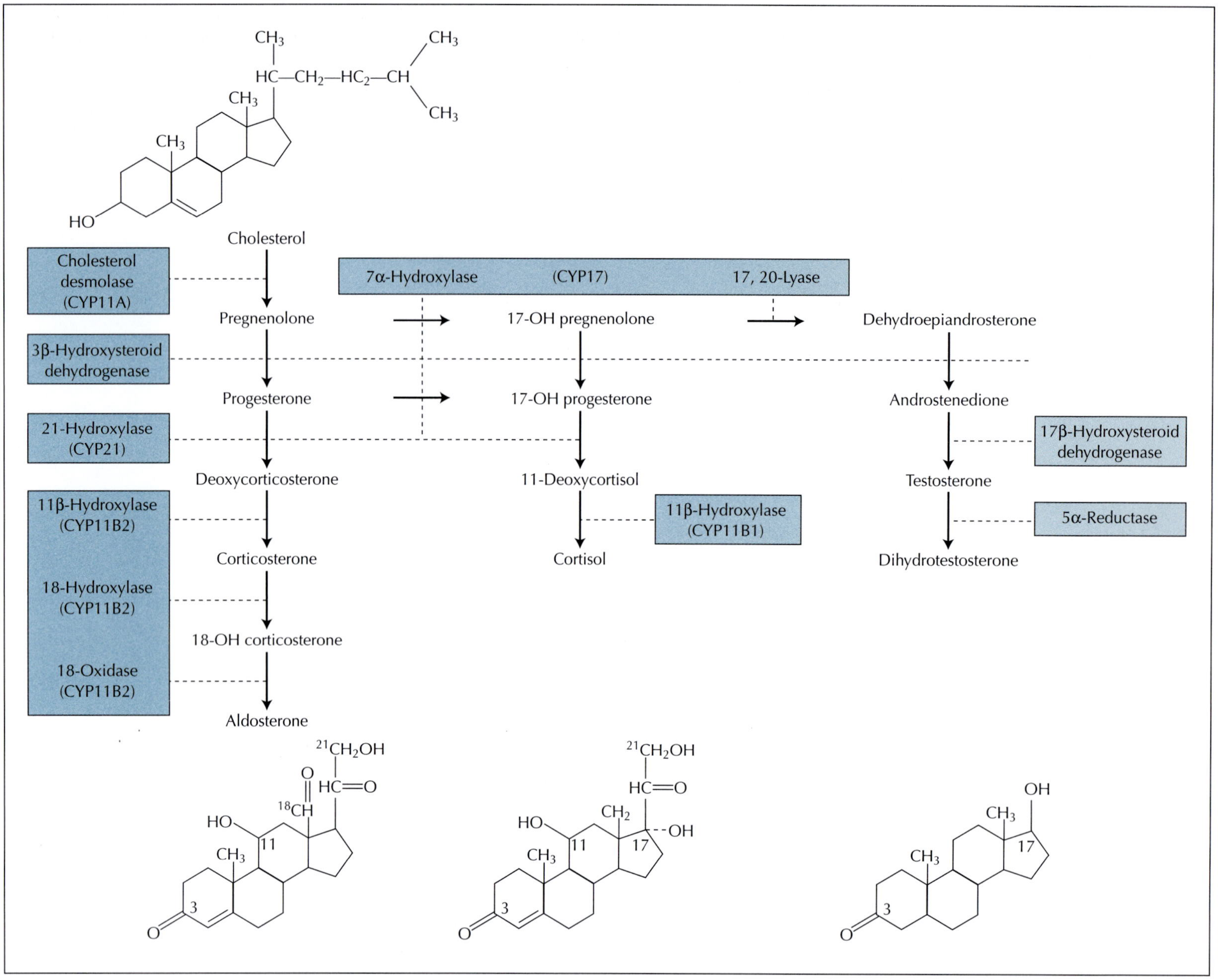

FIGURE 4-6. Biochemical pathways of androgen production.

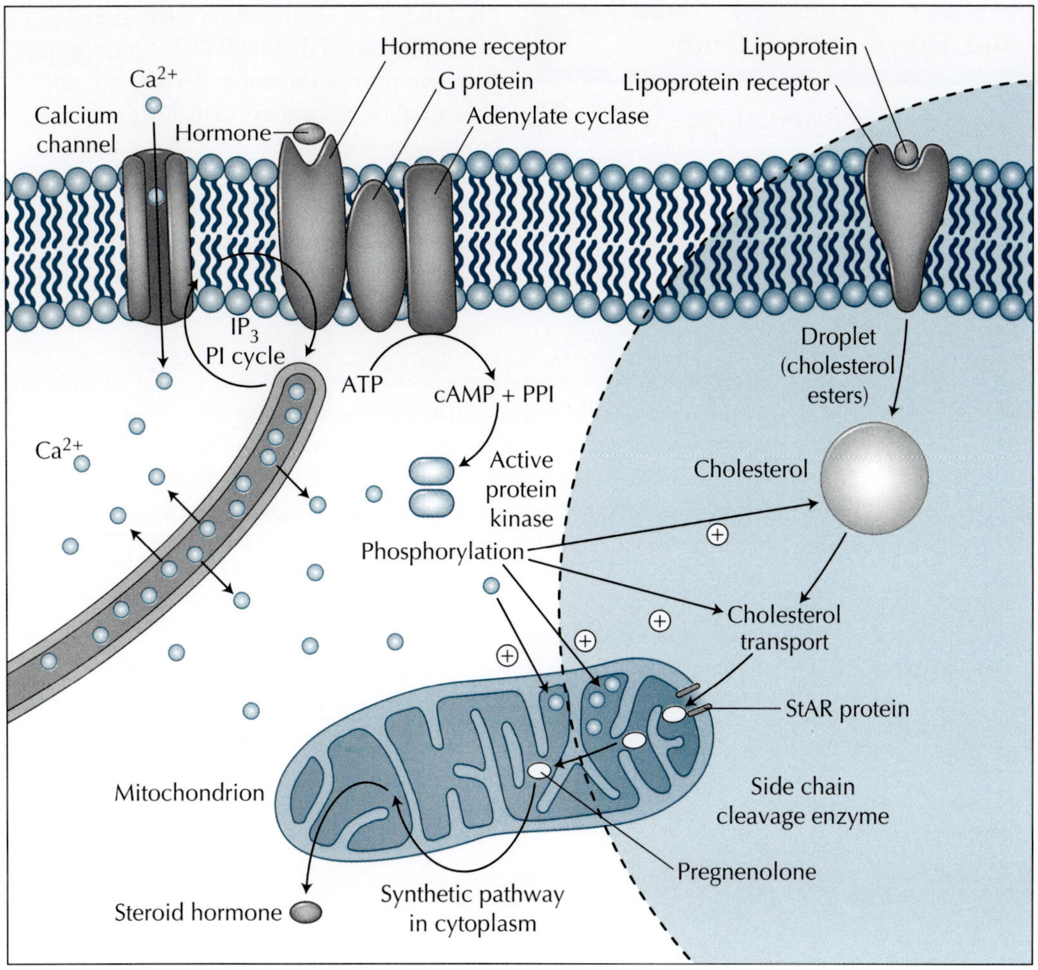

FIGURE 4-7. Testosterone synthesis. This figure shows some of what is understood about the intracellular compartmentalization of testosterone biosynthesis and action. IP3—inositol 1,4,5-triphosphate.

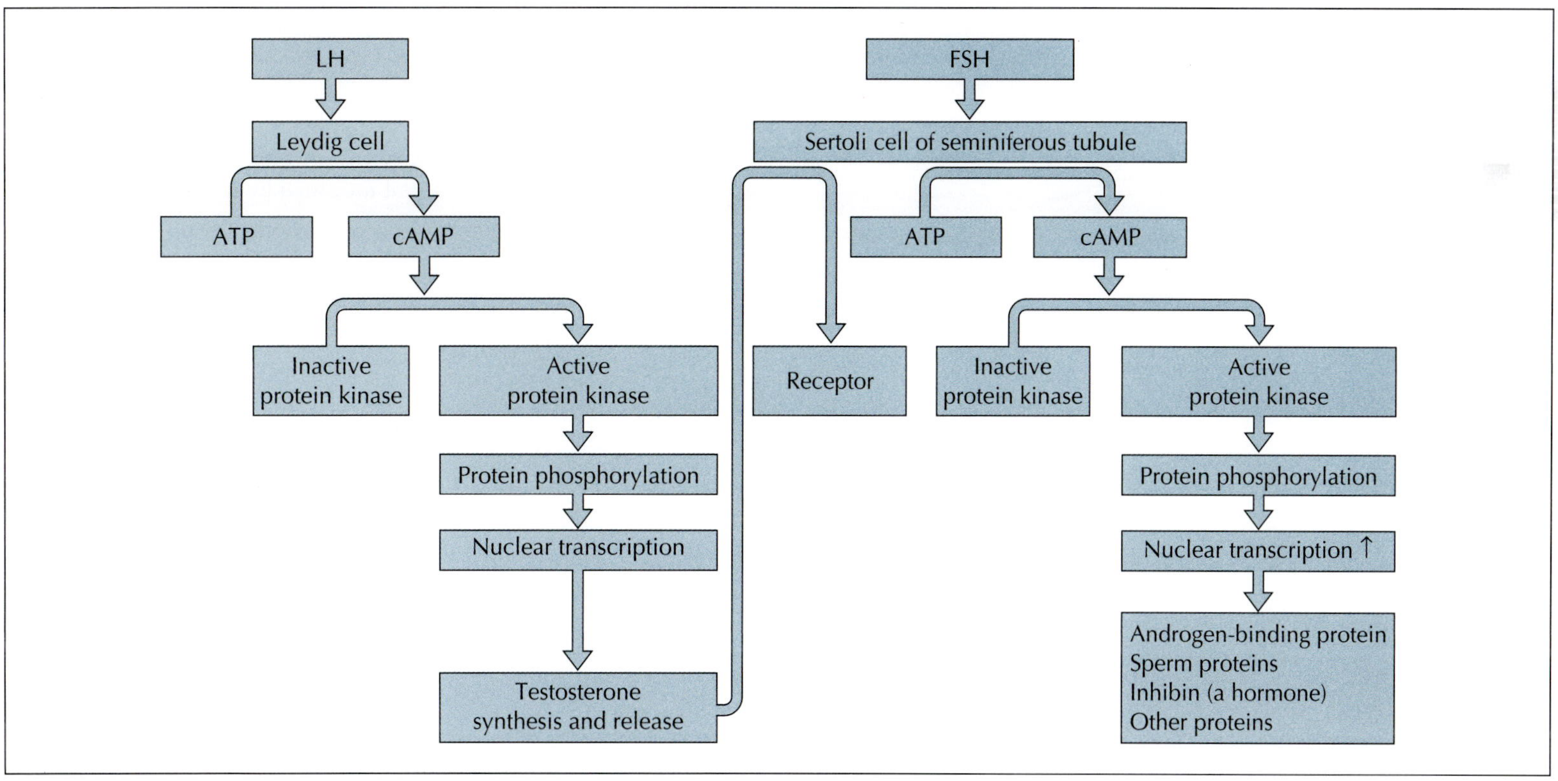

FIGURE 4-8. Testicular actions of luteinizing hormone (LH) and follicle-stimulating hormone (FSH). The significant actions of gonadotropins and testosterone take place in the nucleus where acute as well as long-term (*eg*, transcriptional) effects may be seen. Recent evidence points to the existence of direct vasodilator properties for testosterone.

Comparison of Testosterone and Dihydrotestosterone

	Testosterone	*Dihydrotestosterone*
Concentration in blood	10	1
Potency	1	2
Hormone-AR complex	Less stable	Stable
Affinity for AR	Low	High

FIGURE 4-9. Testosterone versus dihydrotestosterone (DHT). DHT is a more potent androgen than testosterone. Because it is not aromatizable, it is not associated with the production of estrogens. As such it may lack some of the beneficial effects of testosterone (*ie*, bone remodeling). DHT can be considered a selective androgen receptor (AR) modulator.

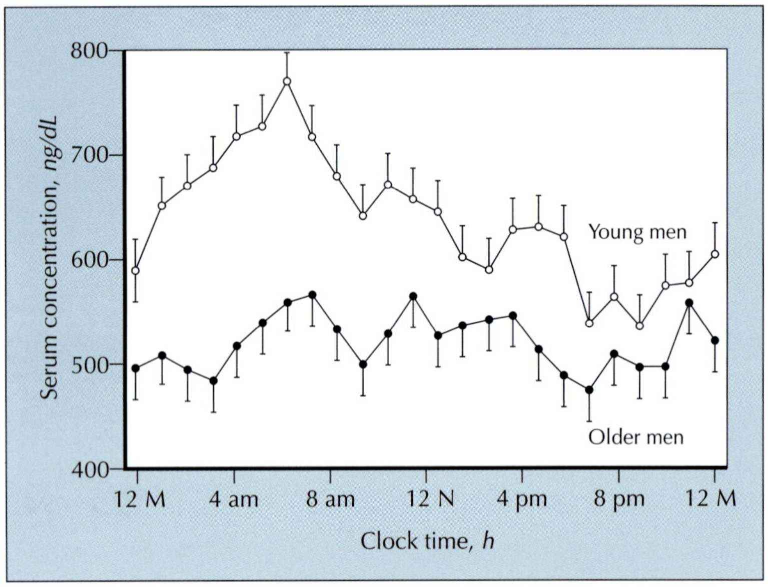

FIGURE 4-10. Diurnal cycle of testosterone. Production of testosterone by the testicles follows a circadian rhythm. In young men, the highest production occurs early in the morning with a nadir around midnight. In older men, the cycle is flattened and the total amount produced in 24 hours is less than in young men. The onset of this decline shows marked interindividual variability but its onset takes place at about 45 years of age.

Measuring testosterone

- Total
- Free
  - Equilibrium dialysis
  - Centrifugal ultrafiltration
  - cFT → *http//issam.ch*
  - Analog ligand assey kits
- Bioavailable
  - Ammonium sulfate precipitation
  - cBT → *http//issam.ch*
- Free androgen index
  - T/SHBG

FIGURE 4-11. Measuring testosterone. There are many methods of measuring serum testosterone. Total testosterone may be misleading because of the amount of sex hormone–binding globulin (SHBG) that renders it biologically inactive. As such, a man with "normal" total testosterone serum levels may be hypogonadal if he has high levels of SHBG. The most reliable indices of androgenicity are bioavailable testosterone and free testosterone; the latter *only* if measured by equilibrium dialysis. A viable alternative is to calculate the "free" testosterone.

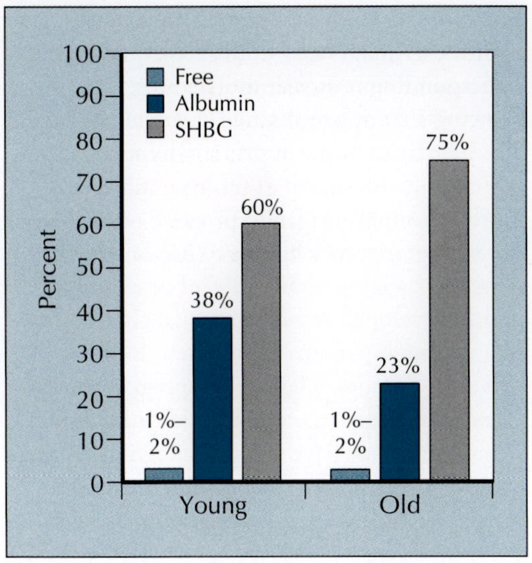

FIGURE 4-12. Testosterone partition in young and old men. This graph shows the physiologic decrease in metabolically active testosterone due to the increase in sex hormone–binding globulin (SHBG) frequently associated with aging. SHBG can also increase in some liver conditions, obesity, and the use of estrogens.

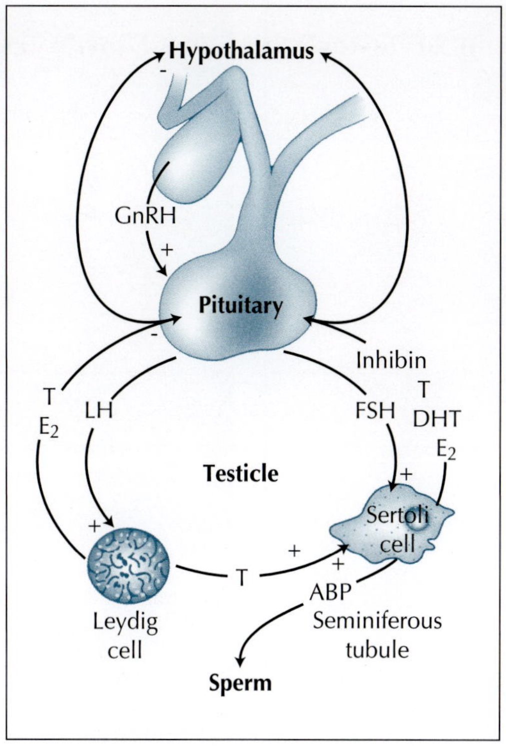

FIGURE 4-13. The hypothalamic-pituitary-testicular axis. (*Adapted from* Dean [1].)

Major Causes of Low Testosterone Production (Primary Hypogonadism)

Orchitis
Cryptorchidism
Radiation
Chemotherapy
Klinefelter's syndrome
Aging (andropause)

FIGURE 4-14. Causes of low testosterone. Primary hypogonadism is caused by intrinsic testicular pathology.

Hormonal levels:
↓T
↑LH
↑GnRH

Causes:
Premature testicular failure
Klinefelter syndrome (*47 XXY*)
Undescended testes
Orchidectomy
Injury
Testicular cancer
Radiation
Chemotherapy
Virus
Alcohol

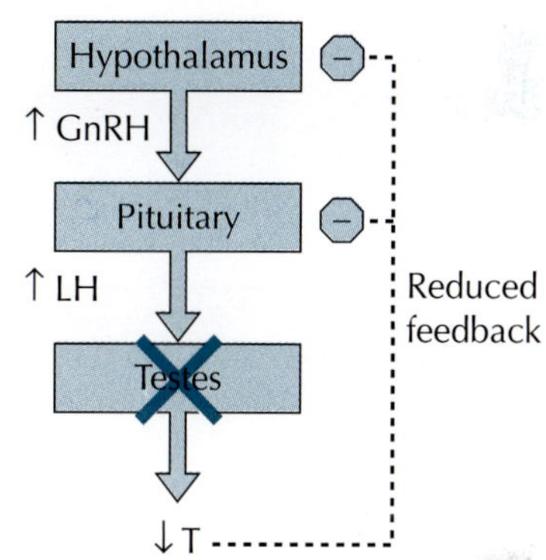

FIGURE 4-15. Pathophysiology of testosterone (T) deficiency. Typically, primary hypogonadism is characterized by low levels of serum testosterone. The hypothalamus and pituitary respond by increasing levels of gonadotropins in an attempt to stimulate the Leydig cells. GnRH—gonadotropin-releasing hormone; LH—luteinizing hormone.

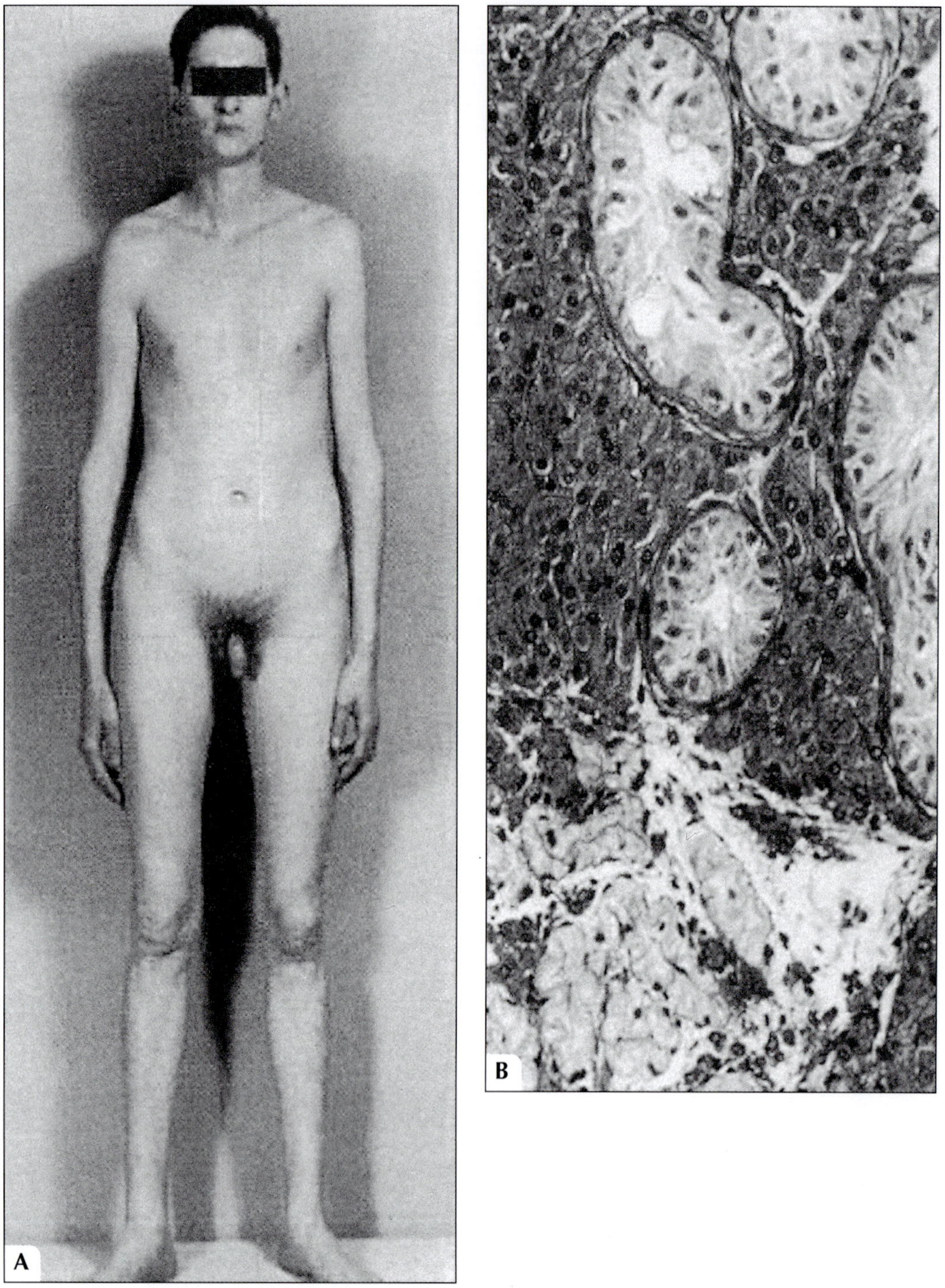

FIGURE 4-16. The typical body habitus of a man with Kleinfelter's syndrome (**A**) and the corresponding testicular morphology (**B**) showing a complete absence of spermatogenesis. The genetic example of primary hypogonadism is seen in about one in 1000 male subjects. Testes are small and fail to produce normal levels of testosterone, which leads to breast growth (gynecomastia) in about 40% of cases and to poorly developed secondary sexual characteristics, although patients may present in the fifth and sixth decades. There is no spermatogenesis. These male subjects are taller and thinner than average and may have a slight reduction in intelligence quotient. Very rarely, more extreme forms of Kleinfelter's syndrome occur.

PATHOPHYSIOLOGY

Causes of Low Testosterone Production (Secondary Hypogonadism)

Hypothalamic or pituitary tumor
Hyperprolactinemia
Exogenous sex steroids
Hypercortisolemia
Certain drugs (*eg,* opioids)
Obesity
Aging (andropause)

FIGURE 4-17. Secondary hypogonadism. Secondary hypogonadism is caused by disease or injury that reduces the testosterone output of the testes as an indirect consequence.

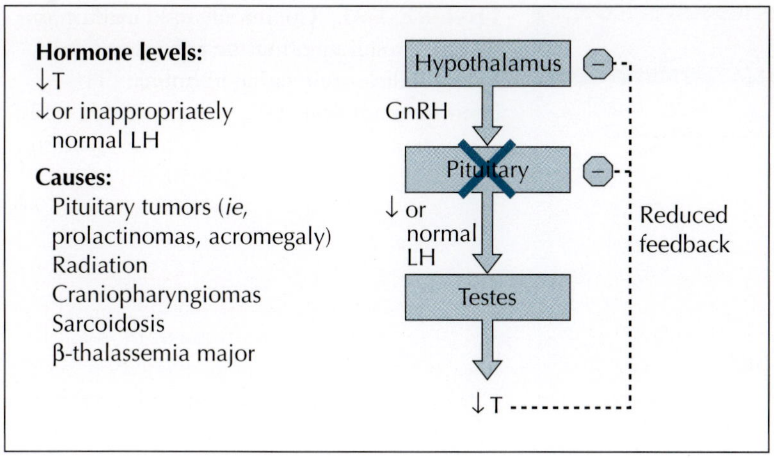

FIGURE 4-18. Pathophysiology of testosterone (T) deficiency: secondary hypogonadism (pituitary dysfunction). Secondary hypogonadism occurs when the anterior pituitary is unresponsive to stimulation by the hypothalamus. Commonly the serum levels of luteinizing hormone (LH) are low or normal in the presence of low serum levels of testosterone. The levels of hormones depend on the time from onset of the disease, but in general, the gonadotropin-releasing hormone (GnRH) pulses will be absent and all other hormone levels low.

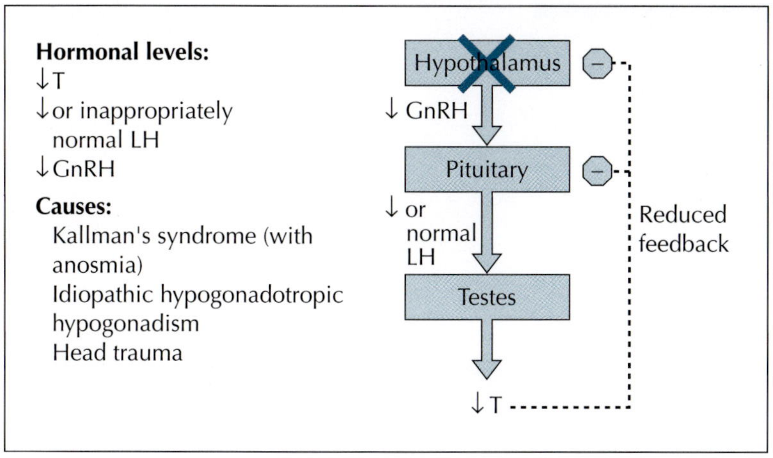

FIGURE 4-19. Pathophysiology of testosterone (T) deficiency: secondary/tertiary hypogonadism (hypothalamic dysfunction). Central dysfunction causes secondary (pituitary) or tertiary (hypothalamic) hypogonadism. Here, in addition to low serum levels of testosterone, there is no compensatory increase in luteinizing hormone (LH) or follicle-stimulating hormone. Secondary and tertiary hypogonadism can be differentiated biochemically by the levels of gonadotropins. The levels of hormones depend on the time from onset of the disease, but in general the gonadotropin-releasing hormone (GnRH) pulses will be absent and all other hormone levels low.

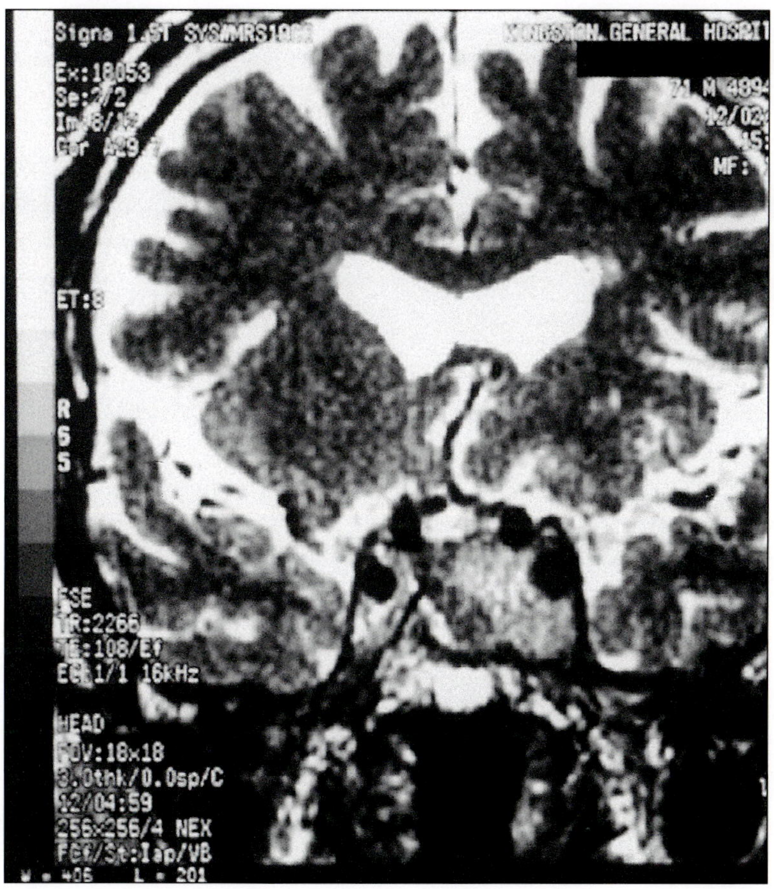

FIGURE 4-20. Pituitary adenoma. An uncommon but important cause of hypogonadism and sexual dysfunction is hyperprolactinemia. Prolactinomas, the common explanation for clinically important hyperprolactinemia, generally respond well to medical treatment, and the patients experience an improvement in sexual function. The associated hypogonadism, however, may require supplemental testosterone treatment.

Drugs Decreasing Testosterone Bioactivity

Drugs	*Mechanism of Action*
Digoxin	Increases estrogen-like activity
Spironolactone	Androgen receptor blocker
Ranitidine	Inhibit cytochrome P450
Cimetidine	Inhibit cytochrome P450 and androgen receptor blocker
Omeprazole	Inhibit cytochrome P450
Cyproterone acetate	Androgen receptor blocker
	Suppressor of LH and FSH production

FIGURE 4-21. Commonly used medications that may result in iatrogenic hypogonadism. FSH—follicle-stimulating hormone; LH—luteinizing hormone.

Systemic Diseases Negatively Affecting Testosterone Action

Disease	*Mechanism of Action*
Cirrhosis	Multifactorial and incompletely understood
Renal failure	Multifactorial, often with disturbances in hypothalamic-pituitary-gonadal function sometimes associated with hyperprolactinemia
Androgen receptor abnormality	Genomic
Complete androgen insensitivity	
Minimal (partial) androgen insensitivity	
Kennedy disease	

FIGURE 4-22. Systemic diseases negatively affecting testosterone action.

TESTOSTERONE AND THE AGING MAN

Reduced Bioavailable Testosterone in the Aging Male

Decreased LH pulse, frequency, and amplitude
Increased SHBG production
Decreased testicular responsiveness to LH (HCG)
Decreased testicular Leydig cell numbers
Increased conversion of testosterone to E_2 in obesity (increased aromatase)
Intercurrent disease

FIGURE 4-23. Reduced bioavailable testosterone in the aging male subject. Aging men frequently suffer from hypogonadism. Often more than one mechanism is operating in this situation. Endocrine causes may be central or peripheral. Commonly, however, there is a primary testicular failure (of variable degree) associated with a diminution of cell numbers (apoptosis?) in the hypothalamus. HCG—human chorionic gonadotropin; LH—luteinizing hormone; SHBG—sex hormone–binding globulin.

A. Hypothalamic-pituitary-testicular Axis in Aging Men

Altered hypothalamic secretion of GnRH
Altered signal to pituitary to release LH
Altered signal to testes
Low testosterone levels

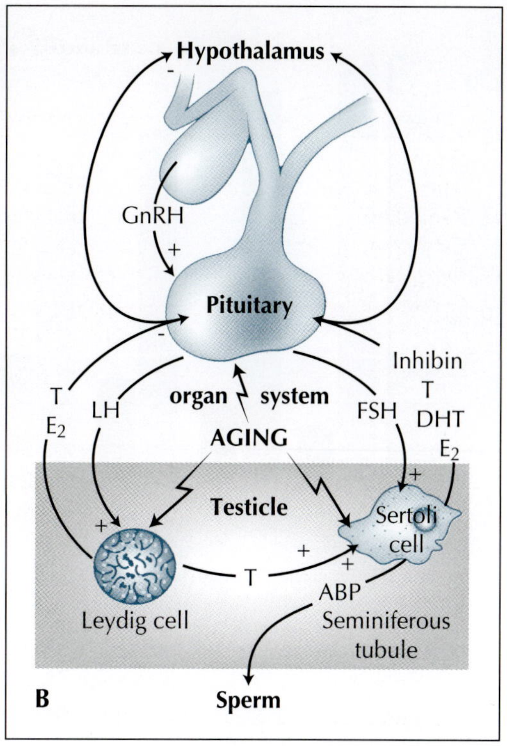

FIGURE 4-24. **A** and **B**, Hypothalamic-pituitary-testicular axis in aging male subjects. The central causes of hypogonadism are most commonly associated with aging. The distinction is of interest but not relevant from the practical point of view. The importance of determining the cause resides in the possibility that a permanent correction is feasible (but not likely) and important for research purposes. In late-onset hypogonadism, the hypothalamic-pituitary-gonadal axis functions with altered sensitivities and responses. GnRH—gonadotropin-releasing hormone; LH—luteinizing hormone.

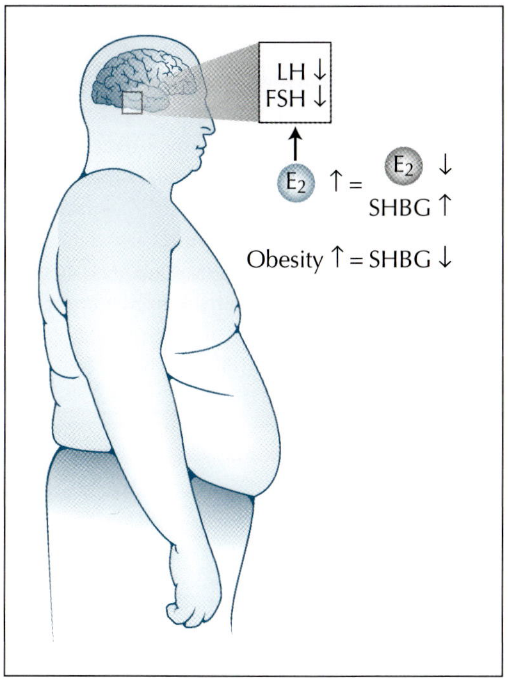

FIGURE 4-25. The role of obesity in sexual performance. Obesity is a particularly detrimental condition for adequate sexual performance. These men have significant endocrinologic alterations (diabetes, hypogonadism), mechanical difficulties in achieving vaginal penetration, and difficulties in administering medications. E_2—estradiol; FSH—follicle-stimulating hormone; LH—luteinizing hormone; SHBG—sex hormone–binding globulin.

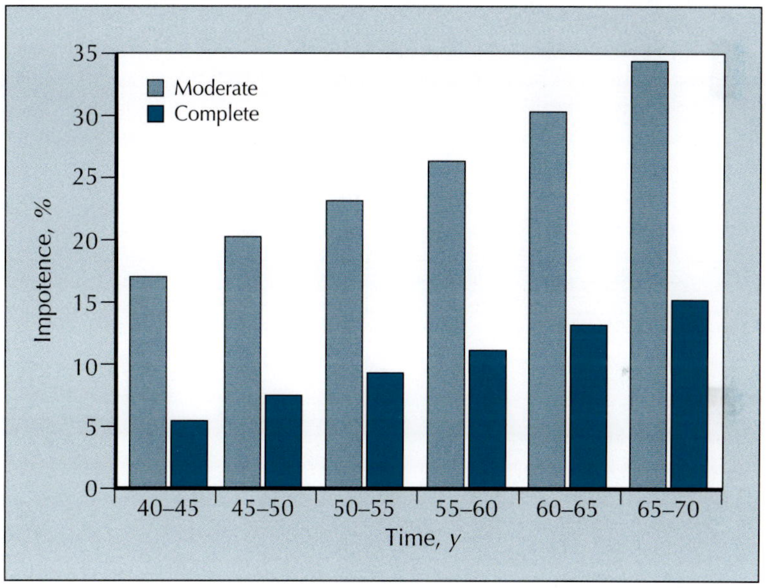

FIGURE 4-26. The Massachusetts Male Aging Study (MMAS): age-related changes in erectile status. The MMAS found age to be the most important correlate of erectile dysfunction.

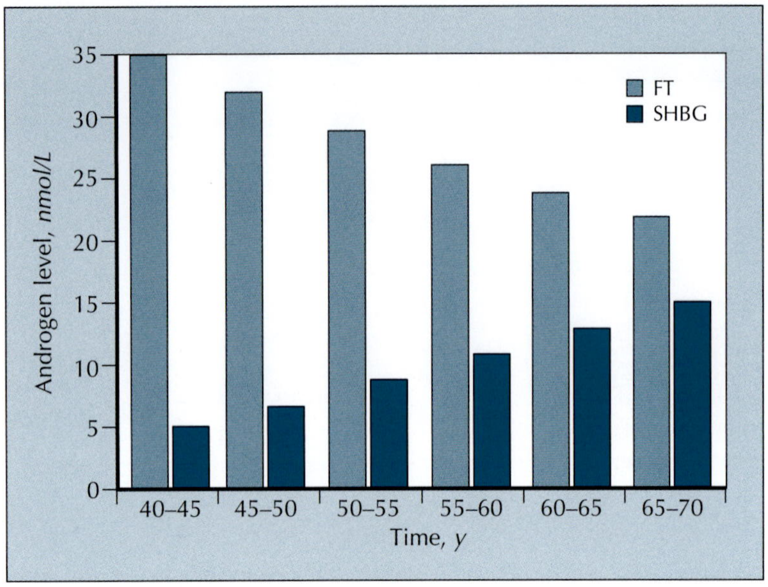

FIGURE 4-27. Age-related changes in androgen status. Interestingly, as age increases and sexual dysfunction becomes more common, the levels of circulating androgens decrease in harmony with the increase in sex hormone–binding globulin (SHBG). FT—free testosterone.

Testosterone, Sex, and Aging in Men

Testosterone is required in many cell systems for normal function, *eg,* the enzymes of penile vasodilation

Castration (adult) causes:

- Rapid loss of measurable testosterone
- Loss of ability to have erection in more than 80%*
- Rapid loss of desire

Low sexual desire and erectile dysfunction occur with low testosterone; however:

- Hypogonadal men may have sexual erections
- Hormonal therapy to normalize testosterone values does not always result in restoration of libido and erection

***However, fetuses, children, and castrati can have erections.*

FIGURE 4-28. Testosterone, sex, and age in men. Adequate levels of testosterone are essential for appropriate sexual function. The key here is that the adequate or "normal" level of testosterone for normal sexual function for any specific individual is unknown. There are large interindividual variations in the levels required. Severe hypogonadism is associated with loss of nocturnal erections but sexual erections may be preserved even in the presence of marked hypogonadism. Hypogonadal men receiving adequate testosterone substitution do not always regain erectile function. There are many comorbidities associated with erectile failure (primarily vascular and neurologic) that are not corrected by administration of androgens. The erroneous belief that testosterone is a panacea for sexual dysfunction has been rejected for decades, but the myth persists.

DIAGNOSIS

Factors Contributing to Sexual Dysfunction in Aging Men

Aging of the hypothalamic-pituitary-gonadal axis
Atherosclerosis
Medical comorbidities
Medications
Depression
Partner status

FIGURE 4-29. Factors contributing to sexual dysfunction in aging men. Many causes other than hormones operate in variable degrees to affect sexual performance. Generally more than one cause is apparent, and frequently all of the ones listed can be elicited in men complaining of sexual inadequacy.

Clinical Diagnosis

History and physical examination
Biochemical determinations: bioavailable T, cFT (see Fig. 4-11)
Questionnaires

FIGURE 4-30. Clinical diagnosis. The first step in the diagnosis of sexual dysfunction is a thorough physical examination. As mentioned previously, an appropriate biochemical evaluation is fundamental to rule out the presence of hormonal abnormalities. Several questionnaires are available for screening for hypogonadism. They are often used, erroneously, as diagnostic tools.

The Androgen Deficiency in Aging Males Questionnaire (Screening)*

1. Do you have a decrease in libido (sex drive)?
2. Do you have a lack of energy?
3. Do you have a decrease in strength and/or endurance?
4. Have you lost height?
5. Have you noticed a decreased "enjoyment of life?"
6. Are you sad and/or grumpy?
7. Are your erections less strong?
8. Have you noticed a recent deterioration in your ability to play sports?
9. Are you falling asleep after dinner?
10. Has there been a recent deterioration in your work performance?

**Positive questionnaire result is defined as a "yes" answer to questions 1 or 7 or any 3 other questions.*

FIGURE 4-31. The ADAM (Androgen Deficiency in Aging Males) questionnaire (screening). This questionnaire is useful as a screening tool. It was not designed and should not be used as a diagnostic instrument.

Current Treatments

	Generic name	*Dosage*
Injectable	Testosterone cypionate	200–400 mg every 2–4 wk
	Testosterone enanthate	200–400 mg every 2–4 wk
Oral	Fluoxymesterone*	5–20 mg/d
	Testosterone undecanoate	10–30 mg/d
Transdermal	Testosterone patch	120–240 mg/d
	Testosterone gel	2.5–5 mg/d
	Testim (Auxilium Pharmaceuticals, Inc., Norristown, PA)	50–100 mg/d
	AndroGel (Solvay Pharmaceuticals, Inc., Baudette, MN)	5–10 g/d

**As 17α-alkylated testosterone products, both fluoxymesterone and methyltestosterone are associated with serious liver toxicity.*

FIGURE 4-32. Commonly available forms of delivery for testosterone. With the notable exception of the methylated (alkylated) ones (fluoxymesterone and methyltestosterone), all are safe and effective when used appropriately by competent physicians.

	Initiator	Conditioner	Other
Central	Apomorphine PT-141	Testosterone	Counseling Prosthesis VED
Peripheral	PGE_1 (ICI, TU) Triple mix (ICI)	Testosterone PDE5 inhibitors	

FIGURE 4-33. Treatment strategies. Testosterone can be shown to modulate almost every level of the control systems for erections. It will correspondingly have an impact on any attempt at pharmacologic therapy. Unless otherwise indicated, the testosterone milieu should be optimized as pharmacotherapy is implemented.

The Main Concerns of Androgen Replacement Therapy

Unresolved issues on prostate safety
Undefined effect on lipid profile
Erythropoietic effect
Induction of fluid retention
Sleep apnea (controversial)
Behavioral changes (controversial)
Liver function (no longer a concern)

FIGURE 4-34. The main concerns regarding testosterone administration. The most prominent concern relates to prostate safety. Much less concerning are the possible detrimental effects in the lipid profile and the increase in hematocrit. The latter is of significant and often overlooked concern in aging men.

Sexual Manifestations of Testosterone Deficiency

Sexual dysfunction
- Low libido
- Poor erectile quality
- Reduced spontaneous and nocturnal erections
- Reduced sexual performance
  - Sexual activity
  - Sexual frequency

Reduced muscle mass and strength
Increased body fat (visceral)
Fatigue
Depression and negative effect on mood and cognitive function
Increased risk of osteoporosis/fractures
Reduced red blood cell volume

FIGURE 4-35. Manifestations of testosterone deficiency. The sexual manifestations appear in a prominent position because they are readily recognized and occur early. The nonsexual manifestations are less evident and may remain undiagnosed for years. (*Data from* Morales *et al.* [2] and Matsumoto *et al.* [3].)

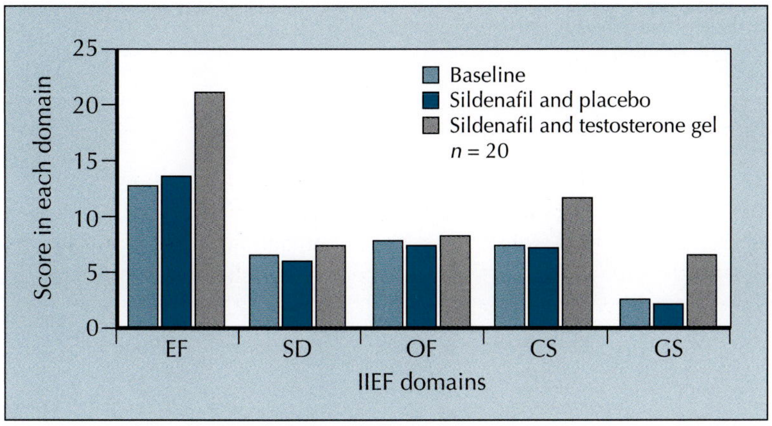

FIGURE 4-36. Testosterone and sildenafil: changes in International Index of Erectile Function (IIEF) domains. Evidence is beginning to appear suggesting that coadministration of testosterone with a phosphodiesterase-5 inhibitor offers therapeutic synergism. Further research on the subject is underway. To date the most comprehensive study is that of Aversa (Unpublished abstract). The number of men treated in this fashion is small and the follow-up short. CS—intercourse satisfaction; EF—erectile function; GS—overall satisfaction; OF—orgasmic function; SD—sexual desire.

Sildenafil and Testosterone

IIEF	*T-gel and Sildenafil*	*Placebo and Sildenafil*	*P value*
Erectile	5.65	2.97	0.03
Orgasmic	4.53	0.36	0.01
Desire	0.44	0.00	0.21
Satisfaction	1.21	0.70	0.25
Overall	1.62	0.61	0.04
Total	10.44	4.62	0.02

FIGURE 4-37. Further study results on testosterone and sildenafil. Support for the Aversa study is coming from various quarters. This study (not yet published in complete form) suggests that hypogonadal men in whom sildenafil treatment has failed can be helped with the administration of transdermal testosterone. The effect appears to be of short duration. IIEF—International Index of Erectile Function.

Study of 24 Men on Sildenafil and Testosterone

Single arm, open label
Response
Sildenafil = 0
T (AndroGel) = 0
Sildenafil + testosterone = 22 (92%)

FIGURE 4-38. Another preliminary study of sildenafil and testosterone with amazing results. Only proper trials will establish the efficacy and safety of this combination. The use of this combination is rational where testosterone can be shown to be subnormal.

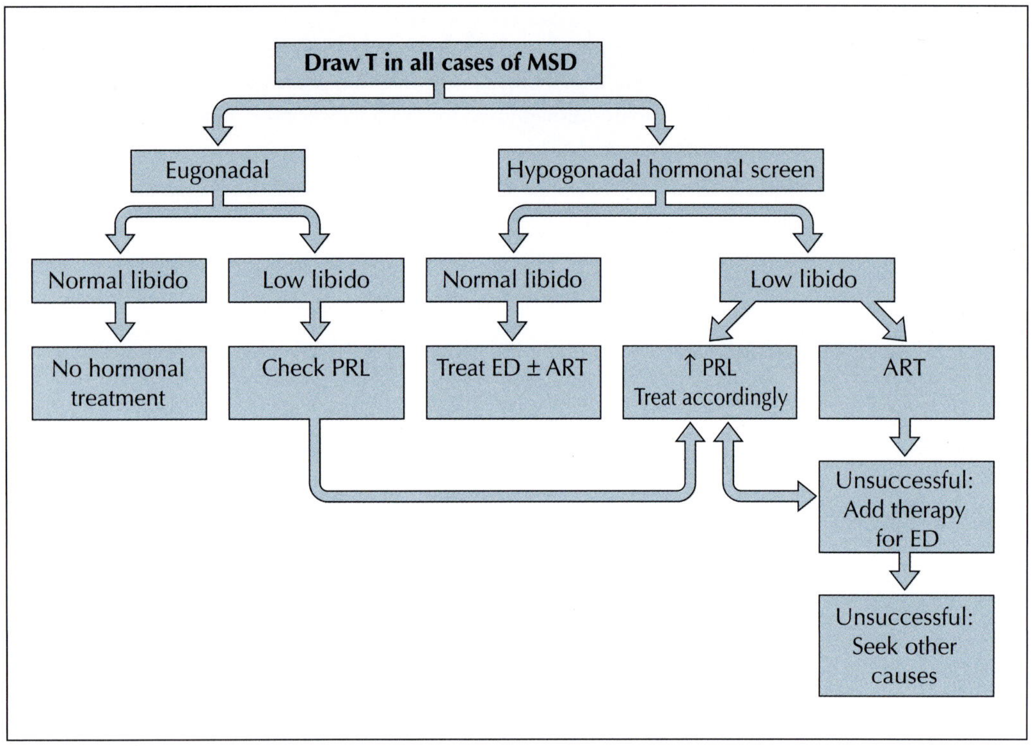

FIGURE 4-39. At the Consultation on Sexual Medicine (Paris, June 2003), there was agreement that a hormonal evaluation is indicated in men complaining of erectile dysfunction (ED). This algorithm, adapted from the forthcoming publication, provides a recommendation in this regard. ART—androgen replacement therapy; MSD—Male Sexual Dysfunction; PRL—prolactin; T—testosterone.

REFERENCES

1. Dean W: *Vitamin Research News* 2000. Accessible at http://www.vpr.com.
2. Morales A, *et al.*: *Aging Male* 2001, 4:151–162.
3. Matsumoto AM: *J Gerontol* 2002, 57A:M76–M99.

A Psychiatric Perspective on Psychogenic Erectile Dysfunction

5

Stephen B. Levine, MD

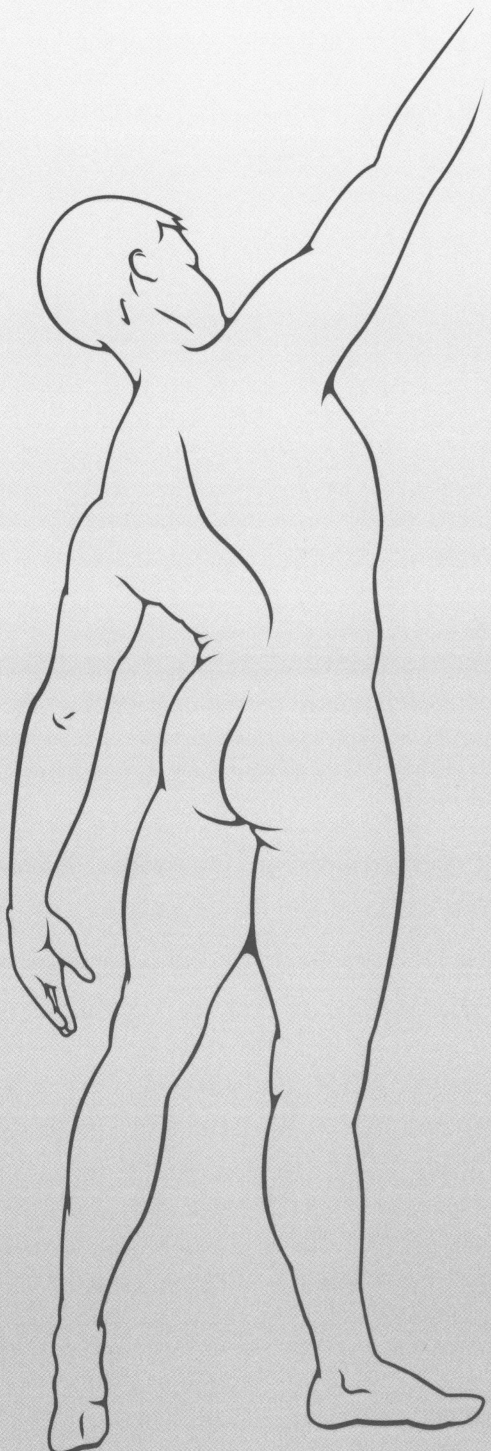

Medicine's basic algorithm for determining treatment is best suited for physical diseases. When we can assume a complaint is a symptom of a specific disease, we construct a differential diagnosis and use further history taking, physical examination, and laboratory tests to confirm the diagnosis. We then direct treatment as best we can to the underlying pathophysiology.

We often modify this basic scheme for psychologic and mixed biologic and psychologic conditions. In these many states, we often cannot identify the biologic disease let alone understand the pathophysiology of its symptoms. When we think that symptoms are primarily caused by life processes (stress), we may privately classify our patients as "worried well," "stressed," "anxious," or "depressed." These labels often mean that we are uncertain about the sources of a patient's complaints. Although we might work up their complaint further, we usually do not because making a definitive diagnosis may be cost prohibitive, ethically unjustifiable, or unreimbursable.

In the situation of erectile dysfunction (ED), recent advances in therapy have allowed us to further modify the basic scheme. The release of a new, safe, and effective oral agent for ED in 1998 created a paradigm shift. ED, a symptom of diverse processes, now can be successfully treated in about half the cases without certainty about its actual pathophysiology. ED had been the subject of concentrated urologic research and strategic pharmaceutical industry medical education for almost 20 years. Some of this work—the role of nitric oxide in vasodilatation—led to our understanding of how sildenafil creates erection and was so important as to be honored with a Nobel prize [1].

Every major account of the causes of ED from ancient to modern times has emphasized that both physical disease and mental life can create the symptom. The impressive progress in biologic therapies for ED, however, has led to a de-emphasis on the psychologic causes of ED in favor of an assumption of a macro- or microvascular cause. Many physicians now prescribe a PDE-5 inhibitor as a first step, thus bypassing the search for a specific cause [2]. The treatment paradigms have changed rapidly [3], far more quickly than anyone can reasonably expect the psychosocial causes of ED to have evolved.

Many patients have completely overcome their ED with the help of mental health professionals. Long before the modern scientific era, 20th century psychiatrists restored potency with psychosocial interventions. Seventy-five years ago, Stekel [4] described many case examples of cures. Masters and Johnson [5] reported that 69% of their sample of 213 men remained functional for 5 years after treatment. A colleague and I followed up on sixteen couples whom I treated with the sex therapy techniques of the mid-1970s and demonstrated fluctuating degrees of erectile success [6]. This same fluctuation was later noted in a 2.5- to 4-year follow up of 99 German couples. In that study, 80% were functioning much better than before therapy [7]. A new technique, creative-dynamic image synthesis, has been shown in a 6-month placebo-controlled follow-up to have enhanced erectile function for 15 of 20 men [8]. Their results are consistent with most published results of other treatments—that is, regardless of the techniques used, many report approximately 75% improvement.

Of course, there are unsolved problems with the evaluation of any therapy, either biologic or psychosocial [9]. Many patients are improved but not restored to premorbid sexual function of younger days. Many are either lost to follow-up or, with time, acquire new psychosocial and biologic factors in their lives that influence their potency—positively or negatively. It is as unreasonable to doubt the impact of psychosocial interventions for carefully diagnosed and selected patients as it is to be uncritical about biologic or mechanical therapies. Each of these three approaches can cure some patients, leave many more improved in a not quite normal state, and fail to be effective for others [10].

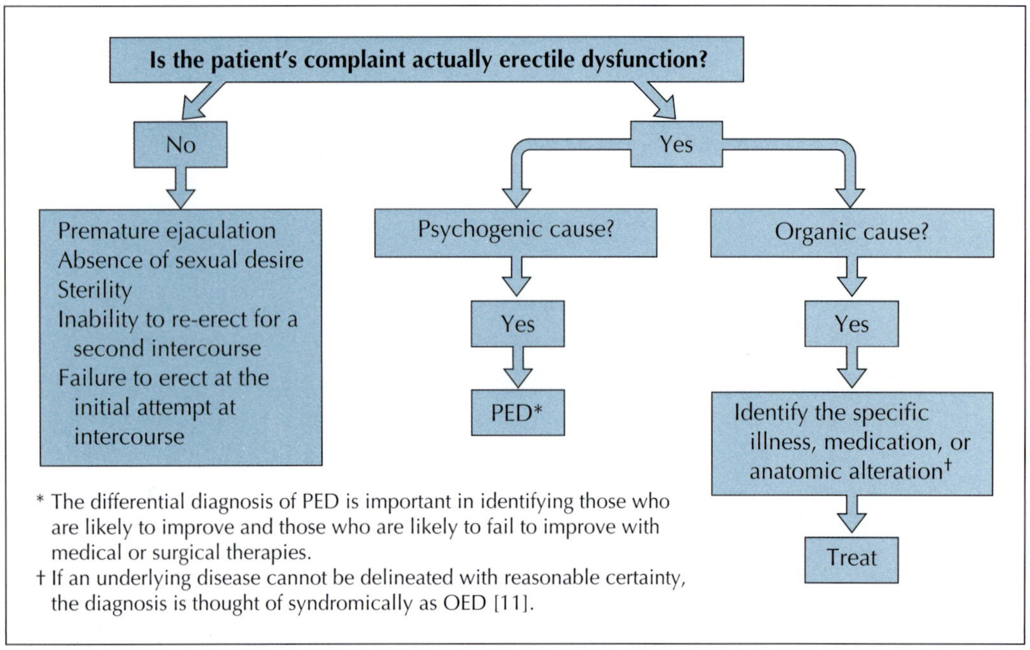

FIGURE 5-1. The urologist's response to the complaint of erection problems. OED—organogenic erectile dysfunction; PED—psychogenic erectile dysfunction.

Three *Syndromes* of Erectile Dysfunction

(Pure) Psychogenic erectile dysfunction (PED)
Organic erectile dysfunction (OED)
Mixed psychogenic and organic erectile dysfunction (MED)

FIGURE 5-2. The three syndromes of erectile dysfunction (ED) [12]. Since the advent of sildenafil, urologists are more apt to diagnose ED syndromatically. Prior to 1998, physicians used far more specialized testing to make a diagnosis. This changed because approximately 80% of patients in the sildenafil trials had improved erections regardless of the pretreatment diagnoses. Now it is apparent that there are three patient groups who are exceptions to this observation: those with diabetes, those with prostate cancer, and those with lifelong PED. Each group has a much lower improvement rate with sildenafil.

There is one uncertainty about this tripartite synthesis. Although cases of pure PED do exist, the ubiquitous psychologic complication of performance anxiety creates an argument that most cases of OED are actually cases of MED. In this chapter, however, I am arbitrarily assuming that the psychogenic factors that are present in MED are those *other than* performance anxiety.

TEN CONCEPTS FOR UNDERSTANDING PSYCHOGENIC ERECTILE DYSFUNCTION

1. Three Basic Principles of Psychosexual Life

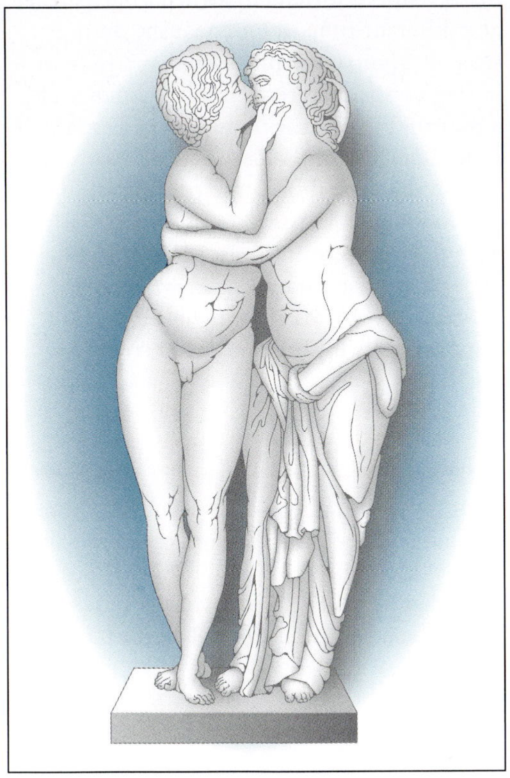

FIGURE 5-3. Psychologic forces inherent in every sexual act. Psychologic forces are inherent in every sex act: with a partner and during masturbation, whether or not the sex is dysfunctional.

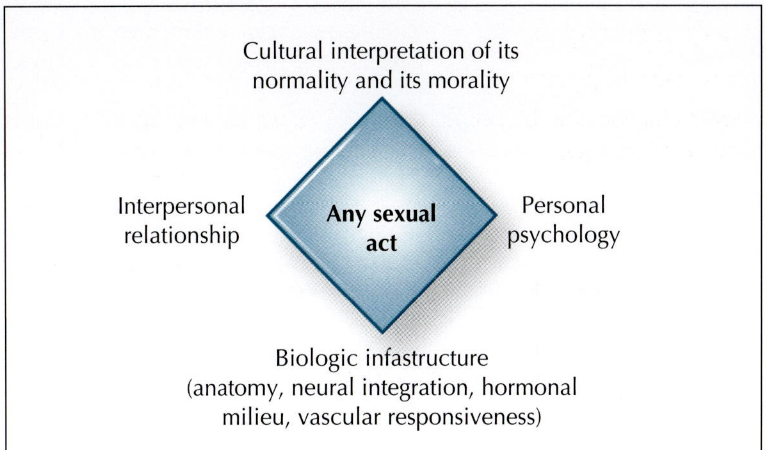

FIGURE 5-4. The four elements in every sexual behavior. Even masturbation conforms to this diamond. It is interpersonal and personal because its accompanying fantasy is usually about another person and reflects the man's private wishes. The man makes a moral judgment about it, *eg*, either it is normal or sinful, and, of course, it rests on his capacity to translate his excitement into penile blood flow, a physiologic process that begins in the structure of the brain [13].

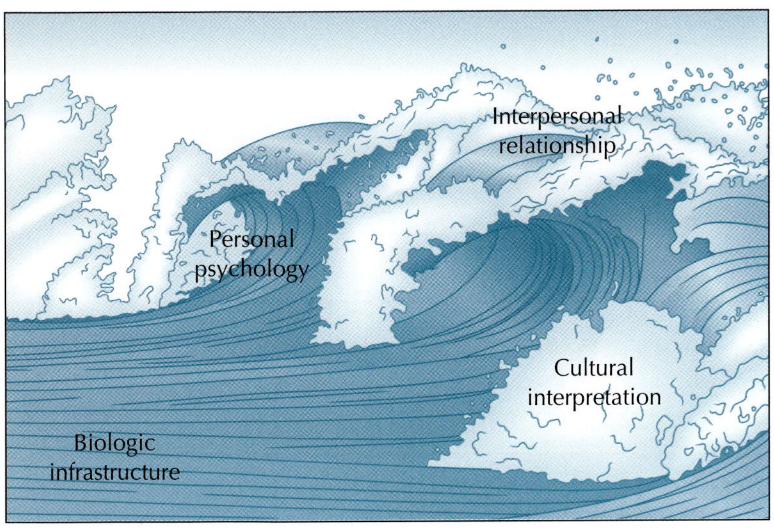

FIGURE 5-5. Sexual life is inherently changeable. The dynamic nature of sexual function is caused by the inherent changeability of each of the four elements (*see* Fig. 5-4).

Patterns of Erections Evident During the Clinical History

Situation	*PED**	*OED*	*MED*
Main partner	Variable	Upper limit seen	Upper limit seen and variable
Other partner	> 8	Upper limit seen	Upper limit seen and variable but may be at times > 8
Masturbation	> 8	Upper limit seen	Upper limit seen and variable
AM erection	Often > 8	Upper limit seen	Upper limit seen and variable
Nocturnal erections	> 8	Upper limit seen	Upper limit seen and variable
Internet/other pornography	> 8	Upper limit seen	At times has > 8
Spontaneous	Variable	Upper limit seen	Upper limit seen and variable

**On a scale of 0 to 10, where < 5 is poor, 5–8 is barely adequate, 9–10 is firm, lasting, adequate.*

FIGURE 5-6. The patterns of erections evident during the clinical history. PED is usually recognized during the history by this pattern: although the patient has difficulty obtaining and maintaining an erection for the completion of a sexual act with the partner of his choice, under different circumstances—masturbation, different partner, same partner at a different time, spontaneously, during sleep or upon awakening—he has a fully firm, lasting consistent erection, often followed by a pleasurable orgasm. This pattern is sometimes reflected in the occurrence of satisfactory intercourse during the time between making the appointment and the first visit with the urologist. It is also reflected in the 15% to 20% spontaneous recovery rates of wait list controls and the high placebo response rates in various clinical trials [14].

The Social History as an Indication of Psychogenic Erectile Dysfunction

Recent Social History	*Acquired PED*	*Lifelong PED*	*OED*	*MED*
Change such as job loss, personal affair, partner's affair, recently separated, recently divorced, recent ill health, partner death, or combination of above	Yes	Not usually	Not usually	Usually

FIGURE 5-7. The social history as an indicator of PED. In the patient with a long history of good potency whose ED occurred soon after a major social change in his life, the chances are good that he has had some evidence of occasionally good erections (*ie*, > 8 on the 0 to 10 scale [15]).

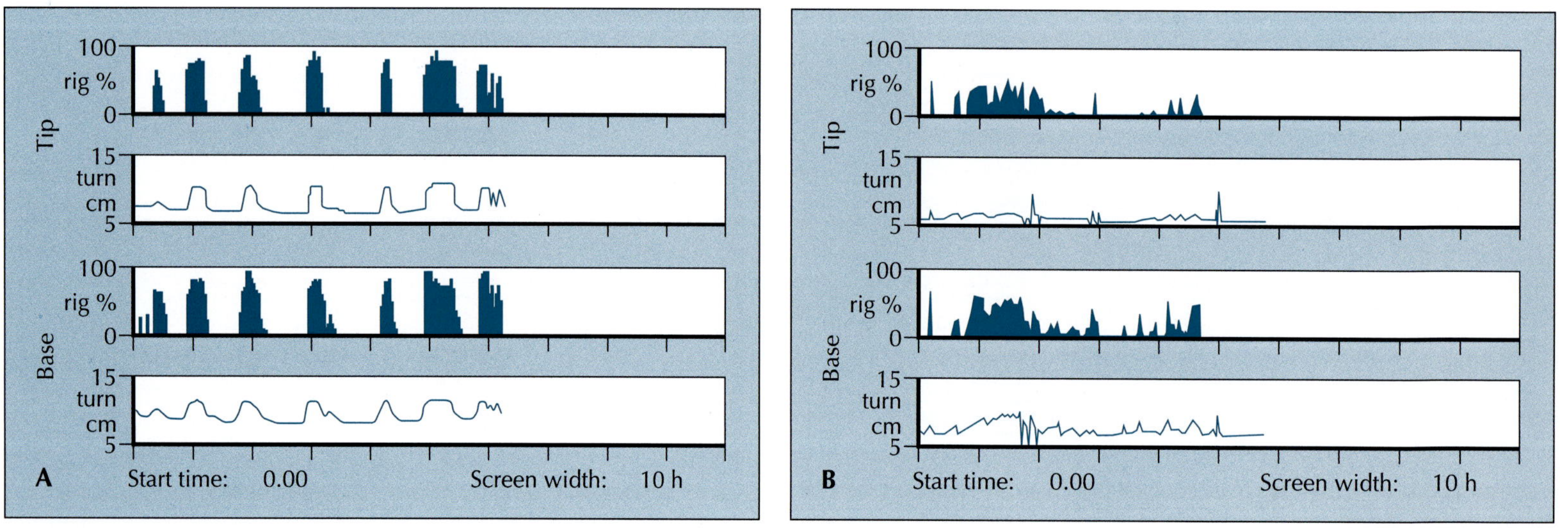

FIGURE 5-8. Normal nocturnal tumescence and rigidity testing that suggests PED. Three methods have been used to demonstrate good nocturnal erectile capacity: evaluation in a sleep laboratory, use of RigiScan (Timm Medical Technologies, Eden Prairie, MN) at home or in the office, and SnapGauge. Each method has its scientific limitations [16], but a normal response indicates a good enough erection to rule out significant organic contributions. **A,** Full psychogenic response on RigiScan with good tumescence and rigidity at base and tip of the penis. **B,** Poor tip and base tumescence and rigidity (organogenic erectile dysfunction).

Organic Contributors to Erectile Dysfunction in Men Younger than 50

Juvenile diabetes
Multiple sclerosis
Paraparesis
Postcolectomy for ulcerative colitis
Recent chemotherapy for cancer
Multiple medications for schizophrenia
Substance abuse

FIGURE 5-9. Younger men usually have PED or MED. In men who do not have PED, the organic contributors as shown in this table are likely to be obvious [17].

Two Questions the Urologist Should Ask Every Patient with Erectile Dysfunction

1. What do you believe is the cause of this problem?
2. Why do you believe this is true?

FIGURE 5-10. Questions to ask the patient about what he feels is the cause of his ED. If the patient has not brought up the subject already, after the urologist is finished with the history, these two questions should be asked. The patient's answers to these questions may reveal something new and relevant that will help to determine the correct diagnosis. They also may demonstrate how he thinks, which will help when discussing treatment options. The patient with PED and MED may reveal to the urologist when previous states of "stress" have caused ED and how they eventually improved when his life improved.

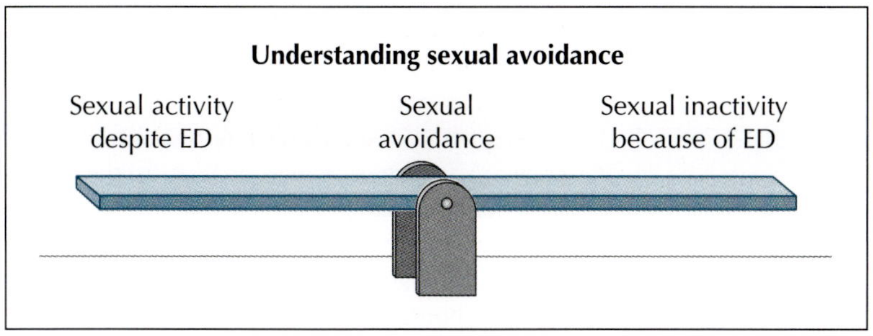

FIGURE 5-11. Looking closely at the years of sexual avoidance. Years without sexual activity with the partner indicate either the man's lack of motivation to gratify his sexual needs with his partner or his partner's disinterest in having him look to her or him for his sexual needs. Although some of this avoidance is a natural consequence of ED itself [18], we must always be suspicious that the ED was actually caused by the psychologic or interpersonal matters that caused sexual avoidance. Many a man, for instance, after an affair is unable to have sex with his wife because of the couple's inability to resolve their feelings about the painful past. Years pass before he seeks a urologic consultation. By this time, he seems to be avoiding sex because he is not confident that he can maintain an erection. The couple may have difficulty using a PDE-5 inhibitor over time.

3. Two Psychologic Requirements for Potency

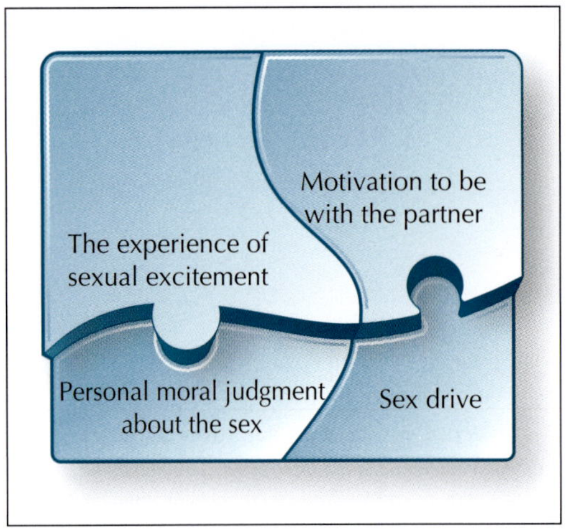

FIGURE 5-12. The two requirements for potency and how they fit together. Sexual excitement is an emotion that is generated from the anticipation of being with a partner and the actual physical experience with that particular partner. Motivation to be with the partner is manifested by his willingness to bring his body to that person for sex. Some PED is in fact an unwillingness to do that. We often say he is lacking motivation or has sexual disinterest.

4. The Cause of Psychogenic Erectile Dysfunction from Three Time Periods

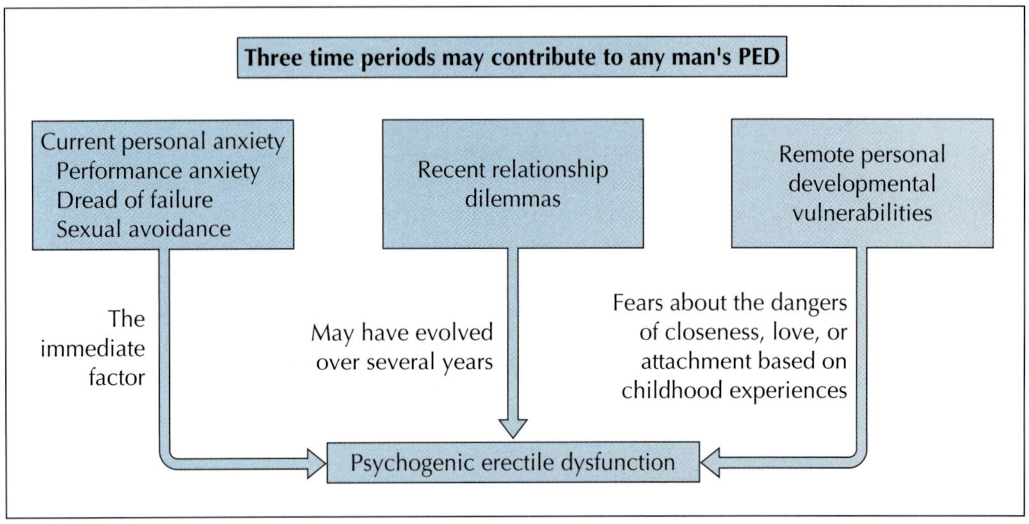

FIGURE 5-13. Three time periods that may contribute to any man's PED. The psychopathogenesis of any case of PED may be quite complicated because it derives from the obvious immediate experience of erectile failure *and* from the current situation that may have set up the feelings that attenuate the feelings of sexual excitement with the partner *and* the youthful experiences that create individual vulnerabilities to anxiety about sexual closeness. Thus, three time periods may contribute to PED and MED.

A. Explanations of Psychogenic Erectile Dysfunction will be "Fuzzy"

Tentative
Nonexclusive
Culture-bound
Era-bound
Ideology-bound
Speculative

Attributions of cause through the ages

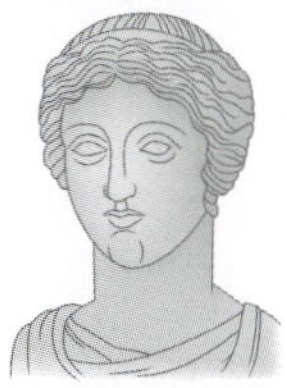

Ancient history

ED caused by excessive masturbation/intercourse; differential diagnoses included imagination, bad habits, mental mechanisms, curses, witches, negative childhood experiences [25]

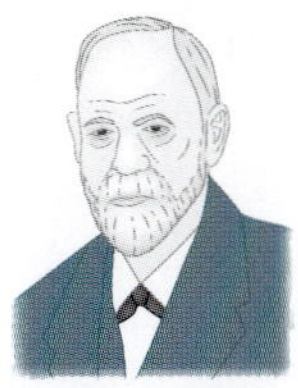

19th century

Sexual dysfunctions were called "venereal diseases"
Urologists were the experts
Most treatments were physical
Until about the mid-1970s, most ED cases were assumed to be entirely psychologic

B

FIGURE 5-14. Attitudes on erectile dysfunction through the ages. **A,** Explanations of PED will be fuzzy. *Tentative* because it takes a long time to discern the subtle contributions from each of the three contributing time periods. *Nonexclusive* because one psychologic explanation does not preclude another and all problems are multifactorial in origin. *Culture-bound* because patients from religious versus secular societies, highly educated versus uneducated societies, rural versus urban societies, and rich versus poor societies tend to regard the causes and treatments of ED somewhat differently. *Era-bound* because until modern times, various societies invoked one of four causes for impotence: curses from God or angry persons; mean, hateful women (witches); adolescent sexual excesses; and negative childhood experiences [27]. Causal ideas evolve over time. *Ideology-bound* because various mental health professionals tend to emphasize different causal forces—*eg*, unconscious forces, conditioning factors, neurotransmitter dysfunction, or only empirically supported explanations. *Speculative* because when explanations are given, regardless of their utility for the clinical situation, there are no means of ascertaining their ultimate correctness.

B, In the 19th century, sexual dysfunctions were called venereal diseases. Urologists were the experts. The term *psychogenic impotence* was not widely used [19]. Most treatments were physical [20]. However, urologists used a psychologic technique to eradicate poor confidence and the anticipation of sexual failure. They cured this mental cause of impotence by convincing the patient to undertake six amatory experiences with the partner without coital connection, a suggestion that originated in the 18th century [21].

In ancient times through the 19th century, the differential diagnoses of impotence included states that depended on the imagination, bad habits, and mental mechanisms. For most of recorded time, and in particular during the 19th century, the two most important causes of impotence were adolescent excesses of masturbation or intercourse [22–24]. Until these causes were rejected as medical "hysteria" in the early 20th century, physicians were uncertain whether these early excesses caused impotence through mental or physical mechanisms [25].

6. Pathogenesis: Why a Man's Psychogenic Erectile Dysfunction Can Be Explained in Numerous Ways

Current Thinking on Psychogenic Erectile Dysfunction

All behavior is created by numerous factors
Longer study of patient's life will lead to more contributions
Various mental health professionals value different forms of explanation [26]
Psychiatric diagnoses/explanations suffer from not being identified distinctly from one another [18]

FIGURE 5-15. This table outlines the current thinking on PED. Regarding our current attitudes, each of the three time periods shown here—immediate, recent, remote—probably make some contribution. Additional factors are provided in the table.

7. Why a Man May Not Be Potent

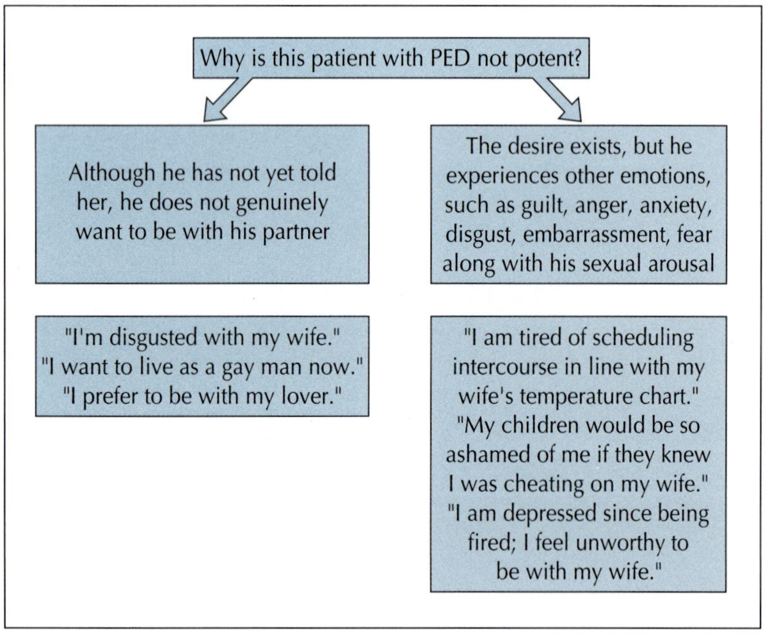

FIGURE 5-16. Men with PED usually fall in two categories: circumstances in which their motivation to have sex with their partner is nil or limited (no corporal nitric oxide secretion), or circumstances in which they feel emotions during lovemaking that attenuate the cavernosal effects of their sexual excitement (insufficient nitric oxide secretion). Some researchers explain PED caused by other emotions as the result of a cognitive distraction from sexual arousal [28].

8. Why Many Cases of Newly Acquired Psychogenic Erectile Dysfunction Have a Good Prognosis

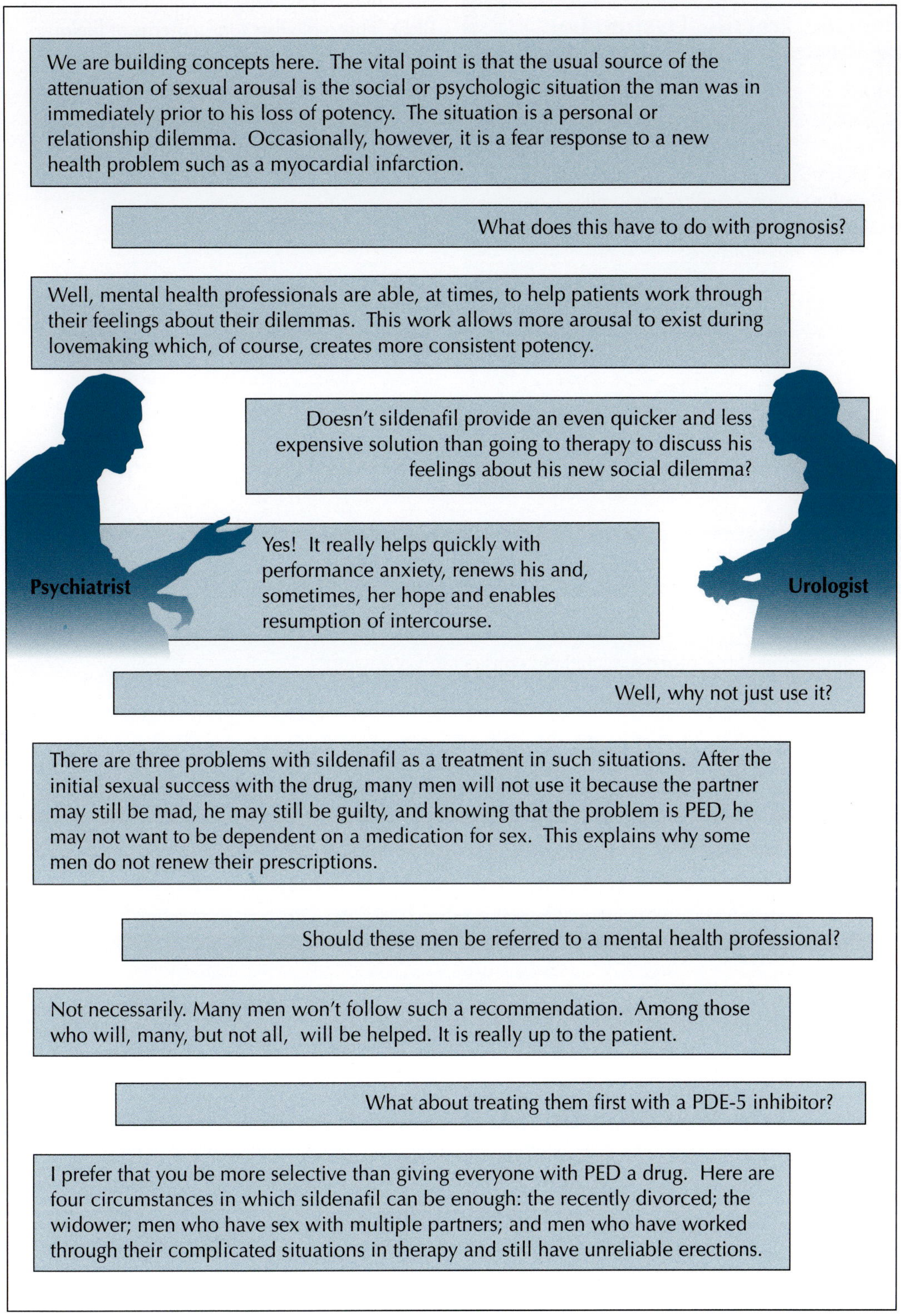

FIGURE 5-17. Interaction between psychiatrist and urologist regarding prognosis of PED. This figure illustrates some psychiatric recommendations for the urologist dealing with PED patients [29]. Many cases of newly acquired PED have a good prognosis [29].

9. Why Most Cases of Lifelong Psychogenic Erectile Dysfunction Have a Poor Prognosis

Four Patterns of Lifelong Psychogenic Erectile Dysfunction

Pattern Type	***Think***
I. Men who have never been potent with a partner	Significant psychiatric illness
II. Men who have repeated failures with only occasional success	Hidden sexual identity issues, *eg*, cross-dressing, homosexuality, paraphilia
III. Men who are consistently potent with a prostitute but not with a "respectable" woman	Long-term traditional psychotherapy after a PDE-5 inhibitor fails
IV. Men who fail at their first intercourse opportunities (probably far more common in countries where strong religious taboos exist [30])	Patient needs support and reassurance by the urologist

FIGURE 5-18. Prognosis of lifelong PED. This table lists four patterns of lifelong PED and what mental health professionals think about them.

10. Criticisms of the Concept of Psychogenic Erectile Dysfunction

Criticisms of the Concept of Psychogenic Erectile Dysfunction

Criticism	***Response***
The explanation of PED addresses psychosocial, not biologic, mechanisms. We do not know how input to the cerebral cortex is translated into lack of motivation and costimulation of attenuating emotions [31]. If we discovered that mechanism, we could deal with PED more effectively.	Yes, elucidation of this process might help considerably. We wait.
Many men in similar circumstances described in this chapter do not have PED	All men do not react the same in the same type of circumstance. This is true as well with organic cavernosal disease. One should remember that every sexual act is constructed by biologic, interpersonal, psychologic, and cultural elements. Similar cases—men having an affair, for example—can be quite different from one another in these other respects.
PED does not seem to be a diagnosis of exclusion	This is a major difference between a psychiatric and a urologic approach. PED as a diagnosis of exclusion is a urologic assumption that exists because PED requires a greater effort at history taking than OED. Urologists, who are understandably not as comfortable as mental health professionals in using the social history, initially used the sleep laboratory or the RigiScan to verify PED. When sophisticated tests of cavernosal function were developed, urologists defined PED by normal responses to these tests. These tests, however, were often cumbersome, difficult for the patient to bear, time-consuming, expensive, and, like all tests, scientifically limited. The mental health professional should refer cases for specific organic diagnosis if the diagnostic criteria for PED are not met during their history of the problem.
PED does *not* mean that there are no organic disease contributions	PED is created by the attenuation or absence of arousal. Although the inciting cause for the PED derives from social, psychologic, or cultural changes in the patient's life, the mediating mechanisms are always biologic. In this sense, PED is organic* [13]. If a diabetic man's ED is relieved with psychotherapy, we would say that his diabetic impairments in cavernosal anatomy and physiology are not yet sufficient to be causal. When we see that they are, we classify his case as *MED*. If his social history is unremarkable and his erections consistently limited, he is diagnosed as having *OED*.
Because the PDE-5s are effective even for some men with PED, we should redefine PED as either PDE-5–responsive ED and PDE-5–unresponsive ED.	This reasoning obscures the concept of PED. It is unwise for medicine to lose the clinical opportunities to restore potency through understanding how psychologic circumstances cause ED and to lose the opportunities to educate the next generation about *all* the mechanisms of ED.

**"Organic" is used in two ways in the ED literature: to refer to 1) the biologic mediation processes of erection [31], and 2) the currently known disease factors that limit erectile capacity.*

FIGURE 5-19. Criticisms and responses regarding the concept of PED.

Psychologic Advantages of PDE-5 Inhibitors with PED and MED

Stops the attenuating effects of performance anxiety and restores confidence
Restores hope to the couple that they can regain a sexual life
Helps people who have processed their painful dilemmas to put their past behind them

FIGURE 5-20. Why a PDE-5 inhibitor works with these conditions. Beyond their effects on the corpora cavernosa, these drugs affect the patient and his partner psychologically.

Limitations of a PDE-5 inhibitor Used in the Setting of PED/MED

Does not enable the man or the couple to deal with the personal, relational, or developmental obstacles to sexual behavior
Does not increase the motivation to be sexual after the first few doses [32,33]
Creates a dependency on the drug that over time will be expensive for many men
May precipitate new problems, *eg,* inability to ejaculate, loss of sexual motivation, vaginal pain on penetration, partner's fear of infidelity

FIGURE 5-21. Limitations of using a PDE-5 inhibitor in the setting of PED or MED.

One Concept of an Ideal System of Care for the Patient with PED/MED

The urologist and MHP work side-by-side in the urology setting
The urologist and MHP separately evaluate the patient and partner at the first visit [34]
Patients who are given prescriptions are also given follow-up visits within 3 weeks to see both professionals

FIGURE 5-22. One concept of an ideal system of care for the patient with PED or MED. MHP—mental health professional.

Correct and Incorrect Understandings Regarding the Treatment of Erectile Dysfunction

These Ideas Used to be Considered True

The differential diagnosis of psychologically induced ED from ancient times to the 20th century included 1) curses from God or an angry person; 2) mean, hateful, or distasteful women (witches); 3) adolescent sensual excesses; 4) negative childhood experiences [25]

During the first 75 years of the 20th century, experts thought that the vast majority of cases of ED were caused solely by psychologic factors [4,5]

These Familiar Ideas are *In*correct

PED and OED are diseases (they are syndromes)

PED is as readily recognized after age ≈ 60 years as it is 30 years earlier despite the obvious differences in the strength of sexual drive. (We are more apt to miss the diagnosis at age 60 than at age 30 because the drive/arousal system is normally weaker.) [35]

Sildenafil made the concepts of PED and MED irrelevant (not unless one does not consider poor rates of continuing to use the drug over time)

Only a highly trained qualified sex therapist should care for men with PED. (PED is often part of a larger emotional dilemma for which many general mental health professionals may be helpful.)

These Ideas are Correct

Success in response to any clinical intervention is an arbitrary distinction somewhere on the continuum between cure and failure; it typically means improvement [36]

The modal age of men with ED who seek help first from a urologist is older than those who seek help from a MHP

Psychosocial therapies for ED by qualified MHPs include individual private conversations with the man, joint conversations with the man and his partner, sensate focus techniques, and more innovative approaches such as hypnotherapy, acupuncture, and creative-dynamic image synthesis.

Methodologically sophisticated comparison studies with large samples are unlikely to exist in the near future to empirically guide the treatment of PED.

Descriptions of psychotherapy approaches to PED in the urologic literature emphasize their empirical support or lack thereof [26]; they do not emphasize the individual differences in every man's PED and the need to individualize the treatment.

It is reasonable to treat some men's PED with psychotherapy and sildenafil, vacuum pumps, MUSE, and so on [37].

FIGURE 5-23. Correct and incorrect understandings regarding the treatment of erectile dysfunction (ED). Figure 5-13 details some of the misunderstandings from ancient through recent times. MUSE—medicated urethral suppository for erections.

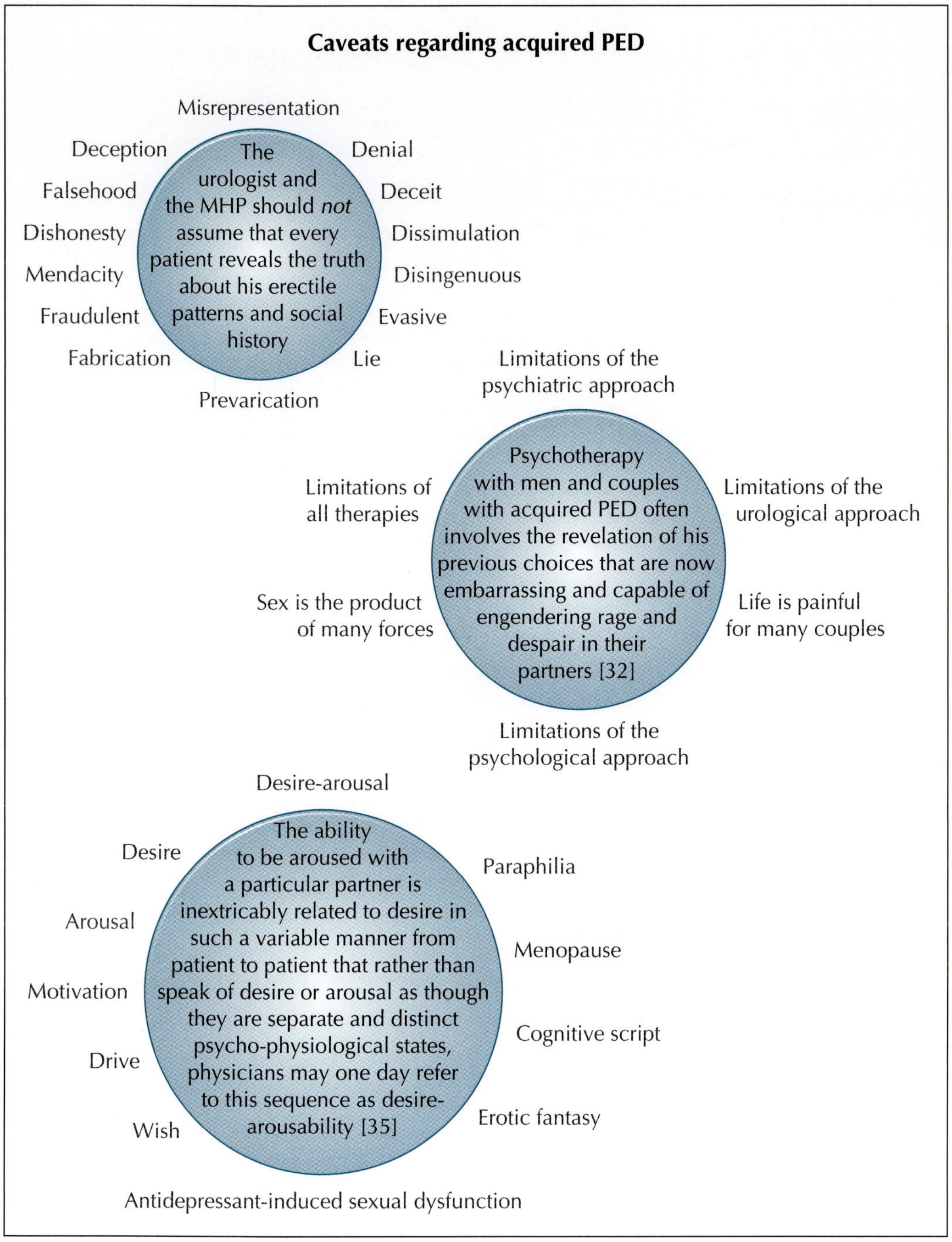

FIGURE 5-24. Three caveats regarding acquired PED.

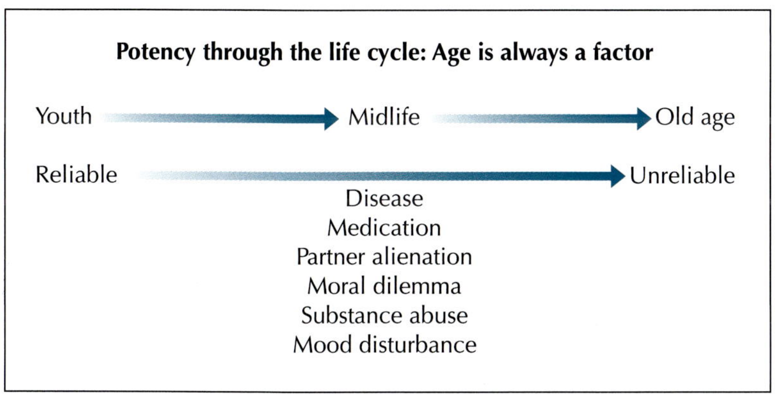

FIGURE 5-25. Potency through the life cycle. Age is always a factor in impotency. Youth's sexual efficiency is high and psychologic factors have less impact on erectile capacity than they will have as the sexual system gradually weakens with increasing age. The clinician, whether a urologist or a mental health professional, always has to be aware that the presenting problem, even when apparently resolved, is probably not completely understood.

REFERENCES

1. Katzenstein L, Grossman EB: Viagra (sildenafil citrate): the remarkable story of the discovery and the launch. New York: Medical Information Press; 2001:90.
2. Basar M, Tekdogan UY, Yilmaz E, *et al.*: The efficacy of sildenafil in different etiologies of erectile dysfunction. *Int Urol Nephrol* 2001, 32:403–407.
3. The Process of Care Consensus Panel: The process of care model for evaluation and treatment of erectile dysfunction. *Int J Impot Res* 1999, 11:59–74.
4. Stekel W: *Impotence in the Male: The Psychic Disorders of Sexual Function in the Male*, vol one. New York: Boni and Liveright; 1927:329.
5. Masters WH, Johnson V: *Human Sexual Inadequacy.* Boston: Little, Brown; 1970.
6. Levine SB, Agle DP: Effectiveness of sex therapy for chronic secondary psychological impotence. *J Sex Marital Ther* 1978, 4235–258.
7. Clement U, Schmidt G: *Short-Term Results in The Treatment of Sexual Disorders.* Edited by Arentewicz G, Schmidt G. New York: Basic Books; 1983:77–122.
8. Sommer F, Obenaus K, Engelmann U: Creative-dynamic image synthesis: a useful addition to the treatment options for impotence. *Int J Impot Res* 2001, 13:268–274.
9. Althof SE, Corty EW, Levine SB, *et al.*: EDITS: development of questionnaires for evaluating satisfaction with treatments for erectile dysfunction. *Urology* 1999, 53:793–799.
10. Turner LA, Althof SE, Levine SB, *et al.*: 12-month comparison of two treatments for erectile dysfunction: self-injection versus external vacuum devices. *Urology* 1992, 39:139–144.
11. Stief C: Is there a common pathophysiology of erectile dysfunction and how does this relate to new pharmacotherapies? *Int J Impot Res* 2002, 14 (suppl 1):S11–S16.
12. Lue TF: Erectile dysfunction [review]. *N Engl J Med* 2000, 342:1802–1813.
13. Sachs BD: The false organic-psychogenic distinction and related problems in the classification of erectile dysfunction. *Int J Impot Res* 2003, 15:72–78.
14. Padma-Nathan H, *et al.*: Efficacy and safety of apomorphine SL versus placebo for male erectile dysfunction. *J Urol* 1999, 161:821A.
15. Levine SB, Althof SE: The pathogenesis of psychogenic impotence. *J Sex Ed Ther* 1991,17:251–266.
16. Levine LA, Elterman L: *Nocturnal Penile Tumescence and Rigidity Testing in Male Sexual Function: A Guide to Clinical Management.* Edited by Mulcahy JJ. Totowa, NJ: Humana Press; 2001:151–166.
17. Aydin S, Unal D, Erol H, *et al.*: Multicentral clinical evaluation of the aetiology of erectile dysfunction: a survey report. *Int Urol Nephrol* 2001, 32:699–703.
18. Althof SE: Therapeutic weaving: integration of therapy techniques. In *The Handbook of Clinical Sexuality for Mental Health Professionals.* Edited by Levine SB, Risen CB, Althof SE. New York: Brunner/Routledge: 2003.
19. Mumford KJ: "Lost manhood" found: male sexual impotence and Victorian culture in the United States. *J Hist Sexuality* 1992, 3:33–57.
20. Sturgis FR: *Sexual Impotence, in Sexual Debility in Man.* New York: EB Treat & Company; 1900:261–297.
21. Hunter J: *Of Impotence, in A Treatise on Venereal Disease.* London: W. Bulmer for G. and W. Nicol; 1810:213–218.
22. Tissot SA: *Onanism.* New York: Collins & Hanney; 1832.
23. Lallemand CF: *A Practical Treatise on the Causes, Symptoms, and Treatment of Spermatorrhea.* Philadelphia: Blanchard and Lea; 1853.
24. Engelhardt HT: The disease of masturbation: values and the concept of disease. *J Hist Med* 1974, 48:234–248.
25. Shah J: Erectile dyfunction through the ages. *Br J Urol* 2002, 90:433–441.
26. Rosen RC: Psychogenic erectile dysfunction: classification and management. *Urol Clin North Am* 2001, 28:269–278.
27. Kendell R, Jablensky A: Distinguishing between the validity and utility of psychiatric diagnoses. *Am J Psychiatry* 2003, 160: 4–12.
28. Cranston-Cuebas MA, Barlow DH: Cognitive and affective contributions to sexual functioning. *Ann Rev Sex Res* 1990, 1:119–161.
29. American Psychiatric Association: *Diagnostic and Statistical Manual, edn IV (Text Revision).* Washington, DC: APA Press: 2000.
30. Usta MF, Erdogru T, Tefekli A, *et al.*: Honeymoon impotence: psychogenic or organic in origin. *Urology* 2001, 57:758–762.
31. Bancroft J: Psychogenic erectile dysfunction: a theoretical approach. *Int J Impot Res* 2000, 12(suppl 3):546–548.
32. Althof SE: When an erection alone is not enough: biopyschosocial obstacles to lovemaking. *Int J Impot Res* 2002, 14(suppl 1): S99–S104.
33. Goldstein I, Lue TF, Padma-Nathan H, *et al.*: Oral sildenafil in the treatment of erectile dysfunction. *N Engl J Med* 1998, 338:1397–1404.
34. Riley A: The role of the partner in erectile dysfunction and its treatment. *Int J Impot Res* 2002, 14(suppl 1):S105–S109.
35. Levine SB: The nature of sexual desire: a clinician's perspective. *Arch Sexual Behav* 2003, 32:279–285.
36. Pallas J, *et al.*: A study using Viagra in a mental health practice. *J Sex Marital Ther* 2000, 26:41–50.
37. Wylie KR, Jones RH, Walters S: The potential benefit of vacuum devices augmenting psychosexual therapy for erectile dysfunction: a randomized controlled trial. *J Sex Marital Ther* 2003, 29:227–236.

Pharmacotherapy and External Devices for Erectile Dysfuncton

6

James K. Kuan
Gerald B. Brock

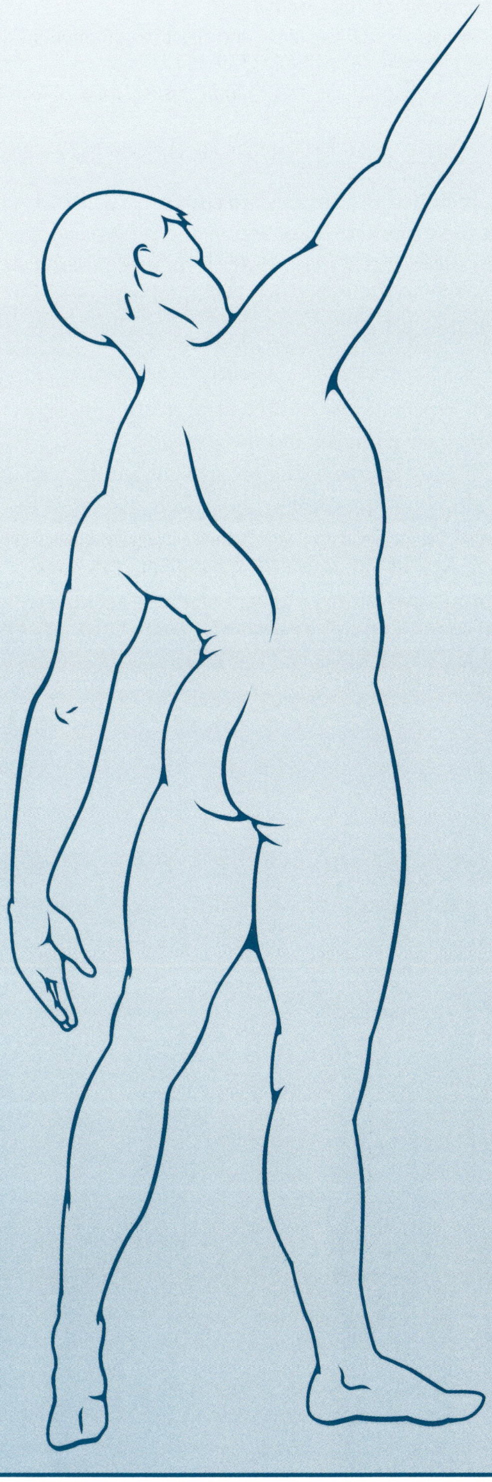

Through history societies have searched for potions, elixirs, and aphrodisiacs, hoping to find a simple, effective means to enhance male sexual performance. Until recently the role of the male sexual health specialist in this matter was limited. Since the elucidation of the NO/cGMP second messenger pathway of cavernous smooth muscle, we have learned that erectile function can be enhanced with inhibition of phosphodiesterase 5 (PDE5) enzyme activity. Sildenafil citrate was the first of such agents available under US Food and Drug Administration approval, now joined by vardenafil and tadalafil. The availability of these agents has ignited a revolution in the management of erectile dysfunction (ED), resulting in the development of drugs that target other important signaling pathways. One such agent is apomorphine, a centrally acting dopaminergic drug. Thus, the previously designated first-line modalities (intracavernous injection, intraurethral suppository, vacuum constriction device) are now considered as second-line and are reserved for those in whom oral agents fail.

Clearly, the current armamentarium represents only the beginning, and the "ideal" drug that is effective, acceptable, and tolerated by all men remains to be discovered. Until then, favorable clinical outcomes are still achievable when patient optimization and targeted pharmacotherapy are used.

Classification of Agents for Erectile Dysfunction

		Initiator	***Conditioner***
Central	***Class***	***I***	***III***
	Target	CNS (dopamine receptors)	CNS (androgen receptors)
	Response	Activation of central biochemical process leading to erection	Promote physiologic environment in CNS that is erectogenic, allowing enhanced initiation by other mechanisms
	Example	Apomorphine sublingual	Testosterone oral/transdermal
Peripheral	***Class***	***II***	***IV***
	Target	Vascular smooth muscle	Penile tissue
	Response	Local activation of erectogenic cascades	Enhancement of local/penile environment to produce erection
	Example	PGE1 VIP Phentolamine Papaverine	PDE5 inhibitors (sildenafil, tadalafil, vardenafil)
Other	***Class***	***V***	
		External devices, surgery	

FIGURE 6-1. Classification of agents for erectile dysfunction (ED). As researchers unveil additional agents for the management of ED, classification of these agents is important. This table shows the proposed format [1]. It uses site of action and whether the agent "initiates" a cascade of events or "conditions" the physiologic environment, making it favorable for erection to occur. Included in the table are currently used and proposed agents with their mechanism of action and pharmacologic response. CNS—central nervous system; PDE5—phosphodiesterase 5, PGE1—prostaglandin E1; VIP—vasoactive intestinal peptide. (*From* Morales and Heaton [2].)

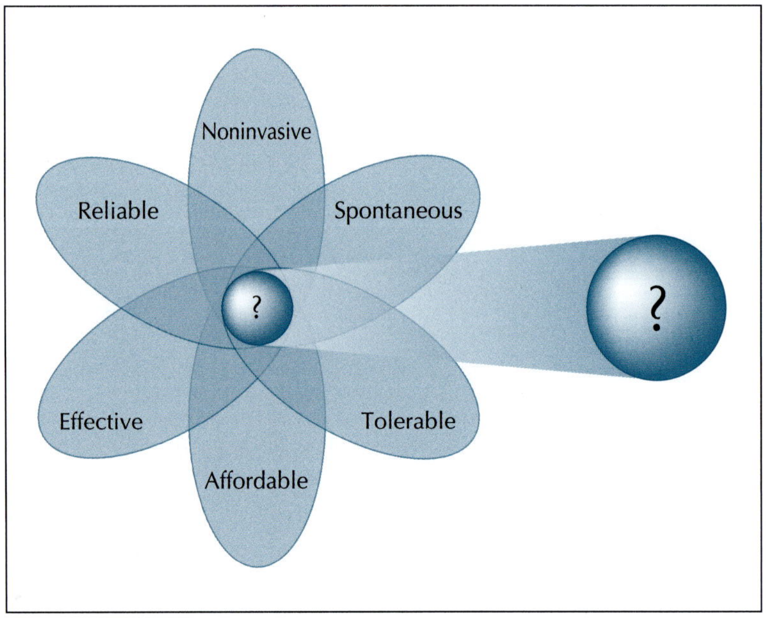

FIGURE 6-2. Goals, expectations, and the ideal treatment. Expectations need to be clearly defined by clinician and the patient prior to initiation of therapy, to avoid disappointment and treatment failure. Because the "ideal" pharmacologic agent likely has yet to be discovered, there should be an awareness of factors that are considered ideal. The advantage of oral therapy over locally delivered therapy is its ease of use and noninvasive nature. Current systemic agents are, however, less selective and may result in more intolerable side effects, potentially limiting use.

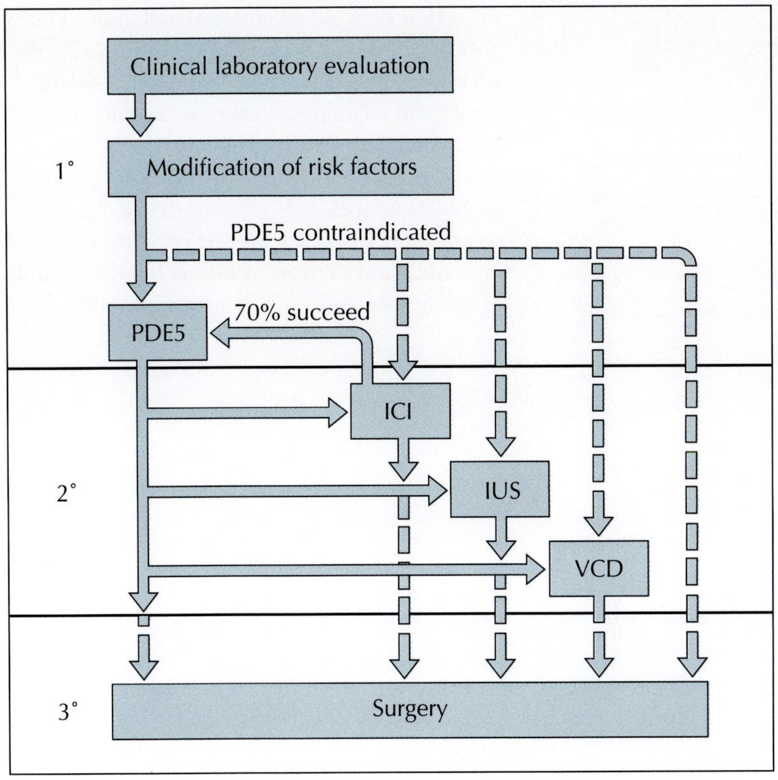

FIGURE 6-3. Pharmacotherapeutic treatment algorithm in eugonadal men. Following clinical evaluation and modification of risk factors, oral therapy with a phosphodiesterase 5 (PDE5) inhibitor should be initiated, unless there are contraindications. In these cases, therapy is initiated with one of the locally delivered options (intracavernous injection [ICI], intraurethral suppository [IUS], vacuum constriction device [VCD]). When ICI has been used in PDE5-naïve patients, these men are offered a trial of sildenafil, with reported success [3]. Failure of primary and secondary modalities necessitates surgical therapy when the patient desires further therapy. Other PDE5 inhibitors, when available, will likely be used interchangeably with sildenafil as primary or salvage therapy.

ORAL AGENTS

Phosphodiesterase 5 Inhibitors

Relative Selectivity of Phosphodiesterase 5 Inhibitors

	Selectivity Ratio vs PDE5		
Isoenzyme	***Sildenafil***	***Tadalafil***	***Vardenafil***
1a	290	20,000	630
1b	1100	21,000	5000
1c	110	11,000	460
2a	19,000	49,000	72,000
3a	12,000	38,000	7700
3b	17,000	18,000	15,000
4a	6000	30,000	46,000
4b	5800	22,000	33,000
4c	5200	23,000	34,000
4d	3600	13,000	16,000
6	6.8	780	2.9
7	22,000	47,000	200,000
8	19,000	30,000	310,000
9	54	19,000	3600
10	3100	9000	12,000
11	1500	14	640

FIGURE 6-4. Relative selectivity of phosphodiesterase 5 (PDE5) inhibitors. PDE enzymes are ubiquitous in human tissue; thus PDE5 agents demonstrate variable patterns of cross-reactivity. This variation may alter the potential side effects experienced by individuals taking them. (Data from Lilly ICOS LLC.) The selectivity ratio is an in vitro assessment of an agent's receptor-binding affinity. Higher values indicate lower cross-reactivity, and lower values represent higher degrees of cross-reactivity.

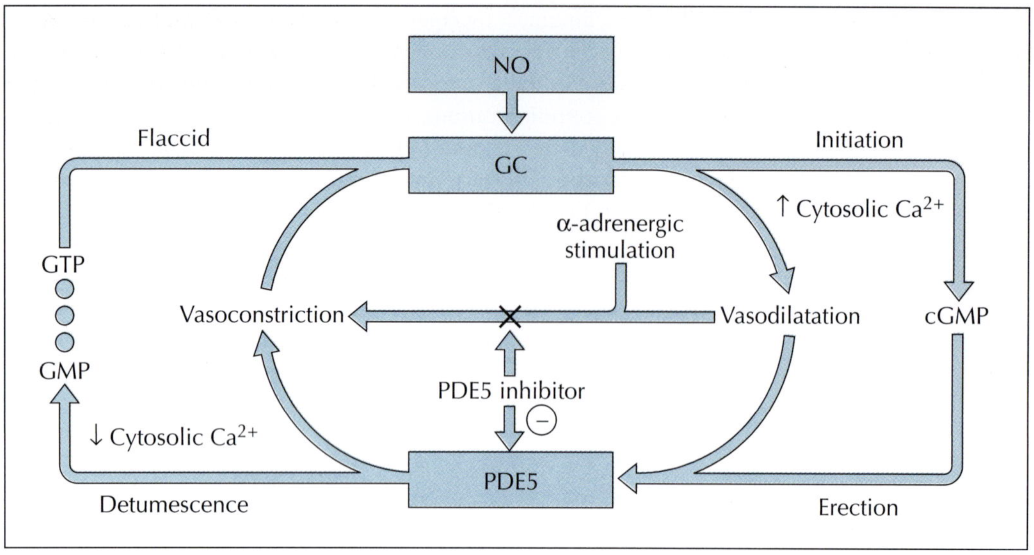

FIGURE 6-5. Mechanism of action of phosphodiesterase 5 (PDE5) inhibitors. Highly selective PDE5 inhibition (sildenafil, tadalafil, vardenafil) facilitates erection by prolonging the erectile response initiated by the NO-GC second messenger cascade, by inhibiting PDE5 degradation of cGMP. Detumescence occurs when α-adrenergic vasoconstriction overcomes the vasodilatory effects of the NO/cGMP couple or in the absence of sexual stimulation [4].

"Comparison" of Available Phosphodiesterase 5 Inhibitors

Inhibitor	*Peak Concentration, h*	*"Advantage"*	*Dose*
Sildenafil	1	Market available Vast clinical experience	25–100 mg (maximum, 200 mg)
Tadalafil	2	Half-life is 17.5 h	10–20 mg (maximum, 100 mg)
Vardenafil	0.7–0.9	Increased biochemical PDE5 potency	10–20 mg (maximum, 40 mg)

FIGURE 6-6. "Comparison" of available phosphodiesterase 5 (PDE5) inhibitors. To date, no randomized, blinded comparison trials comparing any of the current PDE5 inhibitors exist. Thus direct comparison regarding efficacy is not possible. Time to peak plasma concentration, plasma half-life, receptor potency and accumulated clinical experience distinguish each agent from the others. These factors may ultimately define the unique clinical scenarios where a particular agent may be considered as a first-line choice. (*Data from* Pfizer, Bayer, and Lilly ICOS LLC.)

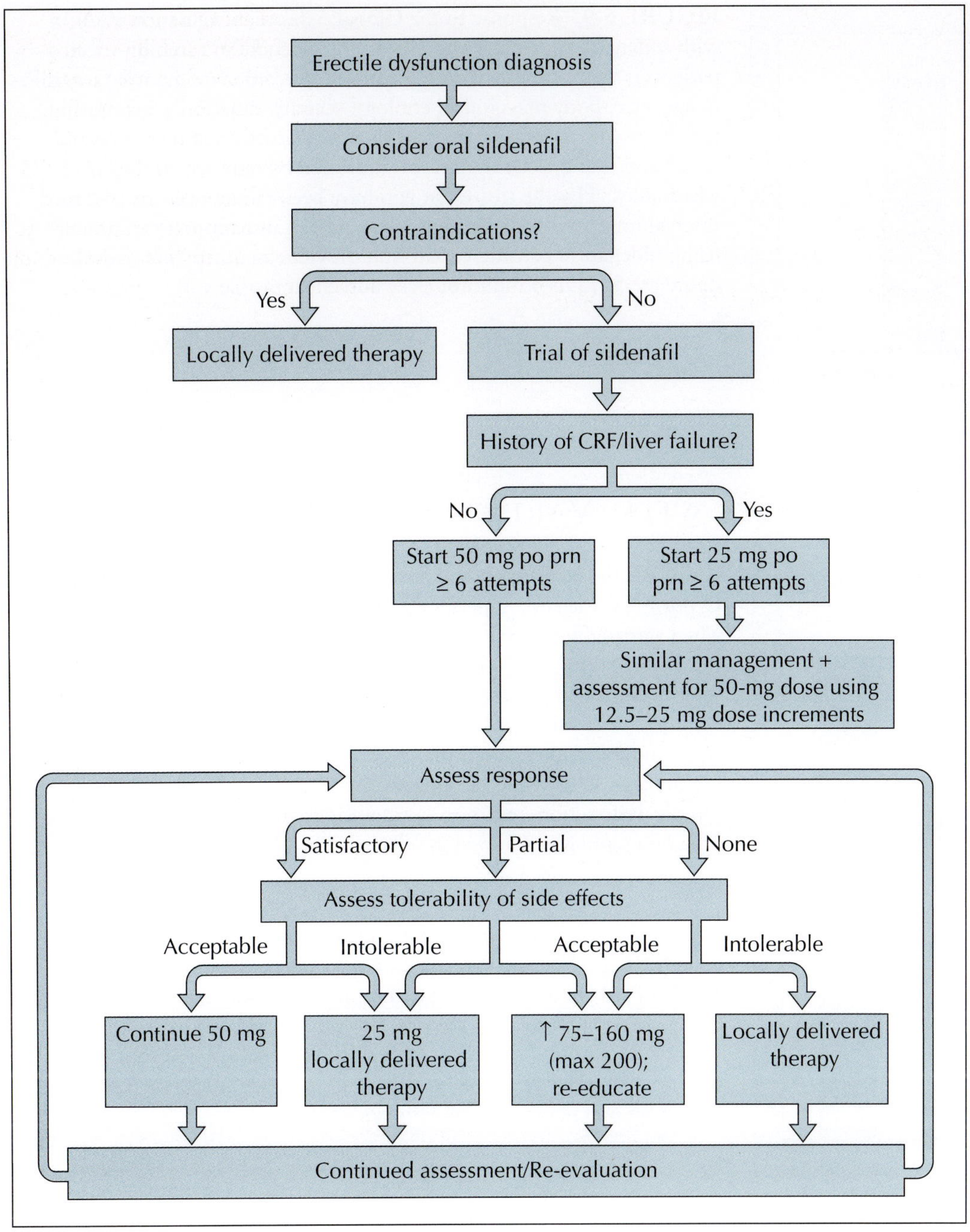

FIGURE 6-7. Initiation and monitoring of sildenafil therapy. When no contraindication (*ie*, hypersensitivity, use of nitrates, undiagnosed chest pain) exists, sildenafil is primary therapy. The initial dose needs to be adjusted down for patients with severe renal or hepatic dysfunction. Patients are encouraged to utilize sildenafil a minimum of six times on an empty stomach before reassessment. Dose manipulation proceeds based on response to therapy and tolerability of side effects, if any. Persistent intolerability of side effects or lack of satisfactory therapeutic response necessitates introduction of re-education (*ie*, ingestion with low-fat meal, peak concentration at 1 hour) or locally delivered therapy. Continued patient–clinician dialogue facilitates therapy that is responsive to the changing needs of the patient and therapeutic options. CRF—chronic renal failure.

Treatment Results with Sildenafil

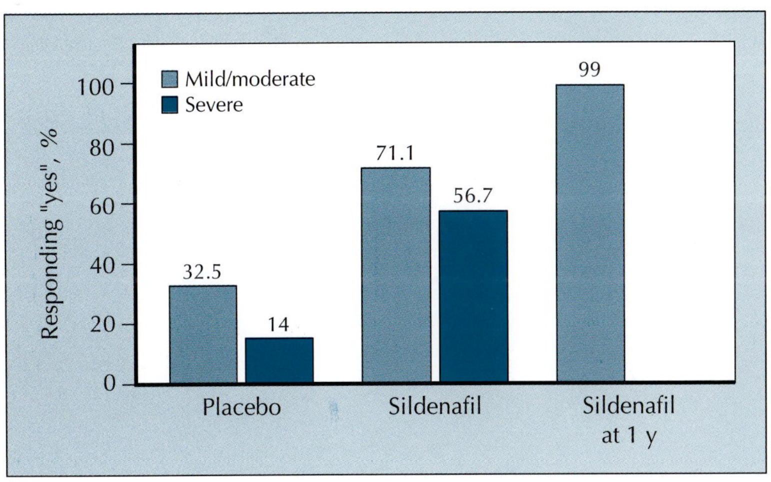

FIGURE 6-8. Response to the Sexual Encounter Profile, question 3 (SEP-Q3) with sildenafil. The introduction of sildenafil revolutionized the management of erectile dysfunction, providing the first reliable, on-demand oral therapy for this common disorder. Millions of men have used sildenafil, and the response to treatment has been favorable. A recent pooled analysis of 11 randomized, double-blind, placebo-controlled trials by Carson *et al.* [5] summarized clinical usage of sildenafil to date. A significant positive response to the SEP-Q3, which asks "Did your erection last long enough to have successful intercourse?" is recorded at all doses of sildenafil when compared with placebo. Durability is reported in three studies, with observation extending to 1 year. In these men, 99% report continued ability to achieve penetrative intercourse using sildenafil.

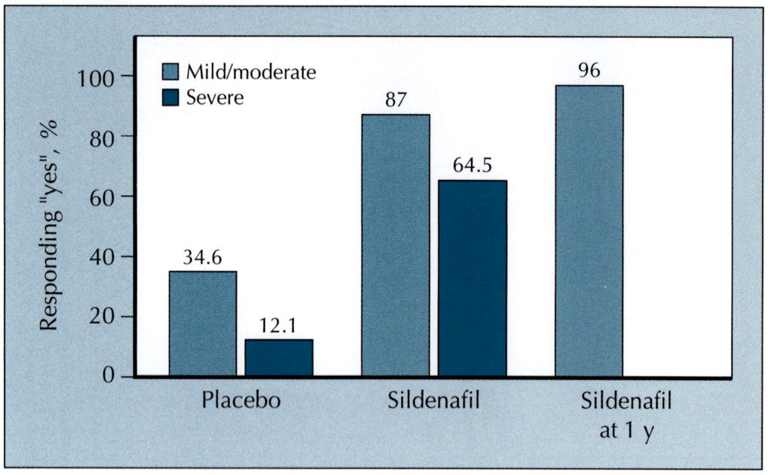

FIGURE 6-9. Response to the Global Assessment Question (GAQ) with sildenafil. The safety and efficacy of sildenafil in carefully selected patients is well established, and improved outcomes are reported regardless of age, race, body mass index, etiology, severity, duration, or comorbidities. Across all of these subgroups, satisfaction with treatment is again noted and found to be significant, indicated by response to the GAQ, which asks, "Has the treatment you have been taking over the past study interval improved your erections? [yes/no]." Contemporary treatment using sildenafil is considered safe and provides an acceptable phosphodiesterase 5 (PDE5) inhibitor class side-effect profile.

Treatment Results with Vardenafil

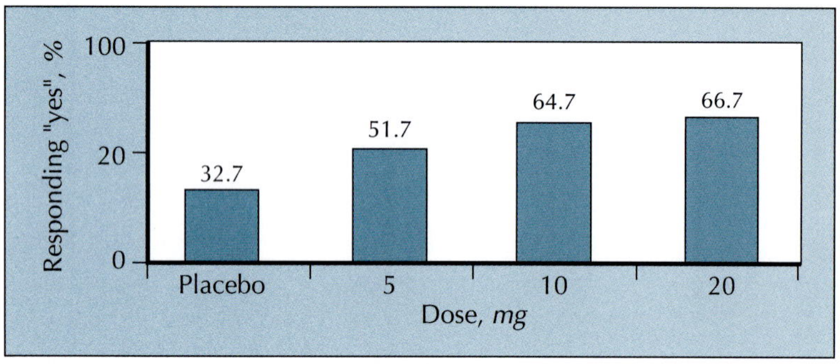

FIGURE 6-10. Response to Sexual Encounter Profile, question 3 (SEP-Q3) using vardenafil. Superior clinical response over placebo is noted when vardenafil is dosed at 20 mg. A randomized study by Hellstrom *et al.* [6] demonstrated a dose-related improvement in 805 men with erectile dysfunction of all causes. The duration of observation was 26 weeks, thus demonstrating vardenafil's durability. The SEP-Q3 was used as a primary endpoint and improvement that increased almost twofold from the initial use to usage at 12 weeks of observation. Depending on baseline levels of erectile dysfunction, return to normal International Index of Erectile Function score was achieved in 39% to 79% of subjects.

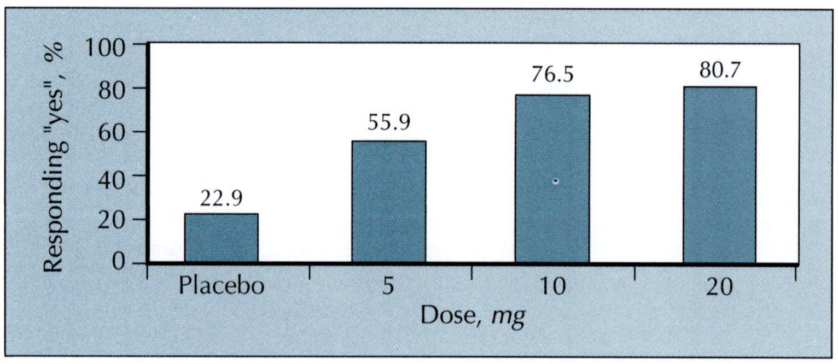

FIGURE 6-11. Response to the Global Assessment Questionnaire (GAQ) using vardenafil. Vardenafil is associated with an acceptable profile of adverse events, citing common phosphodiesterase 5 (PDE5) class symptoms (headache, rhinitis, flushing, dyspepsia), with a few subjects discontinuing therapy. Generally, vardenafil is well tolerated, and patients responded favorably to the GAQ (in a dose-dependent fashion) indicating overall satisfaction with vardenafil.

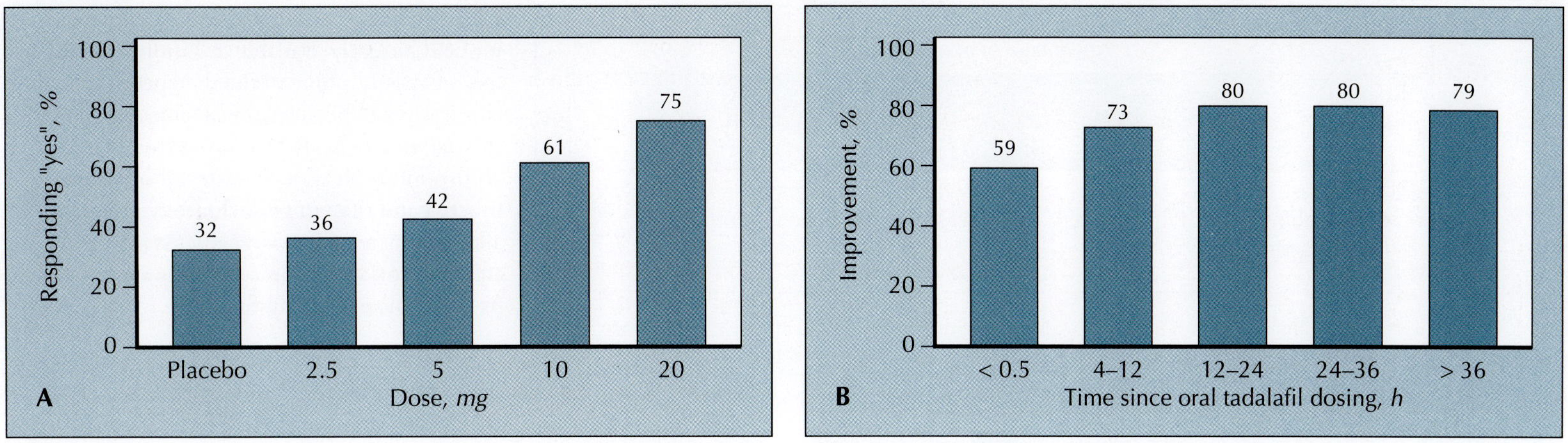

FIGURE 6-12. Preclinical efficacy using tadalafil. An integrated analysis by Brock *et al.* [7] of five randomized, blinded trials with tadalafil involving 1112 men outlines efficacy across a diverse patient cohort. Dose-related improvement in multiple parameters is observed, with the most significant response using 10 or 20 mg. A significant positive response to the SEP-Q3 was noted (**A**). Owing to the unique pharmacokinetics (half-life, 17.5 hours), this response remains durable from 30 minutes to 36 hours after dosing (**B**), allowing successive intercourse attempts.

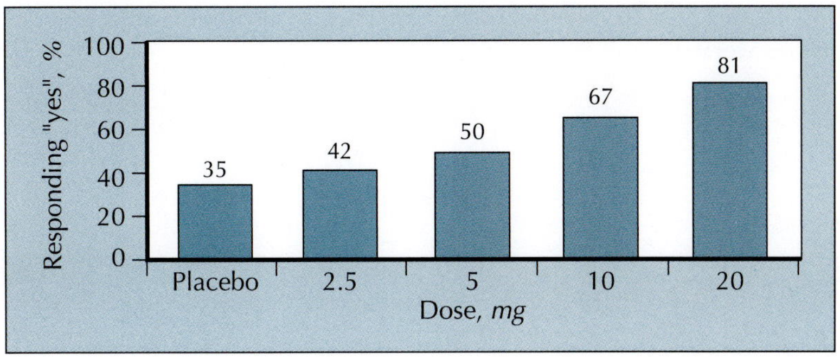

FIGURE 6-13. Response to the Global Assessment Question (GAQ) using tadalafil. A significant positive response is again noted with increasing doses of tadalafil, demonstrating overall patient satisfaction with treatment. During evaluation, concurrent alcohol or fatty food ingestion was not forbidden, thus providing the added benefit of spontaneity. Discontinuation rates were similar for placebo (1.3%) and tadalafil (2.1%). Commonly reported side effects included headache, dyspepsia, back pain, rhinitis, myalgia, and vasodilatation.

DOPAMINERGIC AGENTS

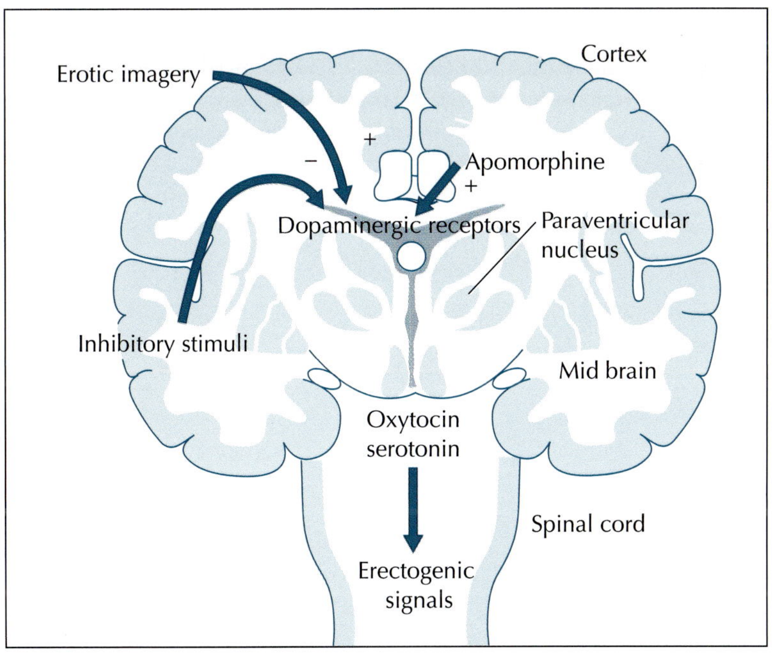

FIGURE 6-14. Mechanism of action of apomorphine. Apomorphine, an agent belonging to the class of central initiators, is a synthetic non-narcotic alkaloid derived from morphine and structurally similar to dopamine. It is rapidly absorbed by the oral mucosa, and in small doses it has an effect in the erectogenic brain nuclei. It is quickly metabolized, working in the central cascade for less than 30 minutes. Its erectile dose falls within a narrow range, and in larger amounts the agent produces adverse effects (nausea and vomiting). Initially, it was used by the subcutaneous route with good erectogenic effects but prohibitive adverse reactions. A new proprietary sublingual formulation has circumvented most of the adverse effects elicited by the drug. This new formulation is undergoing controlled clinical trials at present.
(*From* Morales and Heaton [2].)

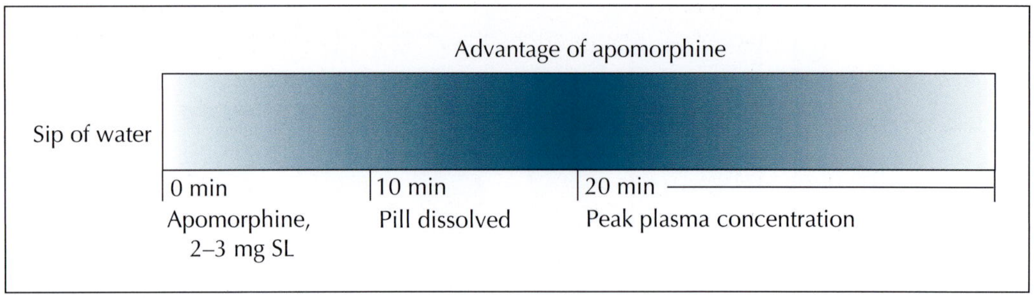

FIGURE 6-15. The advantage of apomorphine. Currently available in Europe, the exact role of apomorphine in the therapeutic algorithm is yet to be determined. The appeal for this agent may likely be derived from its rapid absorption from water-moistened sublingual mucosa and time to peak clinically response, allowing increased spontaneity. As a centrally acting agent, it may become a key agent in psychogenic erectile dysfunction.

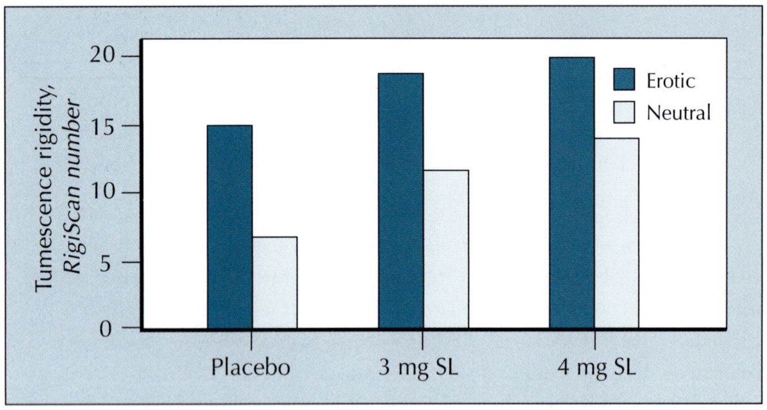

FIGURE 6-16. Effectiveness of apomorphine under laboratory conditions. Under laboratory conditions, apomorphine induces erections with or without erotic stimulation (*ie*, it is not an aphrodisiac). Its effectiveness, however, is enhanced by exposure of the subject to an erotic stimulus. The success rate of apomorphine in patients with a primarily psychologic cause is close to 68%, as assessed by both patients and their partners. The most common side effects, at the 6-mg dose, include nausea (41%), dizziness (29%), sweating (27%), and yawning (19%) [8]. Degrees of tumescent rigidity in RigiScan (Mentor; Santa Barbara, CA) assessment are shown. (*From* Morales and Heaton [2].) SL—sublingually.

LOCALLY DELIVERED THERAPIES

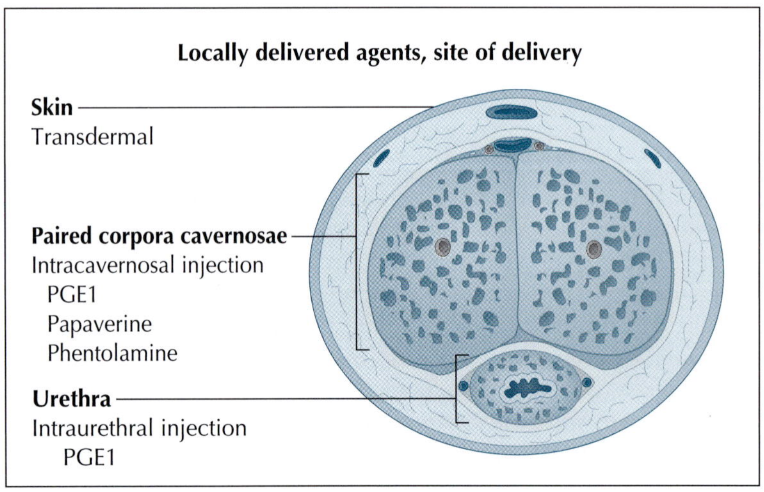

FIGURE 6-17. Agents and sites of delivery. Local delivery of vasoactive compounds lessens the rate of systemic absorption and side effects, which might be experienced if the same agents were used orally. Multiple local agents are reported, with efficacy rates as high as 90%. These include papaverine, prostaglandin E1 (PGE1), moxisylate, and phentolamine. However, only 14% of clinicians use intracavernous injection as their primary modality in the treatment of erectile dysfunction. Fewer use intraurethral suppository delivery or transdermal preparations. An international overview reported by the World Health Organization 1st International Consultation on Erectile Dysfunction, with survey data from over 100,000 patients globally, indicates that PGE1 and triple or multicombination therapy are prescribed most frequently [9]. (*From* Morales and Heaton [2].)

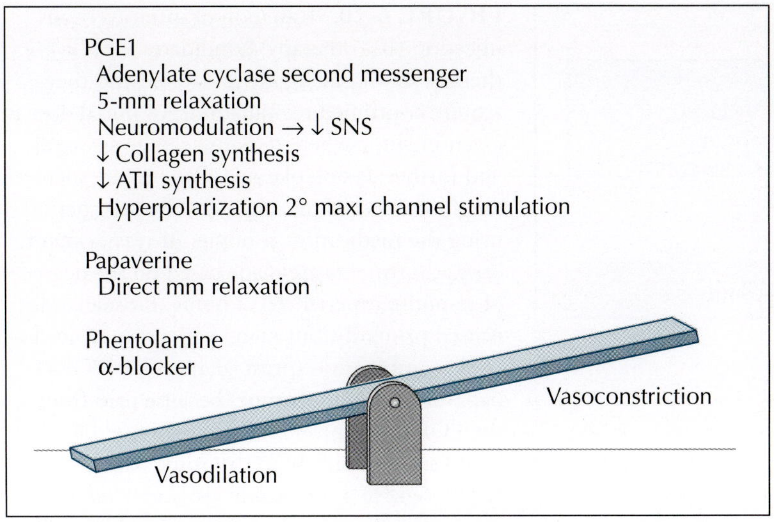

FIGURE 6-18. Mechanism of action. Intracavernous injection of smooth muscle relaxing agents works on the premise that local injection of vasoactive compounds allows targeting of penile vasculature, producing a predictable clinical effect. Following delivery, sexual stimulation must be applied and the use of a penile constriction device may be helpful. Four mechanisms exist by which prostaglandin E1 (PGE1) exerts its relaxant effects: stimulation of adenylate cyclase [10], inhibition of a1 adrenergic stimulation [11], inhibition of angiotensin II secretion [12], and hyperpolarization through Maxi-K+ channels [13]. ATII—angiotensin II; SNS—sympathetic nervous system.

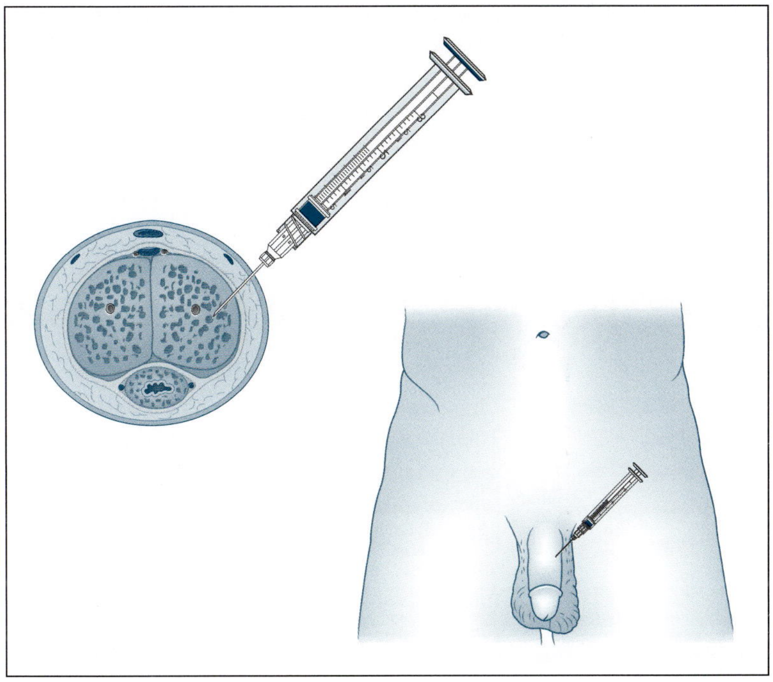

FIGURE 6-19. Technique of intracavernous injection. Care needs to be taken to ensure that self-administration of intracavernous agents by patients is correct. Following cleansing of the skin at the base of the penis with rubbing alcohol, the penis is held on stretch and pivoted onto the needle (30 gauge) at the 2 or 10 o'clock position. When the needle is penetrated to the hub, the medication is injected, activating local smooth muscle resulting in vasodilatation, veno-occlusion, and erection. Misguided injection into the ventral aspect will result in urethral bleeding. (*Adapted from* Lue [14].)

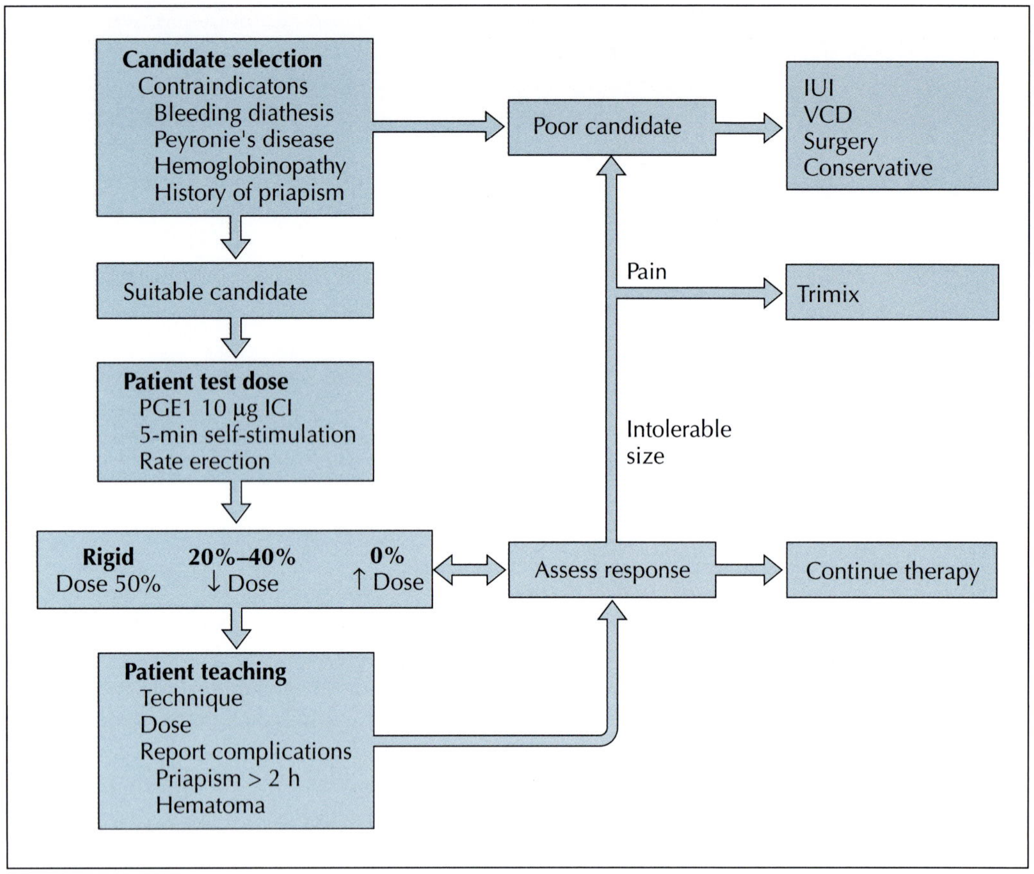

FIGURE 6-20. Initiation of intracavernous injection (ICI) therapy. Candidates for ICI therapy should be highly motivated and they require continued reevaluation. An initial dose is given in clinic where response can be assessed and further dosing planned. Patients are then taught the technique and allowed a trial period using the medication at home. At reassessment, dose adjustments are made based on the degree of response experienced at home. Prostaglandin is used primarily, but many patients may need a triple combination (prostaglandin E1 [PGE1], papaverine, phentolamine) because pain from the PGE1 may prohibit continued use. Despite broad success with ICI [15], some patients (24% to 42% in one study [16]) may require salvage therapies (intraurethral suppository [IUS], vacuum constriction device [VCD], surgery) or opt for no further treatment.

Clinical Experience With Intracavernosal Agents

Drug	*Dose Range*	*Average Success, %*	*Average Dropout, %*
Papaverine	20–80, *mg*	53.9	27.0
Papaverine/phentolamine	7.5/0.25–45/1.5, *mg*	70.8	27.5
PGE_1	5–40, *μg*	73.0	42.3
Papaverine/phentolamine/ PGE_1	8/0.2/10–16/0.4/20*	75.5	24.2

**Dose ranges for papaverine and phentolamine, in mg; for prostaglandin E_1, in μg.*

FIGURE 6-21. Efficacy of common intracavernous injection (ICI) therapies. Prostaglandin E1 (PGE1), 2.5 to 40 μg, achieves a 70% to 80% efficacy rate in unselected patients [17]. Its use is limited by its side effect profile, with study dropout rates ranging from 28% to 67%, and the most common reason was adverse effects: painful penile sensation (10%–20%), penile fibrotic changes (5%–10%), and priapism (<1%). No systemic side effects were reported. Despite the high dropout rate, use of the drug is associated with patient and partner satisfaction, in that a significant improvement in sexual relations, self-esteem, and personality is noticed [18]. The World Health Organization survey, however, indicates that 10% to 50% of patients will seek a change to oral therapy. The combination of papaverine, phentolamine, and PGE1 (trimix) has achieved efficacy as high as 84% [19]. It has been used as salvage therapy in nonresponders to monotherapy and papaverine/phentolamine preparations [20]. The trimix preparation has been shown to have a lower incidence of penile pain (2.1%) [21] compared with alprostadil alone (40%) [22,23]. A slightly higher incidence of priapism was found in those using trimix, but the risk remains low (2.7%). Finally, trimix is superior in the setting of penile scarring or fibrosis. A meta-analysis of 575 patients [24] indicated an overall incidence of 3.3% when compared with rates as high as 10% with PGE1 monotherapy. (*Adapted from* Manning and Junemann [25].)

Pharmacologic Management of Medication-induced Priapism	
Drug	***Usual Dose***
Epinephrine	10–20 μg
Phenylephrine	250–500 μg
Ephedrine	50–100 μg

FIGURE 6-22. Pharmacologic management of medication-induced priapism. (*Adapted from* Lue [14].)

INTRAURETHRAL PROSTAGLANDIN E1 SUPPOSITORY

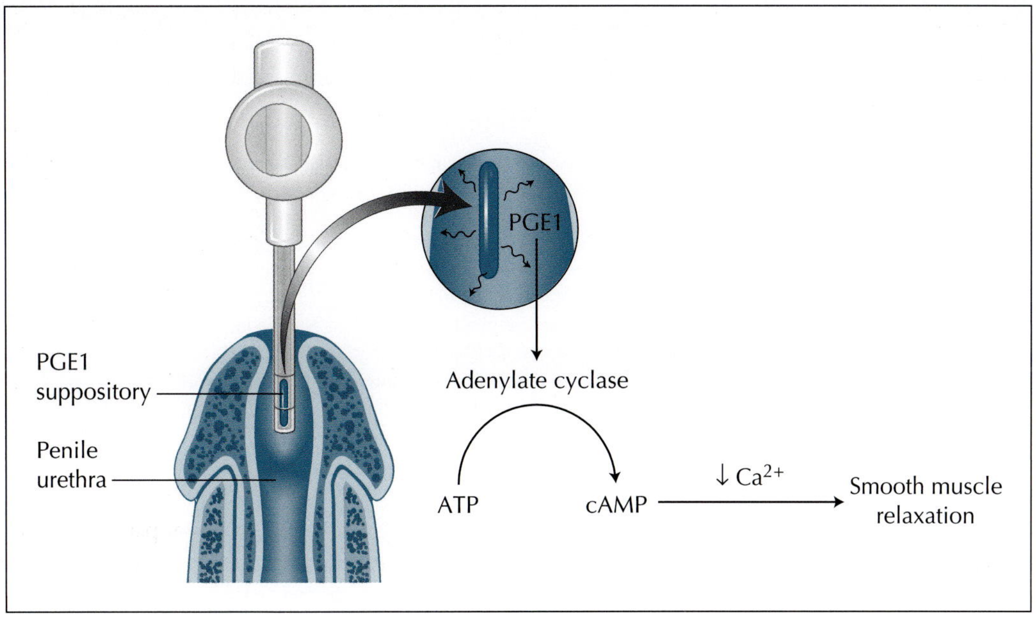

FIGURE 6-23. Results of intraurethral suppository therapy. Delivery of an intraurethral suppository into the fossa navicularis results in diffusion of prostaglandin E1 (PGE1) across urine-moistened epithelium. Coupled with sexual stimulation, erection ensues following activation of the adenylate cyclase second messenger. Syncope can occur with systemic absorption of the prostaglandin, and patients should be warned of this. Padma-Nathan *et al.* [26] published the largest series, reporting an at-home efficacy of approximately 57%. It is contraindicated in men with abnormal penile anatomy, intercourse with a pregnant woman without barrier contraception, and hyperviscosity syndromes. Penile pain is the most frequently reported side effect (12%). Patients may complain of minor urethral bleeding (5%), testicular pain, and dizziness. Penile fibrosis is seen rarely (1.4%). Female partners may report vaginal burning or itching (5.8%) with use of the suppository.

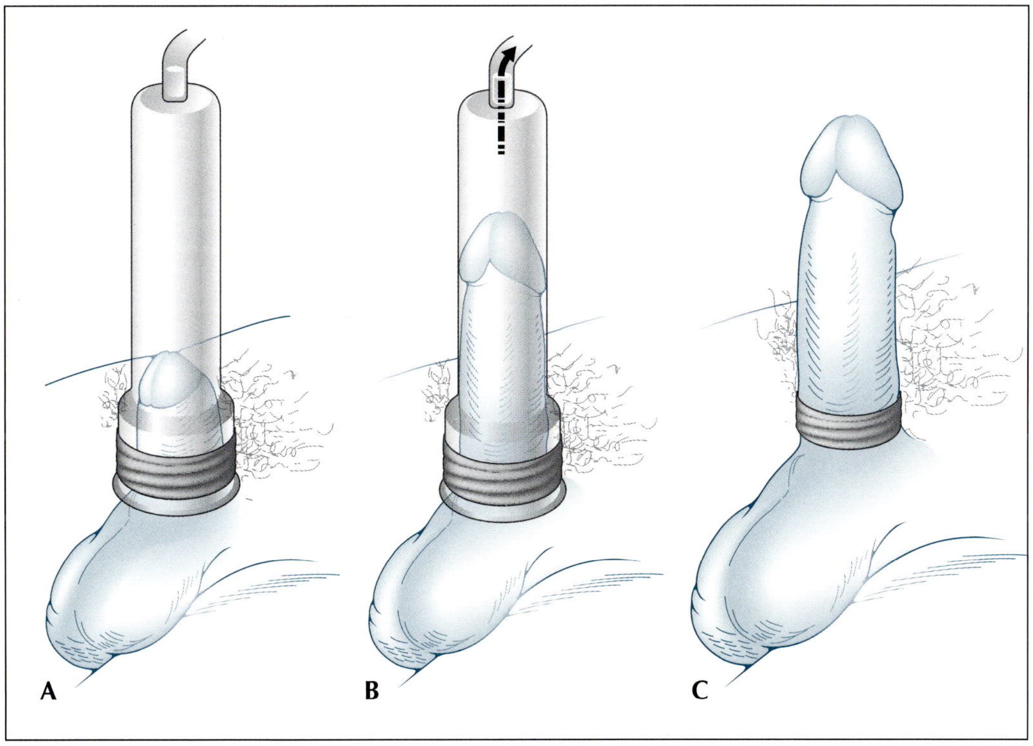

FIGURE 6-24. The use of a vacuum constriction device. Insertion of penile prostheses constitute tissue replacement. The remaining noninvasive therapy, the vacuum device, is based on the principle of trapping sufficient blood in the corpora to produce an erection of adequate rigidity for vaginal penetration. For patients unable to achieve an erection, blood must be carried into the corpora first. The channeling of blood to the corpora can be accomplished by creating subatmospheric pressure in the penis with a vacuum pump (**A** and **B**). Once the desired effect is obtained, blood is kept in the trabecular spaces by a constriction device located at the base of the penis (**C**) [27]. It is reported that about 70% of patients continue using the device beyond 24 months [28]. This figure includes those who agreed to acquire the device and responded to mailed questionnaires. In reality, many patients refuse even to attempt their use initially, a similar situation observed with intracavernosal injections and intraurethral delivery systems.

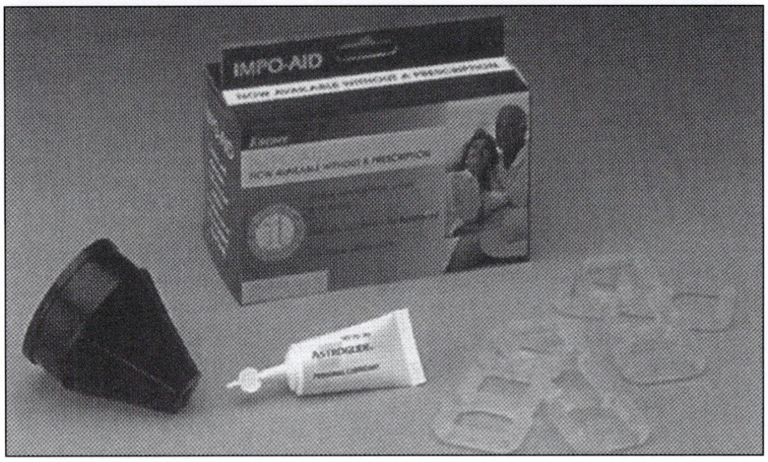

FIGURE 6-25. The IMPO-AID system. Men capable of obtaining a good-quality erection but unable to maintain it may need only the constriction ring at the base of the penis. Such rings are commercially available at much lower cost than vacuum devices. The same precautions regarding time of constriction apply here. The fact that only the distal (extracorporeal) portion of the penis gets rigid may create difficulties for penetration with these systems. (*Courtesy of* Encore, Louisville, KY.)

REFERENCES

1. Heaton JPW, Adams MA, Morales A: A therapeutic taxonomy of treatments for erectile dysfunction: an evolutionary imperative. *Int J Impot Res* 1997, 9:117–121.
2. Morales A, Heaton JPW: Nonsurgical treatments for erectile dysfunction: oral, topical, intracavernous, and vacuum devices. In *Atlas of Clinical Urology*. Edited by Vaughan ED Jr., Perlmutter AP. Philadelphia: Current Medicine, Inc.; 1999:4.1–4.13.
3. Guiliano F, Montorsi F, Mirone V, *et al.*: Switching from intracavernous prostaglandin E1 injections to oral sildenafil citrate in patients with erectile dysfunction: results of a multicenter European study. *J Urol* 2000, 164:708–711.
4. Burnett AL: Nitric oxide in the penis: physiology and pathology. *J Urol* 1997, 157:320–324.
5. Carson CC, Burnett AL, Levine LA, Nehra A: The efficacy of sildenafil citrate (Viagra®) in clinical populations: an update. *Urology* 2002, 60 (suppl 2B):12–27.
6. Hellstrom WJG, Gittelman M, Karlin G, *et al.*: Vardenafil for treatment of men with erectile dysfunction: efficacy and safety in a randomized, double-blind, placebo-controlled trial. *J Androl* 2002, 23:763–771.
7. Brock GB, McMahon CG, Chen KK, *et al.*: Efficacy and safety of tadalafil for the treatment of erectile dysfunction: results of integrated analyses. *J Urol* 2002, 168 (4 pt 1):1332–1336.
8. Heaton JWP, Morales A, Adams M, *et al.*: Resolution of erectile failure after oral treatment with apomorphine. *Urology* 1995, 45:200–203.
9. WHO International Society for Impotence Research: Oral non-endocrine treatment. In *Erectile Dysfunction*. http://www.issir.org.
10. Paoletti R: Biochemistry and pharmacology of prostaglandin E1: introductory remarks. In *Prostaglandin E1 in Atherosclerosis*. Edited by Sinzinger E, Rogatti W. New York: Springer-Verlag; 1986:3–7.
11. Molderings GJ, Van Ahlen H, Gothert M: Modulation of noradrenaline release in human corpus cavernosum by presynaptic prostaglandin receptors. *Int J Impot Res* 1992, 4:19.
12. Kifor J, Williams GH, Vickers MA, *et al.*: Tissue angiotensin II as a modulator of erectile function: I. Angiotensin peptide content, secretion and effects in the corpus cavernosum. *J Urol* 1997, 157:1920–1925.
13. Zhang P, Christ GJ, Brink PR: PGE1-induced alterations in Maxi-K+ channel activity in cultured human corporal smooth muscle cells. *J Urol* 1995, 155 (suppl 6):78A.
14. Lue TF: Male sexual dysfunction. In *Smith's General Urology*, edn 15. Edited by Tanagho EA, McAninch JW. New York: McGraw-Hill/Appleton & Lange; 2001:788–810.
15. Porst H: Vasoactive substances in erectile dysfunction: a survey of 10 years global experience. In *Penile Disorders*. Edited by Porst H. Berlin: Springer-Verlag; 1977:175–196.
16. Bresolle F, Costa P, Rouzier-Panis R, *et al.*: Pharmacokinetics of moxisylyte in healthy volunteers after intracavernous injection of increasing doses. *Eur J Clin Pharmacol* 1996, 49:411–415.
17. Porst H: The rationale for prostaglandin E1 in erectile failure: a survey of world-wide experience. *J Urol* 1996, 155:802–815.
18. Porst H, Buvat J, Meuleman E, *et al.*: Intracavernous alprostadil alfadex: an effective and well tolerated treatment for erectile dysfunction. Results of a long-term European study. *Int J Impot Res* 1998, 10:225–231.
19. Valdevenito R, Melman A: Intracavernous self-injection pharmacotherapy program: analysis of results and complications. *Int J Impot Res* 1993, 150:1822–1824.
20. Goldstein I, Borges FD, Fitch WP, *et al.*: Rescuing the failed papaverine/phentolamine erection: a proposed synergistic action of papaverine, phentolamine and prostaglandin E1. *J Urol* 1990, 143:304A (abstract 463).
21. WHO International Society for Impotence Research: Table 9-3, Incidence of pain with trimix. In *Erectile Dysfunction*. http://www.issir.org.
22. Stackl W, Hasun R, Marberger M: Intracavernous injection of prostaglandin E1 in impotent men. *J Urol* 1988, 140:66.
23. Lee LM, Stevenson RWD, Szadz G: Prostaglandin E1 versus phentolamine/papaverine for the treatment of erectile impotence: a double-blind comparison. *J Urol* 1989, 141:549.
24. WHO International Society for Impotence Research: Table 9-4, Penile scarring with trimix. In *Erectile Dysfunction*. http://www.issir.org.
25. Manning M, Junemann KP: Pharmacotherapy of erectile dysfunction. In *Male Infertility and Sexual Dysfunction*. Edited by Hellstrom WJG. New York: Springer-Verlag; 1997:440–451.
26. Padma-Nathan H, Hellstrom WJG, Kaiser FE, *et al.*: Treatment of men with erectile dysfunction with transurethral alprostadil. *N Engl J Med* 1997, 336:1–7.
27. Lewis R: Twenty years of vacuum therapy for erectile dysfunction in the United States. In *Penile Disorders*. Edited by Porst H. Berlin: Springer-Verlag; 1997:162–174.
28. Nadig PW: Vacuum erection devices: a review. *World J Urol* 1990, 8:114–118.

7

Penile Prostheses

John J. Mulcahy

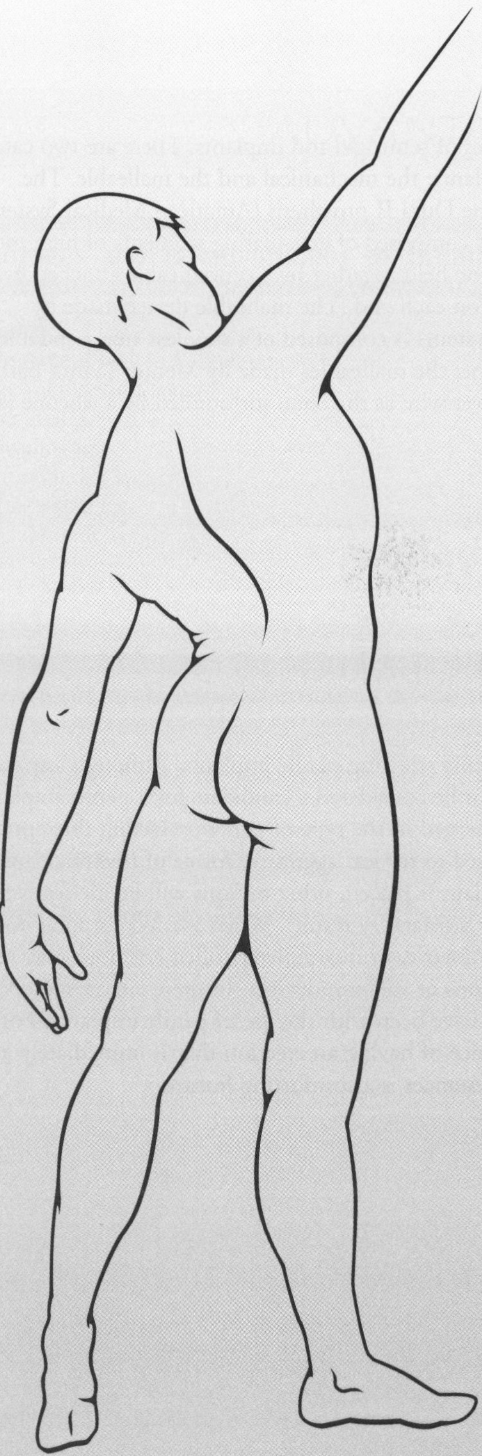

With the introduction of penile prostheses in 1973, interest in erectile dysfunction (ED) increased greatly. Prior to that time, no effective treatments were available and the topic was rarely discussed. Changing sexual customs, beginning in late 1960s, provided a more open forum for discussion and more patients were willing to seek treatment for this common problem. Research on the anatomy and physiology of erections and ED soon followed; investigators sought forms of therapy that were less aggressive and invasive than the surgical placement of prosthetic devices. Highly effective oral, intraurethral, and intracavernous medications have since been marketed, and vacuum erection devices have proven safe, effective, and acceptable to many patients. The growing number of patients opting to treat their impotence problem has, for the most part, selected a less aggressive form of treatment, *ie*, medications and vacuum devices. Penile implant sales, however, have remained stable over the past decade. These devices have provided a predictable and reliable means of restoring erections for many patients, especially for those in whom less invasive treatments have not been effective or in whom scar tissue in the penis has not permitted a satisfactory result with other alternatives.

PREOPERATIVE PREPARATION

Preoperative Preparation

Sterile urine
Cleansing genitalia with a strong soap
Shaving the pubic area in the operating room
Antibiotic prophylaxis
Surgical preparation with an antiseptic solution
Isosmotic filling solutions

FIGURE 7-7. Preoperative preparation. If possible, urine should be sterile. This is sometimes difficult to achieve in patients with neurogenic bladder, and prophylactic antibiotics are frequently given for a week prior to surgery in these patients. Although the urinary tract is usually not entered during placement of a penile prosthesis and urine is not expelled during the procedure, contamination from this source is possible.

Prophylactic antibiotics are usually started with the induction of anesthesia and continued for 48 hours postoperatively. During this period, the wound is open, with complete sealing at 2 days. Continuing antibiotics beyond this period has no advantage [4]. The membranes of the hydraulic devices are semipermeable, and isosmotic filling solutions should be used.

INCISIONAL APPROACHES

Incisional Approaches

Penoscrotal
Ventral penile
Infrapubic
Subcoronal
Perineal
Dorsal penile

FIGURE 7-8. Incisional approaches. A number of incisions may be used for placement of a penile prosthesis. For the three-piece inflatable devices, the infrapubic approach was advocated when these devices were introduced. A penoscrotal incision is also used and requires blind placement of the reservoir through the inguinal canal. The penoscrotal approach is used for the placement of the two-piece device because it allows easy positioning of the pump in the lower scrotum. For placing the rod prostheses, any incision on the penis is convenient; the ventral penile and subcoronal have been the most popular. Although described in the literature, perineal or dorsal penile incisions are rarely used today.

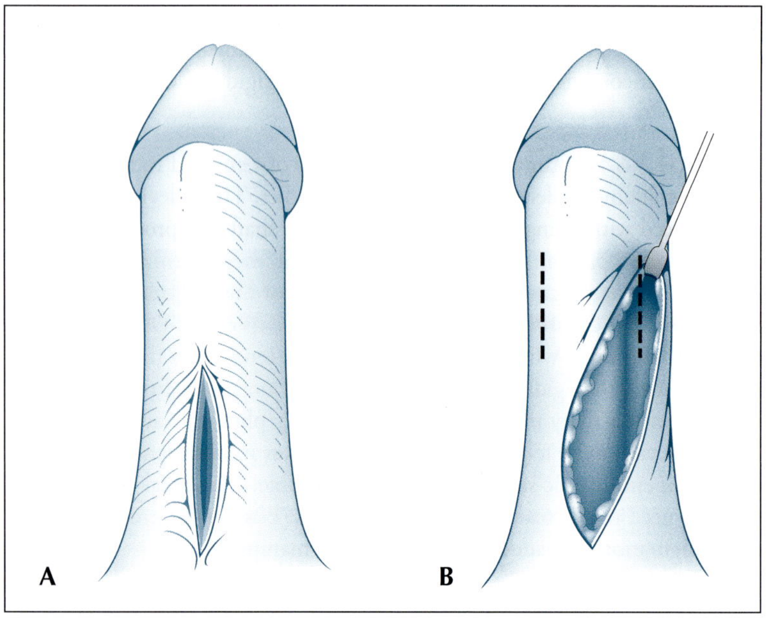

FIGURE 7-9. Ventral penile incision. This incision is useful for placement of semirigid rod devices. It consists of a proximal penile shaft skin incision (**A**) and more distally placed corporotomies [5]. Local anesthesia may be used, semirigid rods can be placed without having to bend the cylinders excessively, and the foreskin may be preserved in the uncircumcised patient (**B**). Incision lines for the skin and corporotomy are not overlying, a feature which reduces the chance of wound contamination and exposure of the prosthesis.

ADMINISTRATION OF ANESTHESIA

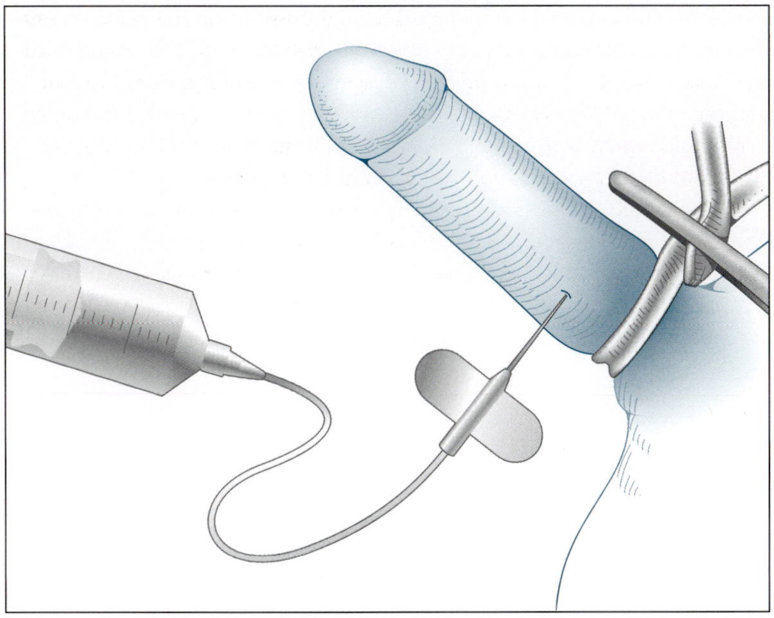

FIGURE 7-10. Technique of administering local anesthesia. A penile block is placed using 1% lidocaine without epinephrine by infiltrating the base of the penis circumferentially adjacent to the tunica albuginea of the corpora cavernosa. A tourniquet is then applied, and about 25 mL of 1% lidocaine is introduced intracorporally as one would perform an artificial erection. In a few minutes the tourniquet is released, and the intracorporal local anesthetic is allowed to flow proximally to anesthetize the whole interior of the corporal bodies.

SURGICAL TECHNIQUE

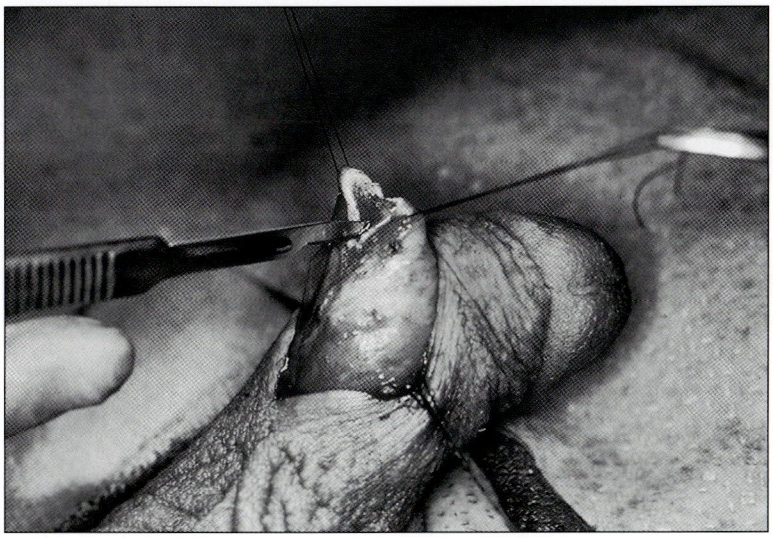

FIGURE 7-11. Corporotomy (ventral penile approach). The skin of the proximal half of the penile shaft is incised. The incision is carried down to the subcutaneous tissues to expose the corpus spongiosum. Buck's fascia and areolar tissue are dissected free from the tunica albuginea of the corpus cavernosum on either side of the corpus spongiosum. Traction sutures are placed in each corporal body and the tunica albuginea is incised using a number 15 blade between the two traction sutures.

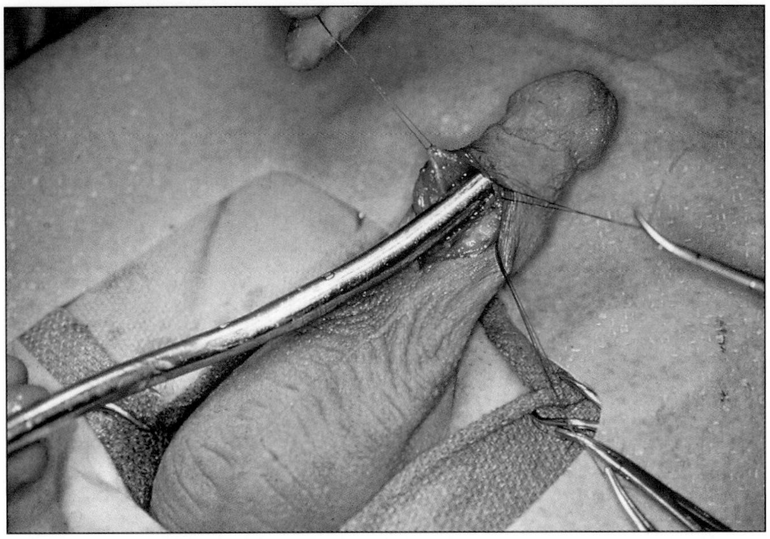

FIGURE 7-12. Dilating the corporal body with Hegar dilators. Initially, the Metzenbaum scissors are passed proximally and distally to create a small plane throughout the corporal body in each direction. Then the Hegar dilators are placed; this pushes the spongy erectile tissue to the periphery and creates a cavity broad enough to position the penile cylinders without difficulty.

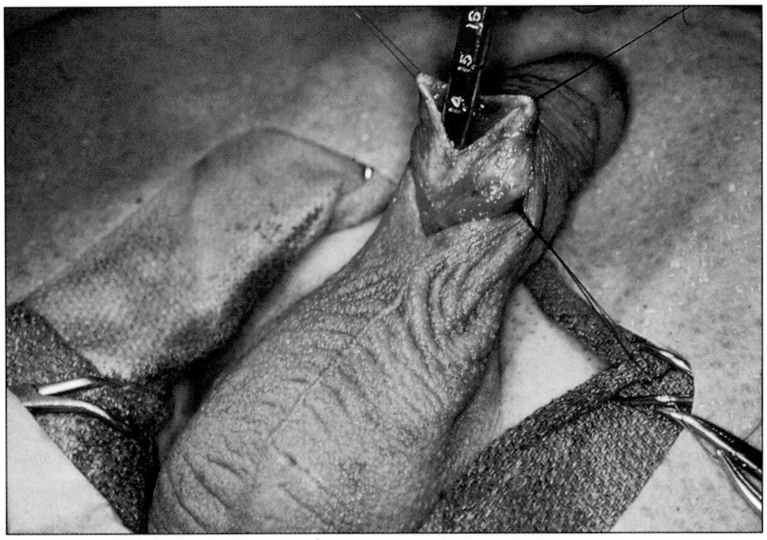

FIGURE 7-13. Measuring the length of the corpus cavernosum with a Furlow introducer. An appropriate measuring tool, such as the Furlow introducer or dialamesensert, is then used to determine the length of the corporal bodies. The measuring device is first placed proximally, with the corporal traction suture used as a reference point. The device is then placed distally, and the two dimensions are added for the total corporal length. For hydraulic cylinders, the length measured should be the length of the cylinder, plus rear-tip extenders, that is inserted. For semirigid rod devices, a length slightly less (≈ 0.5 cm) than the total corporal length will give better bendability to the device without compromising rigidity.

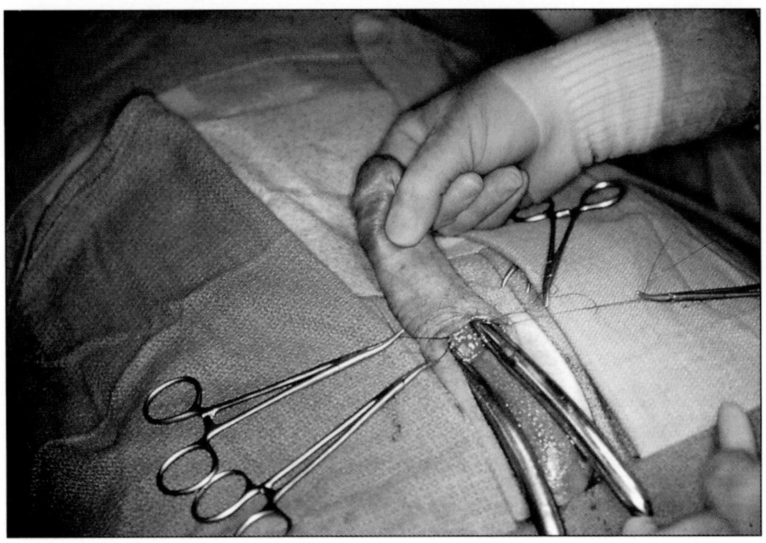

FIGURE 7-14. Width sizing technique for cylinders of fixed girth. The Ambicor, Dynaflex (both made by American Medical Systems, Minnetonka, MN), and semirigid rod devices are sold in sizes of defined fixed girth. To determine which of two or three sizes would be appropriate to insert, two dilators of the smallest available girth are placed simultaneously, distally and proximally, in each corpus cavernosum. When the dilators are positioned, the thumb is apposed to the index finger between the two dilators. If the thumb is easily able to touch the index finger between the dilators, a loose fit will be achieved. An ideal fit would be attained using cylinders of the same size as dilators that separate slightly when the thumb is apposed to the index finger. If no separation occurs with this maneuver, a tight fit would result.

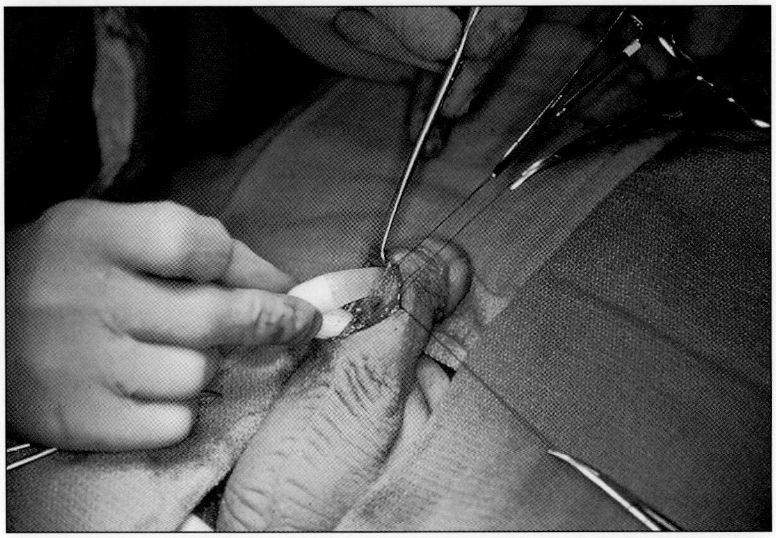

FIGURE 7-15. Distal seating of cylinders by lifting the end of the corporotomy incision over the end of the cylinder with a vein retractor. When the proper-sized length and girth for the cylinder have been chosen, the cylinder is first seated proximally. Because the corporotomy is very near the distal end of the erectile body, the distal end of the cylinder can be easily inserted into the corporal body by lifting the end of the corporal body over the end of the cylinder with use of a vein retractor.

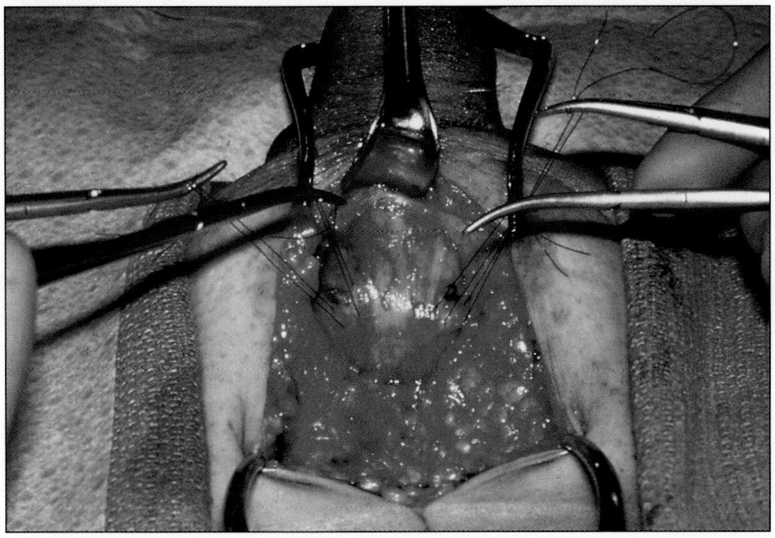

FIGURE 7-16. Longitudinal infrapubic incision for a three-piece inflatable prosthesis. A three-piece prosthesis can be placed infrapubically through a longitudinal or transverse incision. The balloon reservoir is positioned in the prevesical space by an incision in the inferior portion of the linea alba. Care must be taken to place the corporotomies lateral to the dorsal neurovascular bundle to avoid injuries to the nerves contained in this structure. Decreased sensitivity in the glans penis may occur if these nerves are damaged. The pump is inserted in the most inferior portion of the right or left scrotum after a pocket has been created in that area by dissecting from the inferior portion of the infrapubic incision.

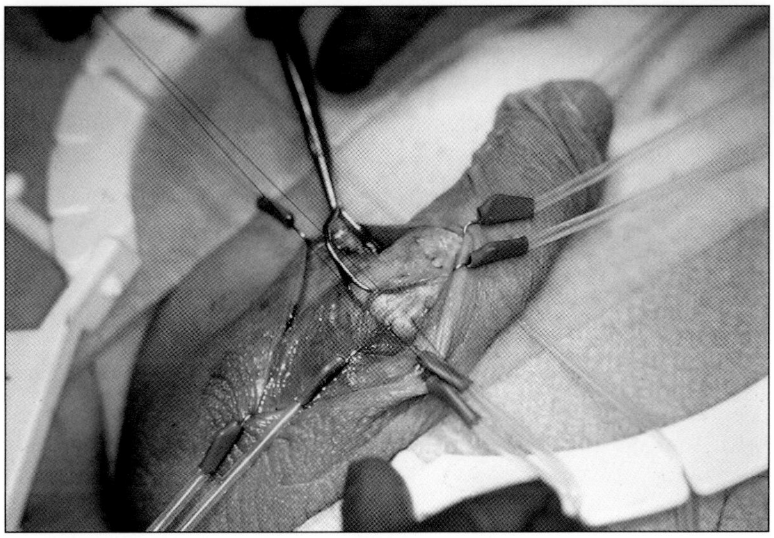

FIGURE 7-17. Penoscrotal incision for placement of three-piece or two-piece prosthesis. A transverse or longitudinal incision may be made in the upper portion of the scrotum for placing a three-piece or two-piece prosthesis. The scar resulting from either incision is imperceptible because it is covered by the rugae of the scrotum. The balloon reservoir is placed through either inguinal canal. Corporal dilation in very obese patients is easier using this approach. The pump may be secured in the inferior portion of the scrotum by sewing scrotal tissue around the tubing adjacent to the pump.

Location of Input Tube Exit from Corpus Cavernosum

Know the range of cylinder sizes and the distance from the input tube to the proximal part of the cylinder of the prosthesis model being implanted

Distance from the proximal end of the cylinder to the input tube

- 5 cm: Ambicor*
- 4 cm: Alpha-1[†] and Narrow Base[†]
- 3 cm: Ultrex*, CX*, and CXR

Total cylinder length = cylinder body size + rear tip extender size

Location of the input tube exit

- Not too proximal: exposure for corporotomy closure will be more difficult
- Not too distal: prepubic pressure during sexual activity will have a shearing effect on the input tube

** American Medical Systems, Minnetonka, MN.*
† Mentor Corporation, Santa Barbara, CA.

FIGURE 7-18. Location of the input tube exit from the corpus cavernosum. In the prototype prosthesis, wearing of the cylinder input tube against the body of the cylinder with eventual erosion into the cylinder was a common problem. Creating a more durable cylinder material and placing a sleeve of teflon around the input tube to reduce friction have greatly reduced the incidence of this problem. It may be totally avoided by placing the exit of the input tube from the corpus cavernosum at its junction with the cylinder. In addition, if the input tube is allowed to run adjacent to the inflatable portion of the cylinder when scar tissue has created a very tight fit, the input tube may be compressed as the cylinder expands. This compression would result in the inability to deflate the cylinder.

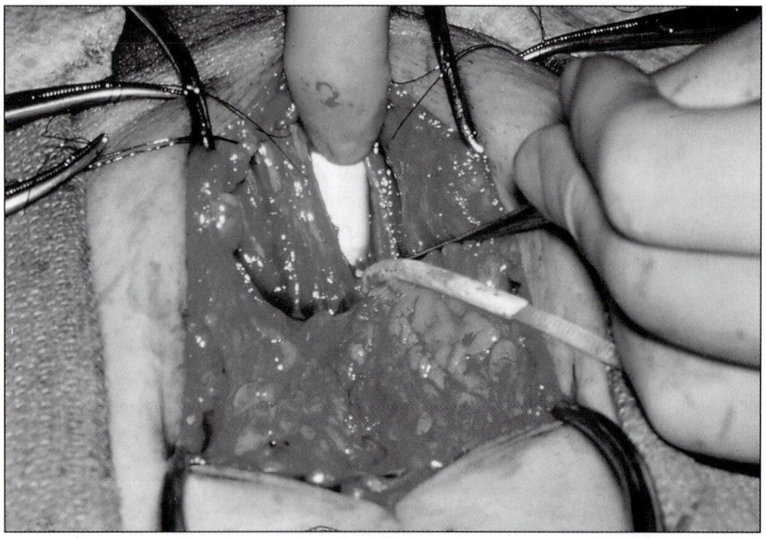

FIGURE 7-19. Exit of input tube from corpus cavernosum. The tunica albuginea of the corpus cavernosum is closed securely around the input tube at the exit as it comes off the inflatable cylinder. Closure in one direction (distally) allows a more secure fit around the tube with less chance of blood oozing from the corporal body following the procedure. Sutures may be preplaced to avoid damage to the cylinder with the needle during closure, or a continuous running suture may be used. The latter is more popular with surgeons because it gives a more accurate corporotomy closure with less risk of bleeding through the suture line.

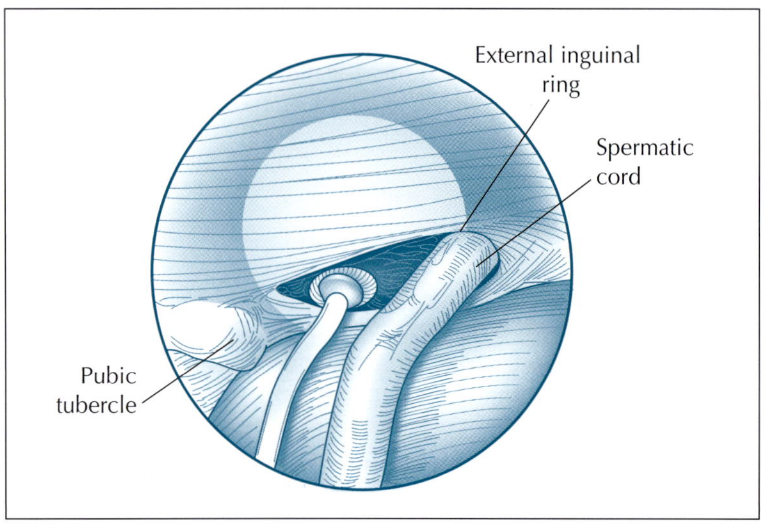

FIGURE 7-20. Reservoir placement through the penoscrotal approach. A Richardson retractor is used to retract the upper portion of the scrotal incision toward the external inguinal ring. The spermatic cord is identified and retracted laterally. A pair of Metzenbaum scissors is used to incise the transversalis fascia over the pubic tubercle, and the index finger is then used to dissect the plane through the inguinal canal to the prevesical space. The reservoir, from which air has been purged, is then wrapped around the index finger and delivered through the inguinal canal to the prevesical space. Fluid is then instilled into the reservoir, and the reservoir is pulled against the internal ring to prevent herniation of abdominal and pelvic contents through the inguinal canal.

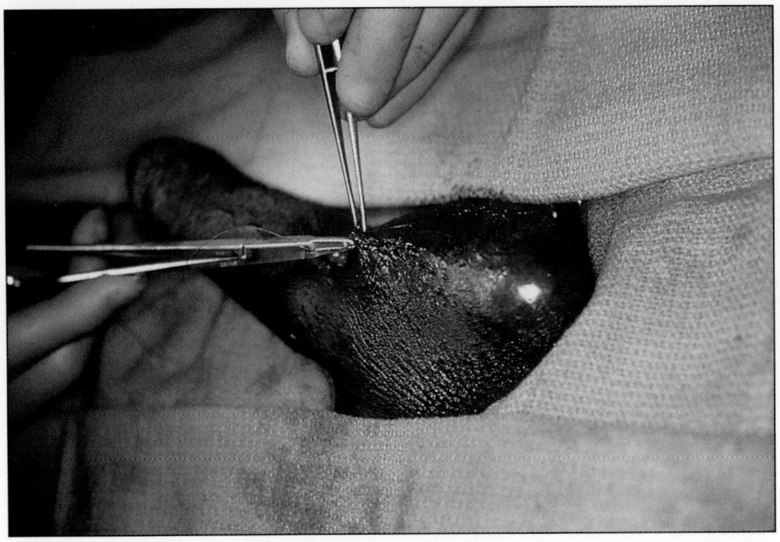

FIGURE 7-21. Placement of a two-piece prosthesis pump. The advantage of using the penoscrotal approach for placing a two-piece prosthesis is that the pump can be readily and simply placed inferiorly within the left or right hemiscrotum.

INTRAOPERATIVE COMPLICATIONS

Urethral Perforation

If accessible in the surgical field
- Close the perforation site
- Irrigate the wound thoroughly
- Continue prosthesis insertion

If inaccessible surgically
- Close the corporotomy
- Leave the opposite cylinder if it is already in place
- Close the wound
- Place the urethral catheter for 3 days
- Return in 2 or more months to reinsert prosthesis

FIGURE 7-22. Urethral perforation. This is an uncommon problem and usually occurs when excessive scar tissue is present within the corporal bodies. In these circumstances, one should use only the tips of the scissors for the initial dilation; the scissors should point away from the urethra and be positioned just under the tunica albuginea dorsally or laterally to help avoid this complication. If perforation does occur and is accessible for closure, the defect should be closed as securely as possible with absorbable suture. It should be assumed that the area is contaminated, and the wound should be thoroughly cleansed with irrigating solution before continuing with cylinder insertion. Success with salvage procedures for infected implants has encouraged use of this approach [6]. If the defect cannot be closed (*eg*, a defect in the fossa navicularis), a cylinder should not be placed in that corporal body.

Crural Crossover

Symptoms
- Different measurement of corporal lengths
- Asymmetric appearance of the cylinders
- Glans tilt to one side of the penis

Solution
- Remove the cylinders
- Place the dilator in one corporal body
- Redilate the other corporal body
- Do not attempt to close the septal defect
- Reinsert the first cylinder while leaving the dilator in the opposite corporal body

FIGURE 7-23. Crural crossover. Perforation of the septum during dilation may occur in up to 25% of penile prostheses. Of itself it is no problem, but if the cylinder migrates or is placed into the opposite corporal body, a less than optimal cosmetic result will occur. After both cylinders have been placed, the surgeon should inspect the corporal bodies thoroughly and be able to palpate a groove between the cylinders as they are inflated in the penile shaft. The tips of each cylinder should be palpated symmetrically under the glans penis. This problem is best managed intraoperatively rather than being brought to the attention of the surgeon by the patient in the postoperative period.

Proximal Crural Perforation

Symptoms
- Large discrepancy in measured proximal corporal length
- Little resistance encountered when dilator is passed proximally

Solution
- For cylinders with input tubes, close corporotomy tightly around input tube to prevent proximal migration
- For unitary cylinders, a cup of synthetic material fashioned around the proximal end of the cylinder is placed in the corporal body with the cylinder and secured with suture to the tunica albuginea of the corpus cavernosum

FIGURE 7-24. Proximal crural perforation. Proximal perforation is usually caused by overzealous dilation or weakened tissue in the region of the ischial tuberosities. If this problem is not attended to at surgery with the unitary devices, the proximal defect will be broadened with the pressure of the cylinder, and soon a ramrod effect will occur and the cylinder will be palpable in the buttocks. Use of a synthetic cup avoids the need for a perineal approach to repair the proximal crural defect.

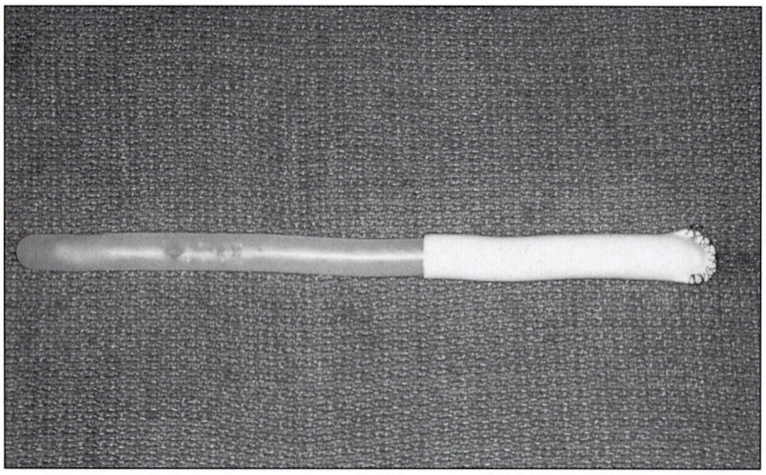

FIGURE 7-25. Synthetic cup fashioned around the proximal end of a semirigid rod. A cup or windsock created from a Gortex (WL Gore and Associates, Flagstaff, AZ) or Dacron (Bard Vascular Systems, CR Bard Co., Billerica, MA) vascular graft can be placed around the proximal end of the cylinder. Natural materials such as cadaver pericardium (Tutoplast, Mentor Corp., Golete, CA) or small intestinal submucosa SIs (Stratasis, Cook Urological, Spencer, IN) may also be used for this purpose. The cylinder with a cup around its proximal segment is then placed into the corporal body and a forceps grasps the edge of the synthetic material and pushes the cylinder toward the distal end of the corporal body under the glans. At this point, the synthetic material is secured to the tunica albuginea of the corpus cavernosum so that the cylinder is properly seated under the glans and will not migrate proximally.

Solutions for Persistent Significant Curvature After Cylinder Insertion

- Modeling
- Multiple incisions in the tunica albuginea on the concave side of the curvature
- One large incision on the concave side of the curve with a synthetic graft to cover the defect
- Nesbit procedure

FIGURE 7-26. Solutions for persistent significant curvature after cylinder insertion. This may be seen when significant scar tissue is present in the penis, as in situations of Peyronie's disease. The initial approach is to inflate both cylinders after corporotomy closure and to clamp the tubing leading from the cylinders. The surgeon then forcibly bends the penis away from the curvature in hope of breaking the scarred area and straightening the penis, a technique called *modeling* [7]. If this is not effective, multiple small incisions or one large incision in the tunica on the concave surface of the curvature may produce sufficient straightening. The Nesbit procedure creates a more secure close of the corporal bodies but will result in some slight shortening of the erection [8].

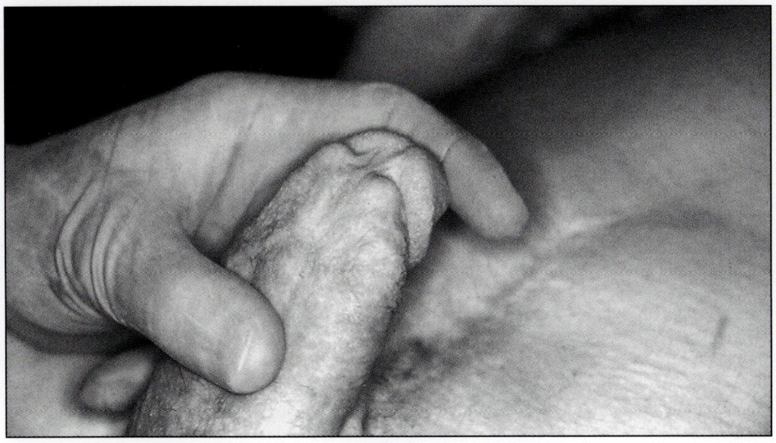

FIGURE 7-27. Hypermobile glans. The prosthesis cylinders reach the end of the corporal body but are not located within the glans. The glans is actually an extension of the corpus spongiosum. The glans may be relatively loosely attached to the end of the penis and, with the prosthesis inflated, may be excessively mobile in a dorsal, ventral, or lateral direction. This condition is seen more commonly in uncircumcised patients with redundant foreskin. The situation may cause difficulty with vaginal penetration if the glans moves off the end of the penile shaft. The glans can be fixed on top of the prosthesis cylinders by placing a permanent suture into the glans substance and into the tunica albuginea of the corpus cavernosum just over the end of the prosthesis cylinder. Tying the suture in place fixes the glans in position [9]. A number of these stitches may be necessary to secure the glans, depending on the degree and the direction of the excessive mobility.

POSTOPERATIVE CARE

Postoperative Care

Prophylactic antibiotics
Dry incision for 10 days
Urethral catheter
Drains
Penile positioning
Operation of device at 6 weeks

FIGURE 7-28. Postoperative care. Antibiotics may be continued for up to 48 hours postoperatively. At this junction the wound is sealed. Patients should avoid soaking the wound for up to 10 days because this may soften absorbable sutures and result in wound separation. Use of drains and indwelling urethral catheters in the immediate postoperative period is favored by some surgeons and not by others. The penis should be positioned in a cephalad direction during the weeks following surgery because scar tissue is being formed during this time. The scar tends to form in the position in which the penis is kept, and a slightly upward-pointing erection is more natural than one pointing toward the toes. By 6 weeks, edema and pain have subsided enough for the patient to comfortably operate the device.

POSTOPERATIVE COMPLICATIONS

Mechanical Problems

Mechanical Problems

Segment wear
Wire breakage
Tubing fracture at fatigue areas
Cylinder or reservoir material fatigue
Pump failure

FIGURE 7-29. Mechanical problems. As with any mechanical device, the penile prosthesis will wear with time, which may lead to malfunctioning, especially from loss of fluid. The more frequently the device is used and the higher the intraluminal pressure achieved during pumping, the more rapidly wear will occur. Tubing adjacent to a connector tends to wear if subjected to unusual angulation. Cylinder creases and weakening of the material at flexion points of the penis, where the device is subject to bending back and forth, and a fold area in the incompletely filled reservoir are common sites where leaks may occur. Wear of the polyethylene segments of the Dura II (American Medical Systems, Minnetonka, MN) results in narrowing of the segments with reduced tension on the springs attaching the cable to the fixed posts. The malleables have been extremely resistant to wear and breakage. Pump malfunction has been very unusual, although slipping of the valves in this area of the prosthesis has occurred.

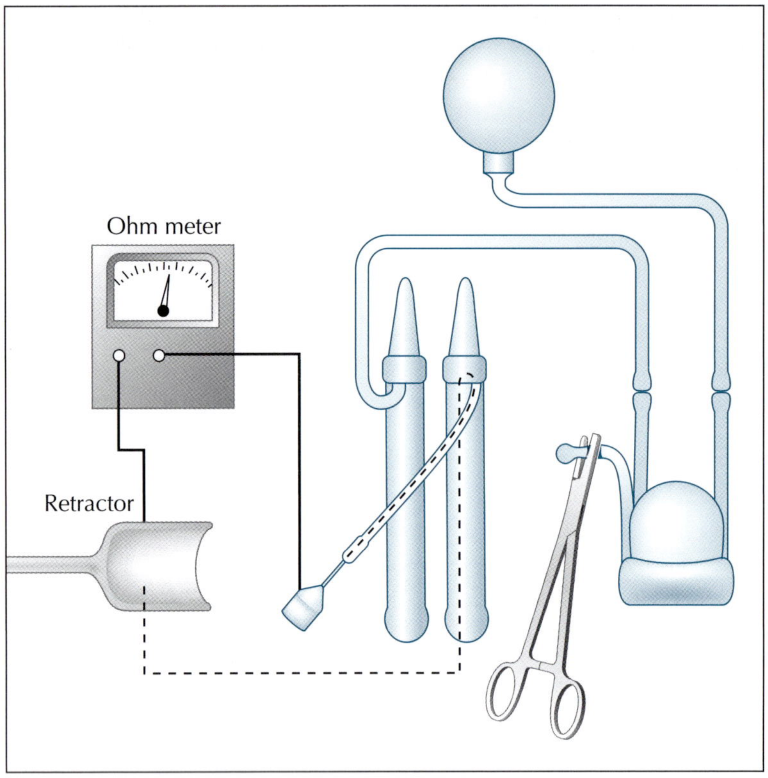

FIGURE 7-30. Prosthesis repair. When a mechanical or malleable rod cylinder malfunctions, a simple replacement of both cylinders is indicated. The site of leakage in a multicomponent prosthesis can be determined using an ohm meter. An intact prosthesis membrane does not allow solute to pass through the walls of the device. A metal blunt needle is placed into the tubing leading to the particular part of the prosthesis to be tested for a leak. After the part is filled with saline, one ohm meter cable is placed on the needle and the other cable on a retractor in any part of the wound. A positive deflection of the ohm meter needle is caused by sodium and chloride ions leaking through the defect in the wall of the part and completing the electrical circuit.

•• Prosthesis Infection ••

Signs and Symptoms of Prosthesis Infection

Erythema
Fever, chills
Persistent or worsening pain
Purulent drainage from wound
Exposed prosthetic part

FIGURE 7-31. Signs and symptoms of prosthesis infection. Despite the use of extreme measures to prevent infection associated with a prosthesis, this unfortunate problem occurs in 1% to 3% of prosthesis operations. It is more common with repairs and reinsertions. Recently, American Medical Systems (Minnetonka, MN) has coated the Ultrex, CX, and CXM prostheses with inhibizone, a combination of rifamycin and minocycline. Mentor Corporation (Santa Barbara, CA) has introduced the Titan, a hydrophilic coating that causes water and antibiotics to adhere to the surface of parts when soaked in an antibiotic solution. It is anticipated that these modifications will further reduce the incidence of implant infections.

Options for Treating Prosthesis Infection

Remove entire prosthesis and all synthetic materials and return for reinsertion after 6 months
Salvage procedure

FIGURE 7-32. Options for treating prosthesis infection. If an infection occurs, it should be treated promptly. The entire device and all synthetic materials can be removed and the patient may return at a later date for reinsertion. Another option that has been gaining popularity is termed a *salvage* or *rescue procedure.* In this approach, all prosthetic parts, foreign material, and permanent sutures are removed. The wound is thoroughly irrigated, and a new prosthesis is inserted at the same sitting. Success rates in eradicating the infection and providing a functioning prosthesis have been achieved in about 85% to 90% of such situations [10]. Virulent organisms, such as *Pseudomonas aeruginosa* and methicillin-resistant *Staphylococcus aureus*, appear to be more difficult to eradicate with a salvage procedure than the more common and less virulent organisms, such as *Staphylococcus epidermidis.*

Sequence of Solutions Used to Irrigate Wound During Salvage Procedure

1. Antibiotics
2. One-half strength hydrogen peroxide
3. One-half strength povidone iodine
4. Pressure wash with Surgilav Plus*; 5-L irrigation solution contains 1 g of vancomycin + 80 mg of gentamicin
5. One-half strength povidone iodine
6. One-half strength hydrogen peroxide
7. Antibiotics

** Stryker Instruments, Kalamazoo, MI.*

FIGURE 7-33. Sequence of solutions used to irrigate the wound during a salvage procedure. Irrigation of the wound with antibiotic solution, hydrogen peroxide, and povidone-iodine has contributed to the high percentage of success with the salvage procedure [11]. To ensure that the solution comes in contact with all parts of the wound, a Robinson catheter is passed to each end of both erectile bodies during instillation of the solutions, and irrigation is carried out through the catheter. Following these irrigations, gowns, gloves, drapes, electric cautery, suction, and instruments are changed prior to insertion of a new prosthesis. No drains or indwelling urethral catheters are left after the procedure and oral quinolone antibiotics are used for 1 month after surgery.

•• Cylinder Extension ••

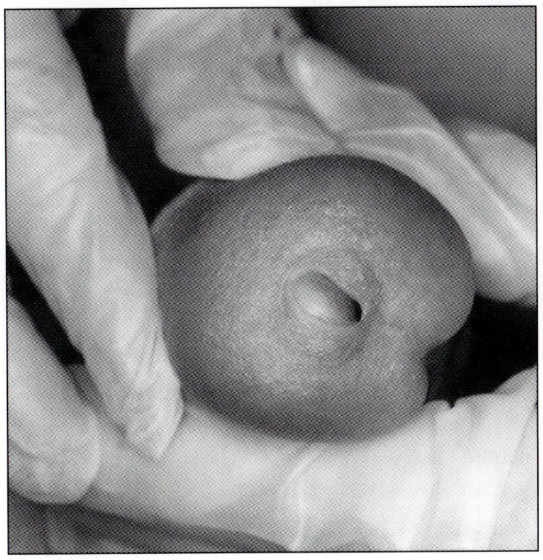

FIGURE 7-34. Distal cylinder extrusion into glans penis. Continued pressure of the end of the prosthesis cylinder against the end of the corporal body or aggressive dilation at the time of insertion may result in perforation of the distal portion of the tunica albuginea of the corpus cavernosum with the cylinder located within the glans. In this position it interferes with urination, resulting in spraying of the stream. The glans offers protection over the ends of the prosthesis cylinder, and extrusion of the cylinder may cause pain for the partner during intercourse. In addition, being precariously close to the skin surface the cylinder is more prone to erosion distally through the end of the penis or into the fossa navicularis.

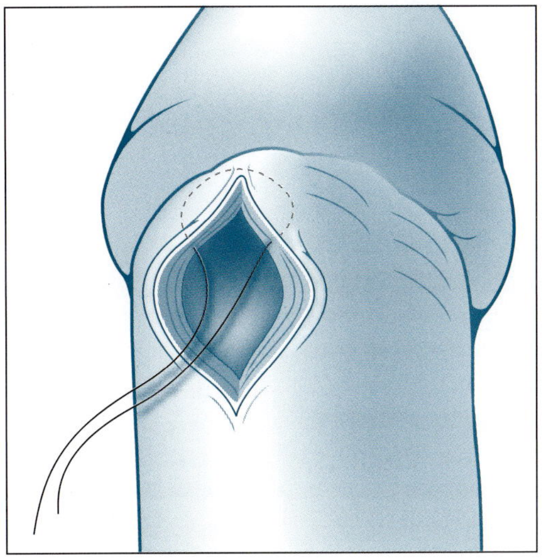

FIGURE 7-35. Repair of distal cylinder extrusion into the glans penis. To repair this problem, adequate exposure to the distal aspect of the tunica albuginea of the corpus cavernosum is gained. The cylinder is removed, and the area of perforation is securely closed with a figure-of-eight or purse-string permanent suture. The cylinder is then reseated in the distal corpus cavernosum, and the corporotomy is closed. After this repair, glans fixation may be necessary.

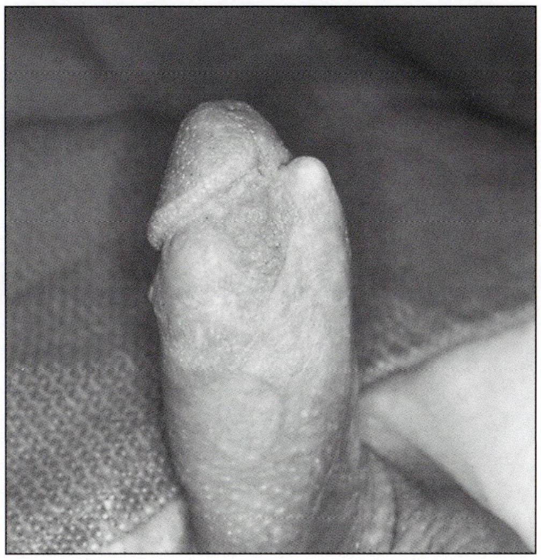

FIGURE 7-36. Lateral cylinder extrusion to the side of the corporal body. Weakening in the lateral wall of the tunica albuginea of the corpus cavernosum may result in cylinder extrusion in this area. This may be caused by aggressive corporal dilation at the time of cylinder placement, excessive pressure exerted in this area by the cylinder, or weakening of the tunica for some other reason. In this location, the cylinder causes discomfort to the patient and the partner during intercourse and is prone to excessive wear, ultimately resulting in erosion through the skin with exposure of the prosthesis part.

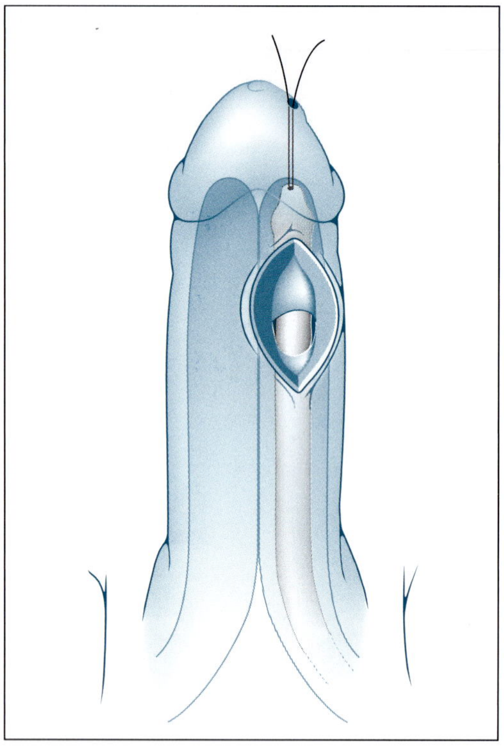

FIGURE 7-37. Repair of lateral cylinder extrusion. To repair the problem, adequate exposure to the distal end of the corpus cavernosum is gained. A longitudinal corporotomy is made over the cylinder, and the cylinder is removed or retracted proximally. A transverse incision using a number 15 blade is made in the back wall of the sheath containing the cylinder. The cavity behind the sheath is dilated with Metzenbaum scissors and Hegar dilators distally to the end of the corporal body, creating a new plane for seating the prosthesis more medially. The prosthesis cylinder is reseated in the new cavity, and the corporotomy is closed, providing two strong layers, the old cylinder sheath and the corporotomy closure, to prevent recurrence of this extrusion [12].

REPAIR RATE OF IMPLANTS

Repair Rate of Implants

Hydraulic
- 5 years = 5% to 10%
- > 10 years—majority of devices will need replacement

Malleable
- Rarely needs replacement

Mechanical
- Higher molecular weight segments of the Dura II* are more durable than the polysulfone segments of its precursor, the Duraphase.†

** Imagyn Urology, Augusta, GA.*
† Dacomed Corp., Minneapolis, MN.

FIGURE 7-38. Repair rate of implants. With the prototype hydraulic prostheses, repair rates of close to 50% within the first few years of insertion were not unheard of [13]. The manufacturers attended to problems of wear, eliminating or reinforcing areas that tended to malfunction. Current-model cylinders have, in many cases, been in place for 10 years or more, and repair rates are acceptable. With hydraulic prostheses, reoperation for mechanical problems within the first 5 years is in the range of 5% to 10% [14–16]. Quantitative figures for repair with the current models beyond this have not been tabulated. With time and frequent use, most models will eventually need to be replaced. Individual wrapping of strands of the malleable prostheses has prolonged the life of these parts.

PATIENT SATISFACTION

Satisfaction with Implants

Patients 80% to 90%
Partners 70% to 80%

FIGURE 7-39. Satisfaction with implants. Three treatments for erectile dysfunction are commonly used—*ie*, medications, vacuum devices, and penile implants. Implants have provided the greatest satisfaction among both patients and partners [17–19]. The fact that the same result is achieved each time and that the erection lasts as long as one wishes, as well as the ease of achieving an erection by simply bending the penis or pumping the prosthesis contribute to this high rate of gratification. When patients are dissatisfied with the results, a shorter penis and lack of spontaneity are the common reasons given. Partners who look less positively upon penile prostheses relate that the erection is now mechanical and that it was not their attractiveness or stimulation that brought about the erection. Better preoperative counseling may avoid some of these unmet expectations.

REFERENCES

1. Mulcahy JJ: Update: penile prostheses. *Contemp Urol* 1994, 6:15–21.
2. Knoll LD: Use of penile prosthetic implants in patients with penile fibrosis. *Urol Clin North Am* 1995, 22:847–863.
3. Eigner EB, Kabalin JN, Dessler R: Penile implants in the treatment of Peyronie's disease. *J Urol* 1991, 145:69–71.
4. Carson CC: Infections in genitourinary prostheses. *Urol Clin North Am* 1989, 16:139–147.
5. Wahle GW, Mulcahy JJ: Ventral penile approach in unitary component penile prosthesis placement. *J Urol* 1993, 149:537–538.
6. Fishman IJ, Scott FB, Selim A, *et al.*: The rescue procedure: an alternative for managing an infected penile prosthesis. *Contemp Urol* 1997, 9:73–80.
7. Wilson SK, Delk JR: A new treatment for Peyronie's disease: modeling the penis over an inflatable penile prosthesis. *J Urol* 1994, 152:1121–1123.
8. Mulcahy JJ, Rowland RG: Tunica wedge excision to correct penile curvature associated with the inflatable penile prosthesis. *J Urol* 1987, 138:63–64.
9. Ball TP: Surgical repair of penile "SST" deformity. *Urology* 1980, 15:603–604.
10. Brant MD, Ludlow JK, Mulcahy JJ: The penile prosthesis salvage operation: immediate replacement of the infected penile prosthesis. *J Urol* 1996, 155:155–157.
11. Teloken C, Souto JC, DaRos C, *et al.*: Prosthetic penile infection: rescue procedure with rifamycin. *J Urol* 1992, 148:1905–1906.
12. Mulcahy JJ: Distal corporoplasty for lateral extrusion of penile prosthesis cylinders. *J Urol* 1999, 161:193–195.
13. Gregory JC, Purcell MH, Standeven J: The inflatable penile prosthesis: failure of rear tip extenders in reducing the incidence of cylinder leakage. *J Urol* 1984, 131:668–669.
14. Daitch JA, Angermeier KW, Lakin MM, *et al.*: Long term mechanical reliability of AMS 700 series inflatable penile protheses: comparison of CX / CXM and Ultrex cylinders. *J Urol* 1997, 158:1400–1402.
15. Kabalin JN, Kuo JC: Long term follow-up and patient satisfaction with the Dynaflex self-contained inflatable penile prosthesis. *J Urol* 1997, 158:456–459.
16. Carson CC, Mulcahy JJ, Grovier FE: Efficacy, safety, and patient satisfaction outcomes of the AMS 700 CX inflatable penile prosthesis: results of a long term multicenter study. *J Urol* 2000, 164:376–380.
17. Fallon B, Ghanem H: Sexual performance and satisfaction with penile prostheses in impotence of various etiologies. *Int J Impot Res* 1990, 2:35–42.
18. Garber BB: Mentor Alpha-1 penile prosthesis: patient satisfaction and device reliability. *Urology* 1994, 43:214–217.
19. McLaren RH, Barrett DM: Patient and partner satisfaction with the AMS 700 penile prosthesis. *J Urol* 1992, 147:62–67.

Surgical Treatments for Vasculogenic Erectile Dysfunction

8

Michael A. Palese
John P. Mulhall
Irwin Goldstein

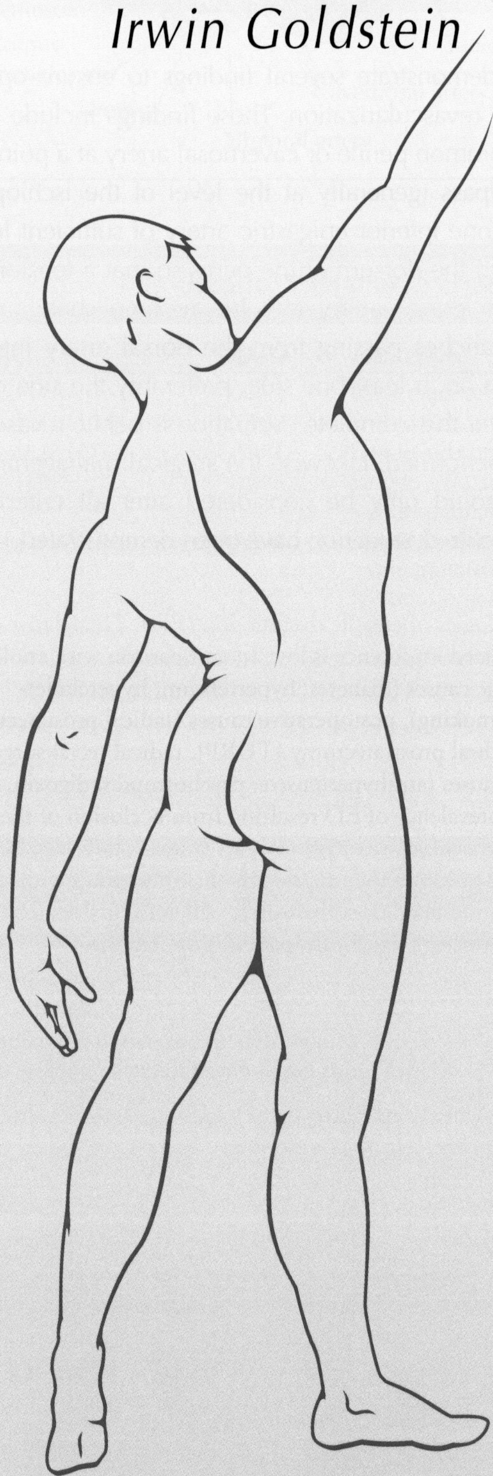

Vasculogenic erectile dysfunction can be corrected, and the options include penile revascularization surgery, crural ligation surgery for the treatment of focal veno-occlusive dysfunction, and the development of pharmacologic and biologic neovascularization agents. During the past several decades, numerous reports in the literature have attempted to detail refinements in all of these techniques.

The overall goal of penile revascularization surgery is to bypass an obstructive arterial lesion in either the common penile or cavernosal artery. The specific objective of this surgery is to increase the blood pressure within the cavernosal artery and therefore the corpus cavernosum. Success rates have been difficult to compare because of the variety of surgical techniques as well as the inconsistent definitions of success among investigators [1–6].

Organic veno-occlusive dysfunction is the result of structural alterations in corporal smooth muscle. The consequence of these changes is the failure to occlude subtunical venous channels, which results in persistent venous outflow. Strategies aimed at improving venous leak have historically involved venous ligation procedures. Generally, most analyses have demonstrated poor long-term results. However, recent interest in crural ligation surgery may hold some promise for select patients with focal venous leak [7–9].

Neovascularization is an attempt to reverse impaired cavernosal artery inflow with the use of angiogenic factors. Tissue hypoxia and inflammatory response are major physiologic stimuli for angiogenesis, but angiogenesis itself is controlled by various factors, which include basic fibroblast growth factor, vascular endothelial growth factor, and hypoxia inducible factor. It is these proteins that induce proliferation and migration of endothelial and smooth muscle cells as well as angiogenesis. At this time, only animal studies have been performed with human clinical trials to follow in the future [10–12]. Nevertheless, preliminary animal data support the need for further assessment of such agents for vasculogenic erectile dysfunction (ED).

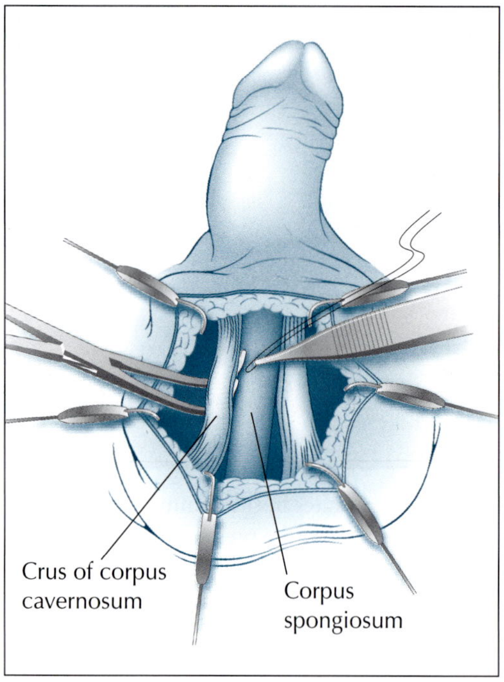

FIGURE 8-20. Crural ligation. The crus is dissected off the periosteum of the ischiopubic ramus through a transverse scrotal incision. The umbilical tape then is passed around the crus.

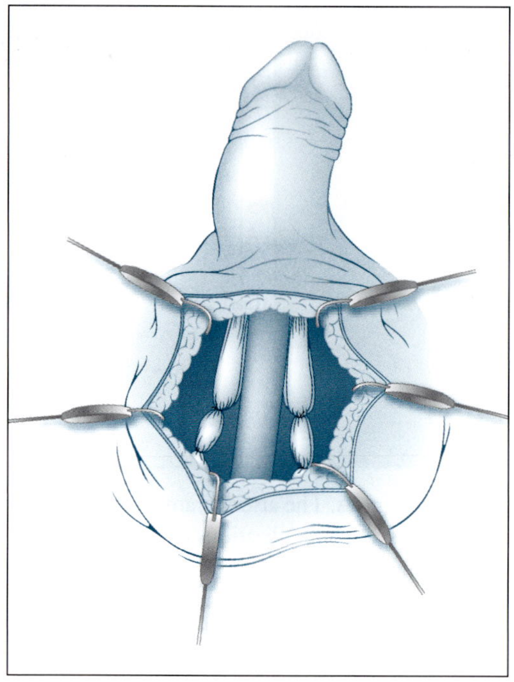

FIGURE 8-21. Crural ligation continued. The crura are ligated at two points on each side, with the umbilical tape dividing the crus into thirds.

Future Techniques: Neovascularization

Angiogenic factors
- VEGF
- bFGF
- HIF

Role of VEGF
- Feasibility of local intracavernosal VEGF injection
- Ameliorating hypercholesterolemia in animals

FIGURE 8-22. Angiogenesis is the growth and proliferation of blood vessels from existing vascular structures. Several angiogenic factors present in the vasculature are mitogens to endothelial cells. These include vascular endothelial growth factor (VEGF), basic fibroblast growth factor (bFGF), and hypoxia inducible factor (HIF). Proper expression of these angiogenic factors is required for normal blood vessel development. In addition, these factors may act as survival factors during endothelial cell injury [22]. The effect of VEGF for augmenting perfusion and stimulating the formation of collateral vessels and smooth muscle has been shown in several animal models [10–12]. In fact, several clinical trials have shown successful induction of collateral vessels in ischemic heart disease [23] and limb ischemia [24]. To date there are no published clinical trials demonstrating neovascularization in the human penis; however, several animal models have shown the feasibility of using local intracavernosal VEGF injection. The effects of hypercholesterolemia on smooth muscle cell content and function in a rabbit model have been ameliorated with VEGF administration [9]. In a rat model of traumatic arteriogenic erectile dysfunction, a single bolus of VEGF improved erectile function [11]. This is a new and exciting area of research that may have many clinical implications in the future.

REFERENCES

1. Zumbe J, Drawz G, Widemann A, *et al.*: Indications for penile revascularization and long term results. *Andrologia* 1999, 31S:83–87.
2. Manning M, Junemann K-P, Pospichal J, *et al.*: Long-term follow-up and selection criteria for penile revascularization in erectile failure. *J Urol* 1998, 160:1680–1684.
3. Sarramon JP, Bertrand N, Malavaud B, *et al.*: Microrevascularization of the penis in vascular impotence. *Int J Impot Res* 1997, 9:127–131.
4. Anafarta K, Aydos K, Yaman O: Is deep dorsal vein arterialization an alternative surgical approach to treat venogenic impotence? *Urol Int* 1997, 59:109–113.
5. Jarow JP, DeFranzo AJ: Long-term results of arterial bypass surgery for impotence secondary to segmental vascular disease. *J Urol* 1996, 156:982–987.
6. DePalma RG, Olding M, Yu GW, *et al.*: Vascular interventions for impotence: lessons learned. *J Vasc Surg* 1995, 21:576–580.
7. Rogers RS, Lue TF: Penile venous surgery benefits patients under 40 years of age. *J Urol* 1999, 161:258–261.
8. Lue TF: Surgery for crural venous leakage. *Urology* 1999, 54:739–741.
9. Mulhall JP, Martin D, Ergin E, *et al.*: Crural ligation surgery for the young male with venogenic erectile dysfunction: technique. *Tech Urol* 2001, 7:290–293.
10. Byrne RR, Henry GD, Rao DS, *et al.*: Vascular endothelial growth factor restores corporeal smooth muscle function in vitro. *J Urol* 2001, 165:1310–1315.
11. Lee MC, El-Sakka AI, Graziottin TM, *et al.*: The effect of vascular endothelial growth factor on a rat model of traumatic arteriogenic erectile dysfunction. *J Urol* 2002, 167:761–766.
12. Gholami SS, Rogers R, Chang J, *et al.*: The effect of vascular endothelial growth factor and adeno-associated virus mediated brain derived neurotrophic factor on neurogenic and vasculogenic erectile dysfunction induced by hyperlipidemia. *J Urol* 2003, 169:1577–1581.
13. Goldstein I: Vascular diseases of the penis. In *Clinical Urography.* Edited by Pollack H. Philadelphia: WB Saunders; 1990:2231–2252.
14. Krane RJ, Goldstein I, Saenz de Tejada I: Impotence. *N Engl Med J* 1989, 321:1648–1659.
15. Michal V, Kramar R, Pospichal J, *et al.*: Direct arterial anastomosis on corpora cavernosa penis in the therapy of erective impotence. *Rozhl Chir* 1973, 52:587–590.
16. Michael V, Kramar R, Pospichal J, *et al.*: Vascular surgery in the treatment of impotence: its present possibilities and prospects. *Czech Med* 1980, 3:213–217.
17. Virag R, Zwang G, Dermange H, *et al.*: Vasculogenic impotence: a review of 92 cases with 54 surgical operations. *Vasc Surg* 1981, 15:9–13.
18. Hauri D: Therapiemoglichkeiten bei der vascular bedinkten erekteilen impotenz. *Akt Urol* 1984, 15:350–354.
19. Crespo El, Bove D, Farrell C, *et al.*: Microvascular surgery technique and follow up. *Vasc Surg* 1987, 21:277–281.
20. Carmignani G, Pirozzi F, Corbu C, *et al.*: Cavernous artery revascularization in vasculogenic impotence: new simplified technique. *Urology* 1987, 30:23–27.
21. Goldstein I: Overview of types and results of vascular surgical procedures for impotence. *Cardiovasc Intervent Radiol* 1988, 11:240–244.
22. Folkman J: Clinical applications of research on angiogenesis. *N Engl J Med* 1995, 333:1757–1767.
23. Losordo DW, Vale PR, Symes JF, *et al.*: Gene therapy for myocardial angiogenesis: initial clinical results with direct myocardial injection of phVEGF165 as sole therapy for myocardial ischemia. *Circulation* 1998, 98:2800–2808.
24. Baumgartner I, Pieczek A, Manor O, *et al.*: Constitutive expression of phVEGF165 after intramuscular gene transfer promotes collateral vessel development in patients with critical limb ischemia. *Circulation* 1998, 97:1114–1120.

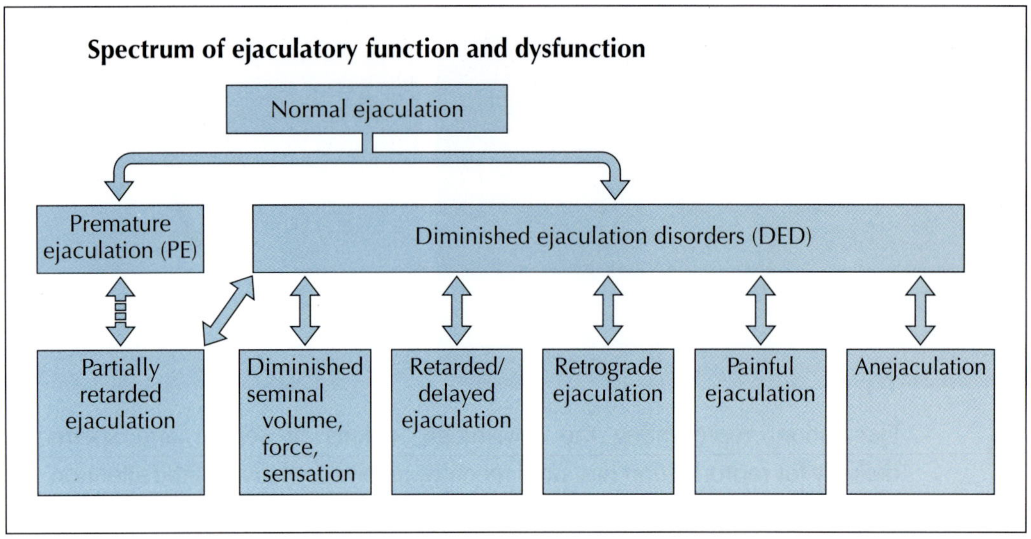

FIGURE 9-1. Spectrum of ejaculatory dysfunction, or male orgasmic disorder (MOD). MOD is a spectrum of disorders that are perceived by the individual as a deviation from an ill-defined "normal" pattern of response. This can be characterized by presence or absence, time and control, pain, volume, or direction of ejaculation. Individuals may experience a variation in their perception of ejaculation over time or with specific sexual encounters or partners. At the very least, a persistent alteration causing distress must be present. Any of these disorders may include an alteration or elimination of the phenomenologic experience of orgasm itself. The acronym "EjD" has been suggested as a less stigmatized term for the specific disorders of ejaculation that are familiar to us at this time. However, it is potentially controversial terminology due to the risk of perceived "commercial exploitation" in a manner that the terms "ED" (erectile dysfunction) and especially "FSD" (female sexual dysfunction) have been recently criticized in the media and elsewhere.

The definitions, prevalence, mechanism of action, etiology, and treatment of these disorders is described in greater detail in the sections that follow.

ANATOMY AND PHYSIOLOGY

Stages of Normal Ejaculatory Physiology

- Emission
  - Bladder neck closure
  - Deposition of seminal fluid into posterior urethra
- Ejection
  - Expulsion of seminal fluid from the urethra
  - Relaxation of the external sphincter
  - Coordinated pelvic floor, bulbospongiosus contraction
- Orgasm
  - A sensory experience associated with these events

FIGURE 9-2. Stages of normal ejaculatory physiology. Ejaculation has been traditionally viewed as a single event comprising emission, ejection, and orgasm; however, these represent distinct events with separate neural pathways. Following a variable period of sensory stimulation represented by the plateau phase from Masters and Johnson [3], a rapid sequence of events ensue. The emission phase begins with closure of the bladder neck followed by deposition of semen from the seminal vesicles and prostate into the posterior urethra. A sensation of "ejaculatory inevitability" arises from the distension of the bulbocavernous and ischiocavernous muscle contraction. Orgasm is a central sensory event that has significant subjective variation. This event can occur independent of emission, ejection, and erection. An ejaculatory bolus is not required for pleasurable orgasm, as evidenced by men with radical prostatectomy.

Volume of ejaculate, semen viscosity, and quality of the central/peripheral sexual stimulation can affect the perception of orgasm. The refractory period is a time of recovery prior to a second ejaculation. The physiologic reason for a refractory period is unknown, and unlike the female, multiple ejaculation/orgasms are rarely encountered. The refractory period lengthens with advancing age and repeated ejaculations.

Orgasm and ejaculation constitute the third phase of the sexual response cycle. Ejaculation is a reflex comprising sensory receptors and areas, afferent pathways, cerebral sensory areas, cerebral motor centres, spinal motor centers and efferent pathways. The ejaculatory reflex is predominantly controlled by a complex interplay between central serotonergic and dopaminergic neurons with secondary involvement of cholinergic, adrenergic, oxytocinergic, and GABAergic neurons. There are three basic mechanisms involved in normal antegrade ejaculation: emission, ejection, and orgasm [4,5]. Ejaculatory dysfunction can result from disruption at any point in this cascade of events. (*Adapted from* Gil-Vernet *et al.* [6].)

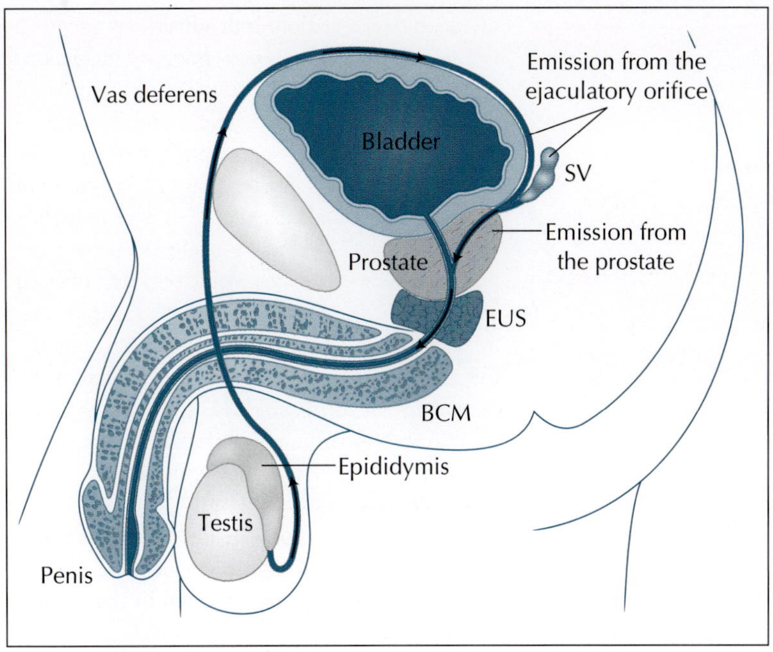

FIGURE 9-3. The physiology of ejaculation. The semen (ejaculatory) volume is derived from the seminal vesicle (50% to 80%), prostate (15% to 30%), Cowper's gland (< 5%) and the testes (< 1%). The total volume and viscosity of ejaculate demonstrates marked variation between individual men and sexual encounters. Infrequent ejaculation is generally associated with increased volumes and viscosity [7,8]. BCM—bulbocavernosus muscle; EUS—external urethral sphincter; SV—seminal vesicle (*Adapted from* Mann [7].)

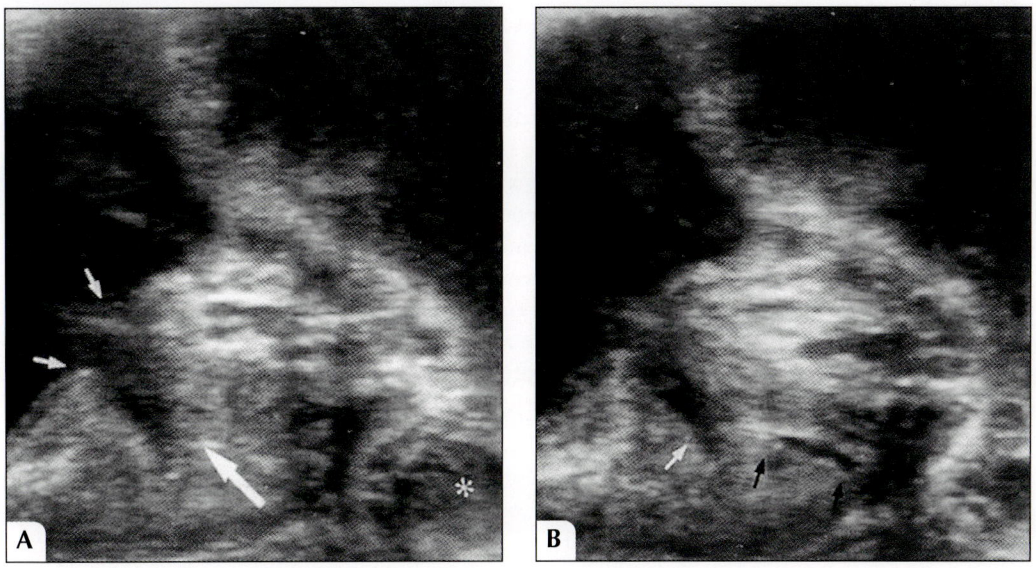

FIGURE 9-4. Transrectal ultrasound during masturbation. **A,** Pre-ejaculatory phase (18 s). The *large arrow* is the prostate. The *small arrows* indicate the bladder neck. **B,** Ejaculation. This real-time transrectal ultrasound recording shows the anatomic and physiologic changes that occur during the pre-ejaculatory phase and ejaculation during masturbation. The inframontanal urethra (*small black arrows*) filling with prostatic fluid during emission and the contracted preprostatic sphincter can be observed. The *small white arrows* indicate the prostatic urethra. (*From* Gil-Vernet *et al.* [6]; with permission.)

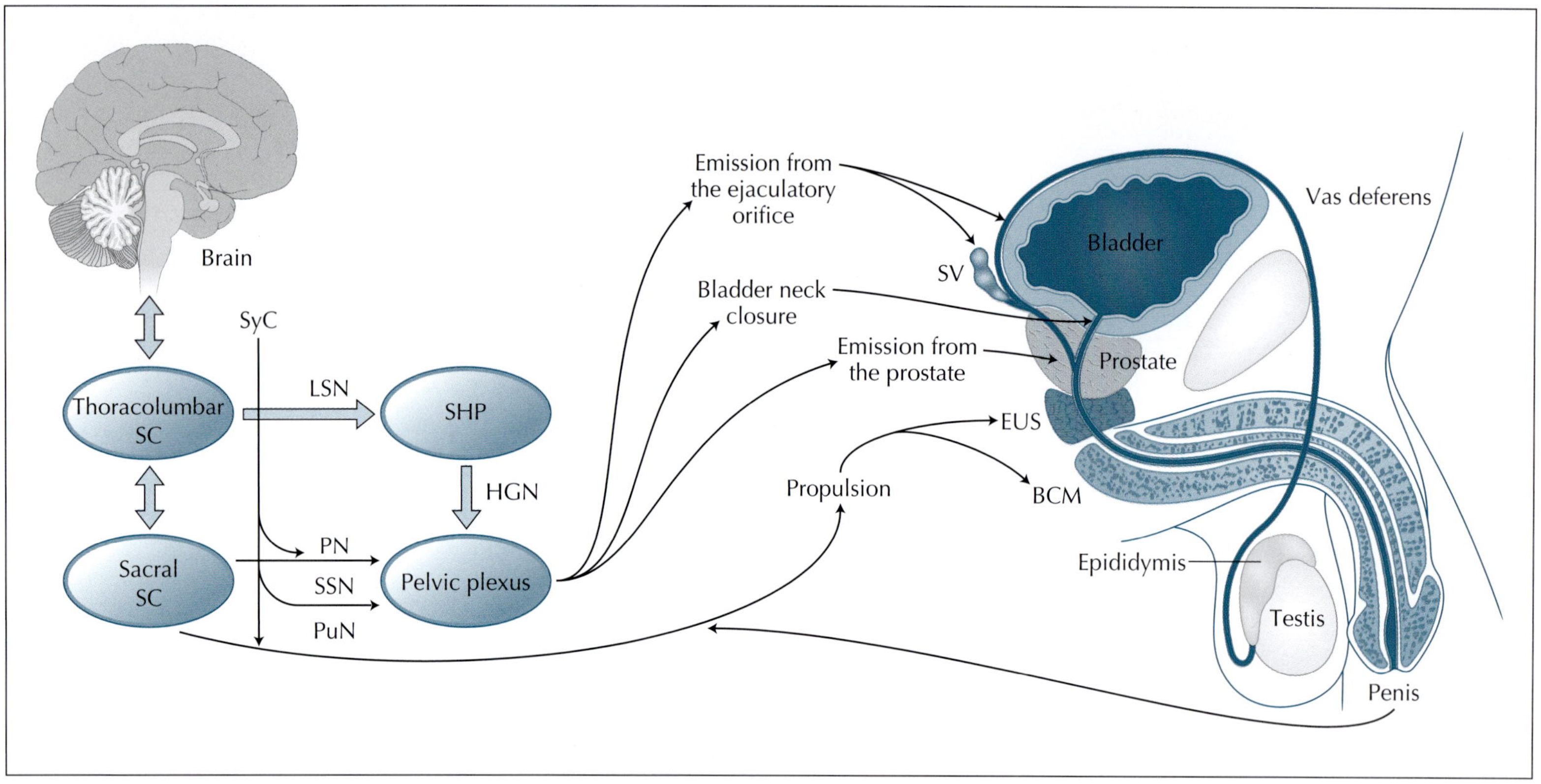

FIGURE 9-5. The neurophysiology of ejaculation. Sensory information from the glans penis travels along somatic afferent pathways within the dorsal nerve of penis to the S4 level of the spinal cord. Seminal emission and ejaculation are centrally controlled by the paraventricular nucleus (PVN) of the anterior hypothalamus and the medial preoptic area (MPOA).

Emission is controlled by the sympathetic nervous system. The cell bodies of the sympathetic neurons are located in the lateral columns of the gray matter in the thoracolumbar segments of the spinal cord. Efferent sympathetic nerves emerge from the ventral roots of the spinal column at Th12-L2 to reach the sympathetic chains bilaterally.

Ejection is controlled by the parasympathetic nervous system. Efferent somatic fibres emerge from the anterior horn of the S2-S4 spinal segments (Onuf's nucleus) and travel in the motor branch of the pudendal nerve to innervate the pelvic floor striated muscles including the bulbospongiosus and bulbocavernosus muscles. Rhythmic contractions of the bulbocavernosus, ischiocavernosus, and other pelvic floor striated muscles propels seminal fluid into the urethra.

Ejaculatory reflexes remain intact in humans and animals with complete spinal transection between cervical level 3 and lumbar level 3.

Thus, ejaculation is mediated by a spinal control center, located in the lumbosacral spinal cord. This spinal control center has been referred to as the spinal ejaculation generator and spinal pattern generator and spinal pacemaker. There are two different afferent pathways to the spinal cord: 1) sensory fibers of the pudendal nerve (dorsal nerve of penis) up to S4, and 2) sympathetic fibers in the hypogastric nerve that transmits information to the spinal cord sympathetic ganglia. Close contact exists between these autonomic and cerebrospinal nervous pathways. BCM—bulbocavernosus muscle; HGN—hypogastric nerve(s); LSN—lumbar sympathetic nerve(s); PN—penile nerve; PuN—pudendal nerve; SC—spinal cord; SHP—septohippocampal pathway; SSN—sacral splanchnic nerve; SV—seminal vesicle; SyC—sympathetic chain.

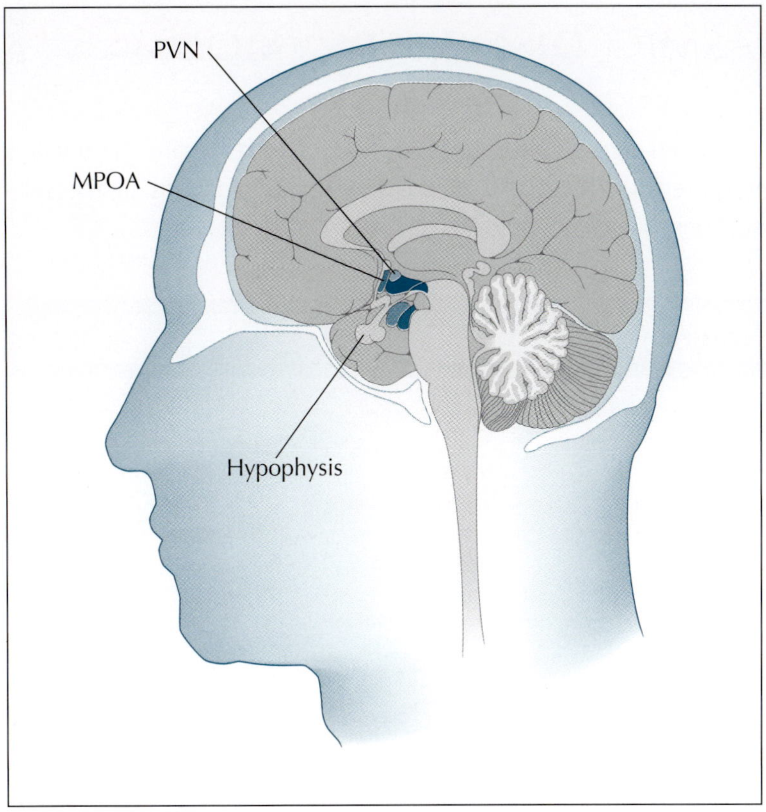

FIGURE 9-6. Cerebral receptor areas. Seminal emission, ejection, and orgasm are integrated into the complex pattern of copulatory behavior by multiple forebrain structures. The medial preoptic area (MPOA), nucleus paragigantocellularis, stria terminalis, amygdala, and thalamus are central to reproductive neurophysiology. Multiple excitatory and inhibitory neurotransmitters are involved including dopamine, serotonin, NO, oxytocin, and GABA. The interaction of individual neural tracts and transmitters has not been fully characterized. Experimental and clinical observations have identified the putative role of central 5-hydroxytryptamine (5-HT). 5-HT has an inhibitory role in sexual behavior in the male. In the rat model, a decrease in central 5-HT neurotransmission decreases the number of intromissions preceding ejaculation and shortens the time to ejaculation. An increase in central 5-HT neurotransmission produces the opposite effect. Administration of different selective serotonin reuptake inhibitors (SSRIs), which results in higher levels of 5-HT, suppresses sexual behavior in male rats [9–11]. PVN—paraventricular nucleus.

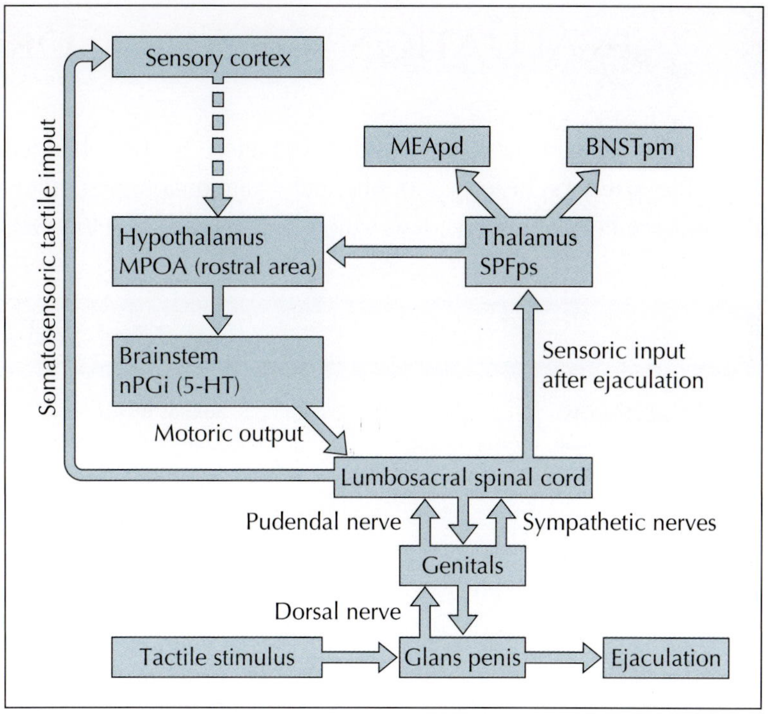

FIGURE 9-7. Central control of ejaculation. Central control of ejaculation is dependent on afferent sensory information and higher cortical areas. It has been observed that the descending serotonergic pathways from the nucleus paragigantocellularis (nPGI) to the lumbosacral motor nuclei tonically inhibit ejaculation; conversely, disinhibition of the nPGI by the medial preoptic area (MPOA) results in ejaculation. Several brain areas are activated after ejaculation by ascending fibers from the spinal cord–posteromedial bed nucleus of stria terminalis, lateral subarea of posterodorsal medial amygdala, and medial parvicellular subparafascicular nucleus of thalamus. These areas have a possible role in satiety and determining the postejaculatory refractory time. BNSTpm—posteromedial bed nucleus of the stria terminalis; MEApd—posterodorsal medial amygdale; SPFPS—medical parvicellular subparafascicular nucleus of the thalamus. (*Adapted from* Waldinger [12].)

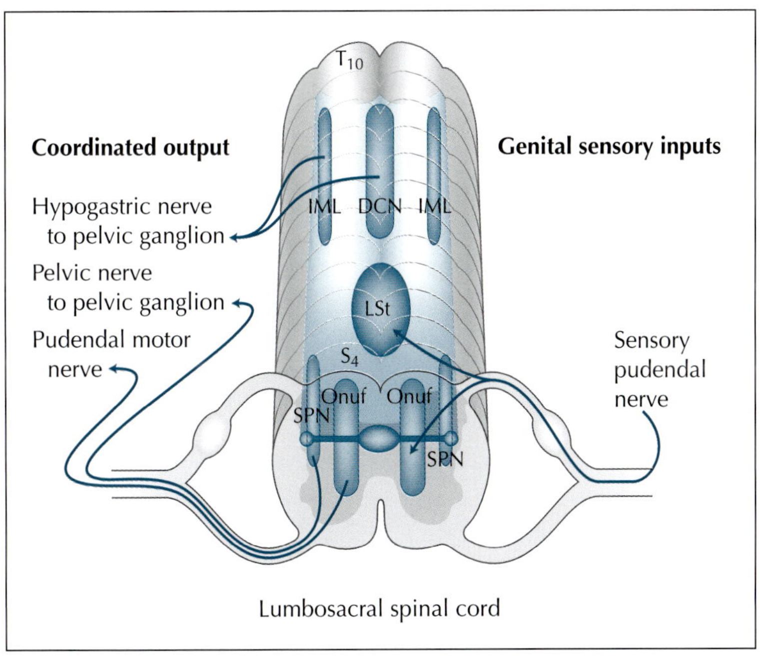

FIGURE 9-8. Efferent pathways. An important secondary ejaculatory center is present in the spinal cord. Ejaculatory reflexes remain intact in humans and animals with complete spinal transection between cervical level 3 and lumbar level 3. Thus, ejaculation is mediated by a spinal control center, located in the lumbosacral spinal cord. This spinal control center area has not been fully characterized and is variously referred to as the "spinal ejaculation generator," "spinal pattern generator," or "spinal pacemaker."

The spinal ejaculation generator coordinates the sympathetic, parasympathetic, and motor outflow needed to induce emission and expulsion. The summation of sensory and cortical inputs activate the spinal ejaculation generator, initiating ejaculation and propagating the coordinated complex outflow patterns. McKenna *et al.* (Personal communications) have speculated on a spinal ejaculation generator that coordinates the sympathetic, parasympathetic, and motor outflow needed to induce emission and expulsion. Additionally, this generator integrates the outflow with sensory inputs during sexual activity. DCN—dorsal column nucleus; IML—intermediolateral cell column of the spinal cord; LSt—lateral striatum; Onuf—Onuf's nucleus; SPN—sacral parasympathetic nucleus.

EVALUATION OF MALE ORGASMIC DISORDERS (MODs)

This section delineates the basic information to be obtained from the patient's history and physical examination, regardless of the specific ejaculatory dysfunction first presented. However, a detailed algorithm for the evaluation of each specific dysfunction is presented along with treatment recommendations in the subsections that follow this one.

Modified Sexual History Outline

Medical History
- Acute or chronic illness injuries
- Surgeries
- Medications
- Drug or alcohol abuse
- Review of systems

History of the present problem
- Date and mode of onset
- Duration
- Situational context
- Exacerbations and remissions
- Effect of any attempted management

Family history
- Family attitudes toward sexuality
- Religious influences

Sexual history
- Early experience
- Level of sexual knowledge
- Past sexual practices
- Cultural myths
- Masturbatory practices: frequency, technique, etc.
- Sexual fantasy
- Homosexual experiences
- History of negative sexual experiences
- Paraphilias

Current sexual interaction or "sex status"
- Assess all four sexual response phases
- Description of recent sex experience (foreplay, intercourse, orgasm)
- Context of recent sexual experience
- Frequency of intercourse and/or orgasm
- Frequency both partners would prefer
- Presence of fatigue or pain during intercourse
- Types of contraception used
- Duration of sex experience
- Assess intrusive antisexual thoughts

Marital history
- Stability of current relationship
- Existence of communication problem
- Current stressors
- Death
- Illness
- Financial concerns
- Occupational worries

Other
- Who initiates and how
- How does symptom vary with different partners
- Awareness of premonitory sensations

FIGURE 9-9. Modified sexual history outline. The diagnostic evaluation of ejaculatory dysfunction focuses on finding potential physical and specific psychological causes of the disorder. A detailed medical and sexual history yields a significant amount of information regarding the impact of the condition on the man's sexual relationship with his partner. Outlined here is information typically contained in a sexual history. The practitioner must identify which variables are most relevant in understanding the etiology of the chief complaint, and focus the interview accordingly. Asking questions in a relaxed, supportive, and nonjudgmental manner with the opportunity for patient expression and expansion will allow global assessment. The health practitioner needs to recognize the significant anxiety that accompanies open-ended questions when exploring a topic that is generally experienced without social reference points. While open-ended questions may be useful, be wary of being too general as such questions may waste valuable professional time, as well as frustrate and embarrass the patient. However, one query provides a valuable shorthand approach to focus the sexual history taking: "Please tell me about your last sexual experience." Using this question facilitates a focused sex history or "sex status" where the critical information is obtained in a reasonable time. The patient can then elaborate upon onset (lifelong or acquired) and occurrence (global or situational). Patient/partner responses help assess the quality of desire, degree and duration of arousal, and orgasm. They also help recognize the intimate relationship between ejaculatory dysfunction and other aspects of the sexual experience. The patient's perception of ejaculatory latency time (ELT) and stopwatch measurement have not been validated, but a good correlation is seen with progressively shorter reported ELT intervals. For many men, absolute duration is not the cause of their sexual dissatisfaction, but rather an impeded sense of ejaculatory control. Assess what previous approaches the patient has used to improve their ejaculatory responses. Many men will have attempted herbal or folk therapies for their condition and the effects of any previous treatments should be assessed. Important information can be obtained from the partner's perception of the problem and their satisfaction with the overall relationship. A significant mismatch may present therapeutic difficulties in achieving a successful outcome. It is important to remember that interviewing conducted at the professional's comfort level is the most critical variable in a successful taking of a sexual history. Therefore, it is essential that the professional monitor their own comfort level while pursuing a detailed analysis of sexual behavior, in order to instill the greatest confidence and resulting openness on the part of the patient. (*Adapted from* Shenassa and Hellstrom [13] and Perelman [14].)

Male Orgasmic Disorders: Specific Physical Examination

Physical signs of chronic systemic illness (bruits, distal pulses, neurologic findings, deep tendon reflexes)
Neurologic examination (gait, muscle strength, reflexes, sacral reflex arc [S2–S4])
Physical signs of endocrine dysfunction (diabetes mellitus, hypoactive or hyperactive thyroid, adrenal, pituitary disease)
Secondary sex characteristics
Testicular examination
Gynecomastia
Structural penile lesions/plaque (Peyronie's disease)
Signs of infection in urethra, prostate, epididymis

FIGURE 9-10. Ejaculatory disorder–specific physical examination. A focused genitourinary sexual examination may identify specific physical findings associated with ejaculatory dysfunction. Additionally concomitant or contributory neurologic, endocrinologic or erectile disorders can be identified and addressed. Particular attention should be given to identifying reversible urethral, prostatic, epididymal, and testicular infections.

Drugs and Ejaculation

Drug Class	*Drug*	*Mechanism of Action*	*Effect on Ejaculation/Orgasm*					
			Decrease Latency	Increase Latency	Absent Ejaculation	Retrograde Ejaculation	Spontaneous Ejaculation	Other
Analgesics								
NSAIDs	Naproxen	Inhibition of cyclooxygenase (inhibition of prostaglandin synthesis)		X	X			
Opioids	Methadone	μ-Agonistic activity (inhibition of activity in locus coeruleus–nucleus related with anxiety and fear)		X	X			
	Morphine	μ-Agonistic activity (inhibition of activity in locus coeruleus–nucleus related with anxiety and fear)		X	X			
Antihypertensives								
α-blockers	Phenoxybenzamine	α_1-adrenergic blockage		X	X	X		
α- and β-blockers	Labetolol	α_1-adrenergic blockage		X	X			
Centrally acting	Clonidine	α_2-adrenergic presynaptic receptors (decrease adrenergic tonus)		X	X	X		
	Guanethidine	Sympathetic blockage (by noradrenaline depletion)		X	X	X		
	Methyldopa	Central α_2- adrenergic agonistic action		X	X			
	Reserpine	Sympathetic blockage (by noradrenaline depletion)		X	X			
Antiparkinsonism drugs								
	Bromocryptine	Antagonism of D_1 receptors		X	X			
	L-DOPA	Agonistic action in dopaminergic	X	X				
		receptors and residual agonist in α- and β-adrenergic receptors	X					
	Pergolide	Potent agonist D_2 action					X	
Appetite suppressants								
	Mazindol	Agonistic action in α- and β-adrenergic receptors					X	
Cytotoxics								
	Methotrexate	?		X	X			
	Vincristine	?		X	X			
Hormone antagonists								
	Cyproterone acetate	Antagonism of prostatic androgenic receptors		X	X			
Hypnotics and sedatives								
	Barbiturates (all)	Increase of GABA-ergic tonus		X	X			
Lithium		Reduction of neuron reaction to α-adrenergic stimulation (blockage of IP_3 production)		X	X			

(*Continued on next page*)

FIGURE 9-11. Drugs and ejaculation [15,16]. MAOI—monoamine oxidase inhibitor; SSRI—selective serotonin reuptake inhibitor.

(*Continued on next page*)

Definitions of Premature Ejaculation (PE)

Defining Source	*Definition*
DSM-IV-R	Defines PE as "the persistent or recurrent ejaculation with minimal stimulation before, on, or shortly after penetration and before the person wishes it. The clinician must take into account factors that affect duration of the excitement phase, such as age, novelty of the sexual partner or situation, and recent frequency of sexual activity. The disturbance causes marked distress or interpersonal difficulty. The premature ejaculation is not due exclusively to the direct effects of a substance (*eg*, withdrawal from opioids)."
ICD-10	In defining PE "the general criteria for sexual dysfunction must be met. There is an inability to delay ejaculation sufficiently to enjoy lovemaking, manifest as either of the following: occurrence of ejaculation before or very soon after the beginning of intercourse (if a time limit is required: before or within 15 seconds of the beginning of intercourse); ejaculation occurs in the absence of sufficient erection to make intercourse possible. The problem is not the result of prolonged absence from sexual activity."
WHO, 2nd International Consultation on Erectile and Sexual Dysfunction	Defines PE as recurrent ejaculation that occurs with minimal stimulation and earlier than desired, before or soon after penetration, which causes bother or distress, and upon which the sufferer has little or no voluntary control.

FIGURE 9-12. Definitions of premature ejaculation (PE). The condition named "premature ejaculation" evokes intense feeling for sufferers. Although there is constant controversy regarding nosology, PE is a well-established term, and there is no question about its meaning, which most men learn during adolescence. Perhaps it is the condition and not the specific name that causes the associated stigma. Any new name would continue to carry a "stigma" because the stigma is attached to the experience of PE. In addition, renaming would cause confusion for researchers, clinicians, and the patient population. Recently "rapid ejaculation" and "early ejaculation" had received some professional use, but historically, the condition has also been referenced in a multiplicity of ways, including ejaculation praecox. A consensus definition of major health organizations (World Health Organization [WHO], American Urological Association [AUA], and Sexual Medicine Society of North American [SMSNA]) should be forthcoming.

The *Diagnostic and Statistical Manual of Mental Disorders* (DSM-IV-R, published by the American Psychiatric Association), the *International Statistical Classification of Diseases and Related Health Problems* (ICD-10) and the World Health Organization 2nd International Consultation on Erectile and Sexual Dysfunction [18] provide definitions of PE. These three sources provide similar though not identical conceptual frameworks for classifying an individual as having PE. Included in these references are three general criteria: short ejaculatory latency, a lack of sexual satisfaction, and a lack of self-efficacy regarding the condition. According to ICD-10, ejaculation must occur "within 15 seconds of the beginning of intercourse." DSM-IV-R is equivocal on duration, stating that "ejaculation occurs with minimal sexual stimulation before, on, or shortly after penetration." ICD-10 makes no mention of voluntary control, while DSM-IV-R notes that ejaculation occurs "before the person wishes." All three nosologies require the man to be distressed (ICD-10 offers a time frame of 6 months; no specific time frame is defined in DSM-IV-R and the WHO definitions). Lastly, both ICD-10 and DSM-IV-R require the clinician to make a judgment regarding the independence of this condition from other mental, behavioral, or physiologic disorders.

Premature ejaculation is a multifactorial diagnosis that has both objective and subjective aspects. Diminished intravaginal ejaculatory latency time (IELT) is an objective finding on which the more subjective aspects of control and personal or relationship distress revolve. It is important to recognize that the absolute measure of IELT may be less important than identifying the distress component, because some relationships have adjusted to the condition. The measurement of time (*ie*, IELT) may be absolute, but should not be the only factor in the definition or diagnosis. In the DSM-IV-R and ICD-9/10, premature ejaculation is considered a psychosexual disorder. The WHO definition does not assign this classification.

Significant limitations of the current definition have made research in PE difficult. Men with PE are not a homogenous group, in that the condition may contain subtypes that would respond to specific therapeutic strategies. The control and distress dimension of the definition await specific validated measurement tools for characterization. As a result, much of the clinical research is often flawed in both assigning of patients and evaluating treatment responses [17–19].

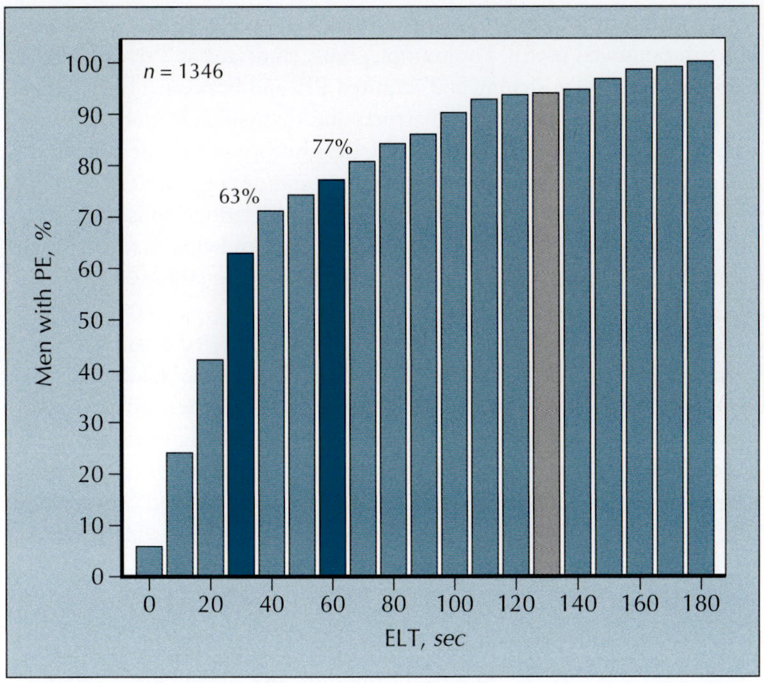

FIGURE 9-13. Intravaginal ejaculatory latency time (IVELT). IVELT is an important objective primary end point for many premature ejaculation (PE) studies. An absolute time threshold for diagnosis has not been established, but in general, a value of less than 2 minutes should provide adequate sensitivity for study inclusion. Waldinger *et al.* [20] reported IVELTs at less than 30 seconds in 77% and less than 60 seconds in 90% of 110 men with PE, respectively. McMahon [21] noted that ejaculation "ante portas" (during foreplay) occurred on the majority of occasions in 5.6% of men with PE. Secondary endpoints or domains are equally important, such as control, satisfaction, and confidence. A major obstacle to our current understanding and application is the lack of normative data for all endpoints of PE research.

Premature Ejaculation: Representative Epidemiologic Studies

Study	*Type*	*Sample Size, PE (%)*
Frank *et al.* (1976)	US couples	100 (42)
Eysenck (1983)	English students	423 (36)
Spector and Carey (1990)	Review	37
Solstad and Hertoft (1993)	Danish	439 (14)
Schiavi *et al.* (1995)	US men	20 (20)
Read *et al.* (1997)	Primary care setting	40 (31)
Lauman *et al.* (1999)	US sample (18–59 years of age)	3159 (29)
Fugl-Meyer and Syogren (1999)	Swedish (18–74 years of age)	4
Simons and Carey (2001)	Review	4
Carson *et al.* (2003)	US men (40+)	1320 (18)
Ho (2003)	Internet population	1239 (15)

FIGURE 9-14. Epidemiologic studies on premature ejaculation (PE). The epidemiology of PE has not been firmly established. A review of studies indicates a trend of decreasing prevalence. Limitations in accuracy of these data revolve around varying ages, definitions, sample population bias, and assessment of erectile functioning. By some estimates PE is a common form of sexual dysfunction, approaching the prevalence of erectile dysfunction, a condition in which it often coexists. PE is probably under-reported and under-treated because no approved therapy exists. The true prevalence of PE is unknown and a large community-based study will be required. Design of this study will require data in the areas of comorbidities, sexual preference, ethnicity, and foreskin status. However, it is currently presumed that the vast majority of men who would meet diagnostic criteria for PE are not being diagnosed or treated [22] (Ho K, Unpublished data on file at Johnson & Johnson.) (*Adapted from* Simons and Carey [23].)

Types of Premature Ejaculation (PE)

Lifelong (primary)
Strong biogenic component
Putative inherited hyper-/hyposensitivity of central 5-HT receptors, interact with psychosocial factors
Variable expression of a psychogenic component

Acquired (secondary)
Psychogenic stressors
Situational
Associated with erectile dysfunction; prostatitis, urethritis; medications

FIGURE 9-15. Types of premature ejaculation (PE). Given the lack of consensus (and supporting data) regarding possible causes of PE, it is not surprising that identification of clear subtypes of PE based on cause has not been successful. Nevertheless, classification of PE into various subtypes based on developmental histories and response characteristics has sometimes proved useful. For example, most clinicians and researchers distinguish between lifelong and acquired PE, and between PE that is limited to specific situations or partners and that which is more global. Knowing that the patient has had a lifelong history of PE not specific to one partner may argue toward a biologic and/or cognitive cause. However, the need to address interpersonal and relationship issues may be less important in these men. In contrast, knowing that the PE is secondary to a specific individual suggests the need to address relationship issues and attend less to a biologic etiology.

Metz and Pryor [25] provided a complex multilayered classification system for PE including multiple "PE types." The physiologic types include 1) neurologic constitution, 2) acute physical illness, 3) physical injury, and 4) pharmacologic side effect. The psychologic types include 1) psychologic constitution, 2) acute psychologic distress, 3) relationship distress, and 4) psychosexual skills deficit. This hypothesized classification schemata, which is thoughtful and elaborate, has not been widely adopted by the medical community [24–25].

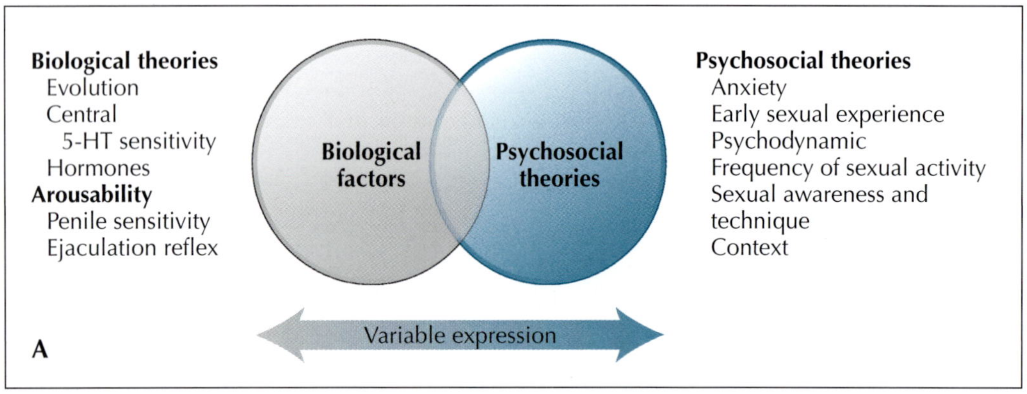

FIGURE 9-16. The multifactorial etiology of premature ejaculation (PE). This figure illustrates the importance of an improved paradigm that recognizes the overlapping interaction of both biogenic and psychosocial factors in understanding the cause of PE. Although the nature of biologic predisposition is not known, it does seem reasonable to conclude that the "threshold" for ejaculatory latency may be distributed along the same bell-shaped normal distribution curve like so many other human variables. Determining whether the exact physiologic mechanism(s) of such a "threshold" are central, peripheral, or some combination, requires further research. However, this pattern of susceptibility presumably interacts with a variety of psychosocial, environmental, and medical risk factors, resulting in a manifest dysfunction for some men. These are many of the same issues that play a significant role in the cause of both retarded ejaculation (RE) and erectile dysfunction (ED) as well.

The etiologic factors involved are outlined in **A** and elaborated in the accompanying table (**B**).

(Continued on next page)

B. Interacting Factors in the Etiology of Premature Ejaculation (PE)

Biogenic

Evolution

PE could result from natural selection. From an evolutionary perspective, copulating quickly was a superior reproductive strategy. Males who copulated more quickly could mate with more females, thus producing more offspring, and passing along a genetic basis for PE.

Central 5-HT receptors

One hypothesized theory of biologic threshold variability is conceptualizing PE as due to central phenomena, specifically, the hypersensitivity of 5-HT1A receptors or hyposensitivity of 5-HT2C receptors, as supported by neuropharmacologic studies. There is alternative evidence for other possible central mechanisms.

Sex hormones

Pirke *et al.* (1979) suggested that men with sexual dysfunction have different levels of LH, free and total testosterone than men without sexual dysfunction. There were no differences between men with ED, RE, and normal controls of any of the three measured hormones.

Arousability

Men with PE might ejaculate rapidly because they become aroused more quickly than other men. Yet, Spiess *et al.* (1984) and Strassberg *et al.* (1987, 1990) found no differences between men with PE and men without PE in their subjectively or objectively measured sexual arousal in the laboratory.

Disease

A variety of diseases may be associated with PE, but chronic prostatitis is most frequently mentioned. It was suggested that possible mechanisms for prostatitis could cause PE: hypersensitive ejaculatory reflex due to chronic inflammation; intentional deferral of ejaculatory control in an attempt to reduce ejaculatory pain by reducing duration of coitus.

Psychogenic

Psychodynamic theories

Unresolved excessive narcissism during infancy could result in exaggerated importance being placed on the penis and the associated pleasure of urination. Result of an unconscious, deep-seated hatred of women. By ejaculating quickly, the man both symbolically "soils" the woman and robs her of her sexual pleasure. There are no empirical investigations of either theory.

Early sexual experiences

Men whose early sexual experiences are characterized by haste and nervousness may be conditioned to ejaculate rapidly. Men may have conditioned themselves to ejaculate quickly due to, for example, their perception that their partner was not sexually interested. No studies have compared the early sexual histories of men with PE with a non-PE control group. It is not known whether these early conditioning experiences are unique to men with PE. Many men's early sexual encounters involve haste and nervousness. Masters and Johnson did not differentiate between primary and secondary PE.

Anxiety

There are multiple theories of anxiety suggesting a relationship between high levels of sexual anxiety and PE.

It has been hypothesized that increased anxiety activates the sympathetic nervous system, the same system responsible for the emission phase of ejaculation (Kaplan, 1974; Williams, 1984; Wolpe, 1982). However, there is also research not supporting a relationship between anxiety and PE. Kockott *et al.* (1980) subdivided men with PE into high anxiety and low-anxiety groups: High-anxiety men showed PE during intercourse and more sex avoidance behavior; low-anxiety men showed PE during both intercourse and masturbation and less sex avoidance. There was no non–sexually dysfunctional control. Anxiety related to interpersonal sexual activity was not measured and there was no objective, physiological measures of anxiety to validate the subjective self-reports. Other speculated that men with high levels of anxiety are distracted during sexual activity from monitoring the level of arousal or attending to the premonitory sensations of ejaculation (Kaplan, 1974, 1989; Zilbergeld, 1978, 1992).

Frequency of sexual activity: Some researchers have found that men with PE have lower frequencies of sexual activity than men without PE (Gospodinoff, 1989; Spiess, 1984). Underlying mechanism and the direction of the correlation is undetermined. Does more frequent sexual activity lead to increased awareness of sensations premonitory to ejaculation, an increased ejaculatory threshold and decreased anxiety. Do men with PE avoid sex because of their anxiety or embarrassment about their lack of control? There is conflicting evidence, although Waldinger's research supports the accepted concept, that increased frequency of sexual activity in general, increases latency to ejaculation.

Sexual technique: ejaculatory control is a result of consciously or unconsciously learning to use techniques that are effective in delaying ejaculation (Zilbergeld, 1978). It seems that all men with primary PE lack rudimentary skill in adequately managing their bodies in response to progressively escalating levels of sexual arousal, regardless of other predisposing etiological factors [14].

FIGURE 9-16. ***Continued*** In conclusion, it seems clear that the causes of PE are frequently multidimensional, most importantly a given individual's biologic predisposition to rapid ejaculatory latency, interacting with intrapsychic and interpersonal issues. The reader should conclude that similar to ED, despite the existence of organic pathogenesis, PE always has a psychologic component—even if the PE is initially the result of constitution, illness, or treatment. 5-HT—5-hydroxytryptamine; LH—luteinizing hormone.

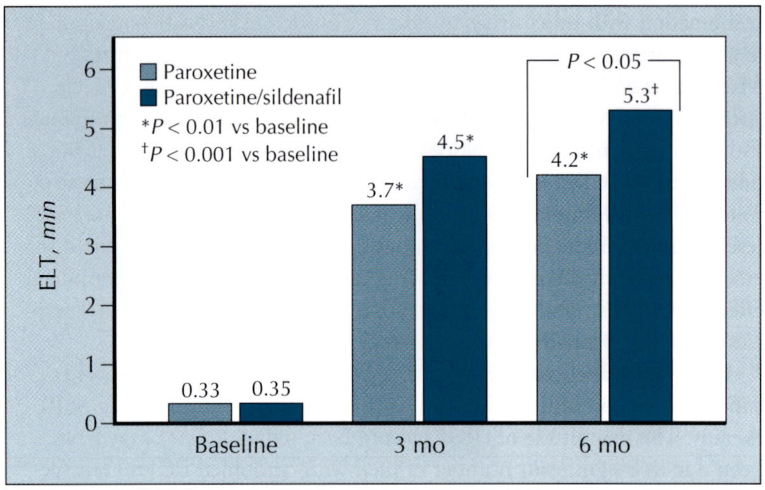

FIGURE 9-29. Intravaginal ejaculatory latency time (IVELT) with paroxetine and sildenafil. In an open-label study of 80 potent men, Salonia *et al.* [39] compared treatment with paroxetine alone, using initial chronic and then "on demand" dosing, with a combination of paroxetine and sildenafil, using the same dosing regimen for paroxetine and sildenafil administered 1 hour prior to intercourse. Both treatments significantly improved the ejaculatory latency time and intercourse satisfaction domain of the IIEF. The combination of paroxetine and sildenafil produced superior results in both end points at 6 months treatment. Additionally, intercourse frequency was higher in the combined treatment group and the authors suggested a possible role of sildenafil in the treatment of rapid ejaculation. The use of combination therapy may have a role in the treatment of PE but comes with an increase in the cost, complexity, and acceptance of therapy. In addition there is exposure to the side effect profile of two drugs along with their specific drug-drug interactions.

Topical Local Anesthetics

Aycokk (1942): dibucaine
Shapiro (1943): nupercaine
Damarau (1963): benzocaine
Berkowicz (1995): lignocaine/prilocaine
Morales *et al.* (2003): Lignocaine/prilocaine
Xin *et al.* (1998): SS cream (royal Chinese remedy)
Limitations
- Difficulty in dosing (easy overdosing)
- Anesthesia to the partner
- Messy

FIGURE 9-30. Topical local anesthetics. Use of penile/glans topical local anesthetic sprays or gels as well as barriers (condoms) are widely used therapies for premature ejaculation that have few controlled studies with evolving efficacy data. The proposed mechanism of action is to lessen penotactile sensations felt during intercourse. This has been demonstrated by decreased amplitude of sensory evoked potentials in a laboratory setting. More recent application of potent prescription topical anesthetic desensitizing creams (Lidocaine, EMLA) and a proprietary SS cream have shown moderate effectiveness in uncontrolled studies. Use of the agents may be limited by penile hyposensitivity and transvaginal absorption leading to vaginal numbness. Additionally, the use of creams and barriers is cumbersome and may increase anxiety with a corresponding decrease in erectile capacity.

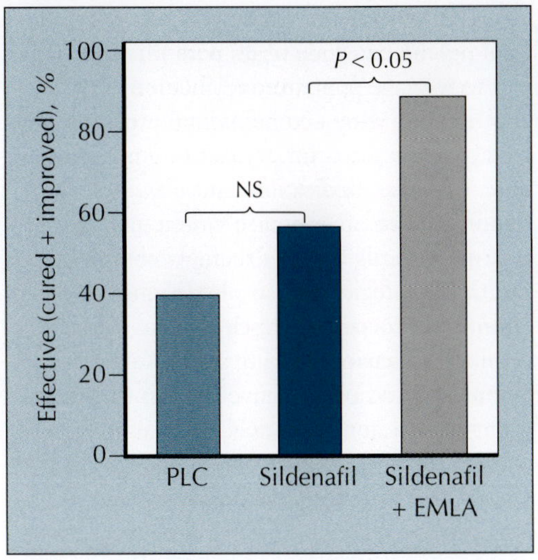

FIGURE 9-31. Sildenafil plus topical EMLA cream treatments for premature ejaculation (PE). Combination therapy of sildenafil has been used in patients. In an open-label study, Tuncel noted no difference in effectiveness between sildenafil and placebo. Combination of sildenafil and EMLA was better than sildenafil monotherapy, but erectile functioning or the effect of EMLA monotherapy was not assessed. (*Adapted from* Tuncel, European Society for Sexual Medicine, PS4-5, Istanbul, Turkey, 2003.)

Level II and III Treatments for Premature Ejaculation

Level II
- Intracavernous Injection Therapy for PE
  - Self injection
    - Alprostadil monotherapy (Caverject, Edex)
    - Papaverine, phentolamine, alprostadil in combination
  - Mechanism of action in PE
    - Augmented erection and improved ejaculatory control in men with PE secondary to ED
    - Sustained erection postejaculation allowing continued thrusting
    - Decreased erectile recovery time allowing rapid achievement of second erection before ejaculatory recovery
  - Risks
    - Pain
    - Priapism
    - Intracavernous fibrosis and penile curvature/deformity
- Intraurethral procedures

Level III
- Penile prosthesis
- Surgery (dorsal neurotomy)

FIGURE 9-32. Level II and II treatments for premature ejaculation (PE). This figure describes the "second line" use of injection therapy for PE. Intraurethral approaches could also be used in this manner, but some of the same risks and limitations apply and the efficacy is probably even poorer. These approaches are not highly recommended.

Level III interventions are equally ill-advised when treating premature ejaculation, albeit researchers and clinicians have reported using such approaches.

Combination Treatment: Integrating Cognitive-Behavioral Psychosexual Strategies with Pharmaceuticals to Manage Premature Ejaculation

- Pharmaceuticals plus psychosocial education
  - Individual procedures
    - Physiologic relaxation training
    - The pubococcygeal muscle control technique
    - Cognitive and behavioral pacing technique
      - Behavioral stop-start technique
      - Sensual awareness training: entrancement arousal vs partner involvement
      - Cognitive arousal continuum technique
- Pharmaceuticals plus psychosocial education
  - Couple procedures
    - Couples sensate focus pleasuring exercises
    - The partner genital exploration relaxation exercise
    - Couple use of the behavioral pacing method: stop-start technique
    - The intercourse acclimatization technique, *eg*, "quiet vagina"

FIGURE 9-33. Integrating cognitive-behavioral psychosexual strategies with pharmaceuticals to manage premature ejaculation (PE). A combination drug and behavioral protocol may best produce the necessary learning needed for a cure, with less medication continuously required. Such an approach would integrate pharmaceuticals with sex therapy; combining multiple strategies such as physiologic relaxation, pubococcygeal muscle training, and cognitive behavioral pacing strategies (stop-start technique) and partner involvement (including intercourse accommodation techniques, *eg*, "quiet vagina"). Relapse prevention strategies should also be incorporated to minimize the amount of medication needed long term and to extend the benefits of treatment. (*Adapted from* Perelman [14], Metz [25], and McCarthy [25a].)

Future Goals for the Treatment of Premature Ejaculation

- Effective new therapies are needed
- Demonstration of clinical effectiveness
- Develop ideal oral pharmacologic agents
- "On demand" treatments
- Further development of a combined pharmaceutical and sex therapy algorithm

FIGURE 9-34. Future goals for the treatment of premature ejaculation (PE). There is a significant need to develop effective new therapies for PE. Further basic research may provide novel therapeutic approaches. More important will be demonstrating clinical effectiveness in all primary and secondary endpoints of PE therapy. An ideal oral pharmacologic agent should have a rapid onset of action and a short half-life without accumulation on repeated dosing. The quantitative increase in IELT should demonstrate significant improvement in the domains of control and satisfaction and be corroborated by both patient and partner. This pharmacokinetic and therapeutic profile provides for "on demand" therapy, which has demonstrated patient acceptance in erectile dysfunction therapy. A number of companies are looking at "on demand" treatments. In fact, Johnson and Johnson have indicated they are currently developing a novel serotonergic agent with rapid onset of action for the treatment of PE that may be used for as needed dosing (Personal communication). These new drugs will provide even greater opportunity for combining both pharmaceutical and sex therapy techniques and procedures in the treatment of PE.

Diminished Ejaculatory Disorders (DED)

Retarded (delayed/inhibited) ejaculation
Anejaculation
Retrograde ejaculation
Diminished seminal volume, force, sensation
Partially retarded ejaculation
Anorgasmia
Painful ejaculation

FIGURE 9-35. Various types of diminished ejaculatory disorders (DED). DED is a collective term for an alteration of ejaculation that involves a delay in time, pain, reduction in sensation, force, or direction of semen. At the extremes are anejaculation (time) and retrograde ejaculation (direction), but more commonly encountered is delayed ejaculation or semen volume reduction. Each of these disorders represent some manner in which the normal stages of ejaculatory physiology are disrupted. While defined independently, these conditions may overlap each other. For instance, diminished seminal volume, force, or sensation may be related to aging or may also be a manifestation of a somatic illness such as diabetes.

Partially retarded ejaculation is sometimes observed in men who attempt to control a rapid ejaculation by suppressing the muscular contractions associated with ejaculation. These men experience diminished pleasure and sensation as semen is released during emission, but the ejaculatory sensations are dulled through over control of striated muscle. This may be observed in men who prematurely ejaculate when they attempt to consciously delay their orgasm but end up experiencing a partially retarded ejaculation.

A final disorder, anorgasmia, refers to a perceived absence of the orgasm experience independent of whether or not any or all of the physiologic concomitants of ejaculation have taken place.

"Retarded Ejaculation" or Delayed Ejaculation/inhibited (RE)

WHO, 2nd Consultation definition: The persistent or recurrent difficulty, delay in, or absence of attaining orgasm, following sufficient sexual stimulation, which causes personal distress.

DSM-IV (1994) definition: Persistent or recurrent delay in, or absence of, orgasm following a normal sexual excitement phase during sexual activity that the clinician, taking into account the person's age, judges to be adequate in focus, intensity, and duration. The disturbance causes marked distress or interpersonal difficulty.

Incidence: RE was considered a clinical rarity reportedly at less than 2%. However, some clinical practices report higher rates in settings of religious orthodoxy.

FIGURE 9-36. The DSM-IV-R definition of retarded ejaculation (RE) or delayed ejaculation/inhibited. Multiple terms are used to describe a delay or absence of male orgasmic response. RE, delayed ejaculation, and inhibited ejaculation as well as idiopathic anejaculation, primary impotentia ejaculations, and psychogenic anejaculation have all been used essentially synonymously to describe this problem in men. Like the term "premature ejaculation," the most commonly used term—retarded ejaculation—is often avoided because of its pejorative associations.

According to the DSM-IV-R, male orgasmic disorder is defined as persistent or recurrent delay in, or absence of, orgasm following a normal sexual excitement phase during sexual activity that the clinician, taking into account the person's age, judged to be adequate in focus, intensity, and duration. The disturbance causes marked distress or interpersonal difficulty. The clinician is to note if the orgasmic dysfunction is not better accounted for by another Axis I disorder and is not due exclusively to the direct physiologic effects of a substance or a general medical condition.

Failure of ejaculation can be a lifelong primary event (*eg*, congenital anorgasmia) or an acquired or secondary problem. It can happen in every sexual encounter or it may be intermittent or situational. It may be caused by organic, psychogenic, or combined factors. Some men can masturbate to orgasm; others, for a multiplicity of reasons, would or could not masturbate. Loss of masturbatory capacity secondary to emotional or physical trauma can be identified. Affected men may report intermittent nocturnal emissions, and others are either unaware of or do not have nocturnal emission/orgasm. Coital anorgasmia is the driver for extremely religious individuals referred for fertility problems, although this is not the case for other men distressed by their inability to achieve orgasm in response to manual or oral stimulation by their partner. Retarded ejaculation has been reported in men utilizing therapies for erectile dysfunction [43]. The presence of a surgically or pharmacologically enhanced erection may reduce the need for fantasy or the pleasure awareness normally required for maintaining the erection and experiencing ejaculation. These men experience an unpleasant prolonging of the ejaculatory interval, particularly if associated with anxiety [2]. There is no standard definition of what length of time constitutes RE, but it is not unusual for sexual irritation or exhaustion to be a primary complaint from prolonged intercourse for the man or his partner.

Etiology of Diminished Ejaculatory Disorders

Anatomic causes: transurethral resection of prostate; bladder neck incision
Neurogenic causes: diabetic autonomic neuropathy; spinal cord injury; radical prostatectomy; proctocolectomy; bilateral sympathectomy; abdominal aortic aneurysmectomy; retroperitoneal lymph node dissection
Endocrine: hypogonadism; hypothyroidism
Medications (iatrogenic): α-methyl dopa; thiazide diuretics; tricyclic and SSRI antidepressants; phenothiazine
Psychosocial causes: psychodynamics, interpersonal, cultural, behavioral, contextual, cognitive

FIGURE 9-37. Causes of diminished ejaculatory disorders (DED). The organic causes of DED are varied but can be placed in several broad categories: anatomic causes, neurogenic causes, endocrine, and medications (iatrogenic). Disruption in bladder neck competence from surgical therapy for prostatic obstruction is a significant long-term side effect that requires careful preoperative discussion. Pathologic lesions of the sympathetic innervation of the coordinated ejaculatory reflex may result in a variable effect on the quality of ejaculation or orgasm. Commonly used medications, particularly the antidepressants, may cause a central inhibition of ejaculation.

In addition to psychodynamic and interpersonal causes for retarded ejaculation, a biologic etiology should also be considered. There is strong likelihood of biologic variability in the threshold of arousal necessary before experiencing orgasm. Furthermore, it seems likely that the dispersal pattern of ejaculatory latency should resemble the same bell-shaped distribution as do so many other human characteristics. Perelman extrapolated from Waldinger's animal model that individuals experiencing either premature ejaculation (PE) or retarded ejaculation (RE) were likely to be biologically predisposed to their symptom [43]. The dysfunction becomes manifest given certain external factors: medications, sexual circumstances, and intra- and interpersonal dynamics, etc. [18,43]. Rowland *et al.*'s [40] data showed that men with RE reported the lowest levels of sexual arousal in the laboratory, compared with men who reported rapid ejaculation, erectile dysfunction, or were normal controls. Their findings suggest that inhibited arousal may be more common among men with RE, who do not manifest other apparent somatic pathology. Perelman [43] speculated that normal variation in the function of the nervous systems responsible for ejaculation could result in a somatically determined variation between men's ejaculatory latency and capacity. He noted that exploration of biologic predisposition is often helpful by itself in reducing patient and partner anxiety and mutual recriminations, while simultaneously assisting the formation of a therapeutic alliance with the health care professional [43].

Masters and Johnson [3] first indicated that RE was associated with orthodoxy of religious belief. Beliefs may limit sexual experience necessary for developing the knowledge necessary to learn to ejaculate or may result in an inhibition of normal function. Perelman [43] observed that regardless of specific religion involved (*eg*, Muslim, Hindu, Jewish), many devout religious men have masturbated only minimally or not at all. Some of these men masturbated for a period of years like their secular counterparts, but guilt and anxiety about "spilling seed" often resulted in idiosyncratic masturbatory patterns, which in turn resulted in RE. These men often had little contact with women prior to marriage. These very religious men may date, but were less likely than their secular counterparts to experience orgasm with a partner, especially through intercourse. Some of these men did sexually experiment with women who they did not marry; however, their cognitions about these women often reflected a "Madonna-whore" split [43].

Multiple explanations for RE have been offered, with unconscious aggression and unexpressed anger recurring as themes in the RE literature.

Additionally, pregnancy fears received emphasis, since the reason for professional referral is often the female partner's wish to conceive. Finally, Bancroft's [41] model of psychogenic factors in erectile dysfunction depends on a delicate balance between central excitatory and inhibiting mechanisms would seem to have potential applicability to the understanding of RE as well.

An excellent critical review of the psychological etiology of RE was provided by Apfelbaum [42], who provocatively first noted the sexual politic surrounding RE and female anorgasmia: "Like the woman who has inappropriately been castigated for willfully depriving her husband of the pleasure of bringing her to orgasm. The retarded ejaculator's own belief that he is withholding is widely endorsed, understandably by his partners and less justifiably by most therapists." Not only psychoanalysts, but sex therapists and behavior therapists as well, seemed to assume the RE patient's orgasm is blocked, rather than the patient's level of arousal being insufficient [43].

Apfelbaum [42] observed that some men appeared able to achieve erections sufficient for intercourse despite a relative absence of subjective arousal. He felt these "automatic erections" were taken as erroneous evidence by both the male and his partner that the man was ready for sex and capable of achieving orgasm. Perelman believed this same process was the likely cause of increased anecdotal clinical reports of RE for patients using popular urologic-based treatments for erectile dysfunction. Urologists received a few early complaints of RE, secondary to successful penile prosthesis surgery and intracavernosal injections (ICI). However, sildenafil brought huge numbers of patients to physicians' offices. Many of these patients experienced restored erections and coitus with ejaculation. Although sildenafil has been used with some success to facilitate reversal of the antidepressant sexual adverse effects, the effect of PDE-5 inhibitors may be bimodal. The phenomena of erection without adequate psychoemotional arousal occurred in some men using sildenafil when they did not experience sufficient erotic stimulation before and during coitus. These men confused their erect state as an indication of sexual arousal when it merely indicated vasocongestive success [2,43].

Apfelbaum [42] coined autosexual orientation to describe men with RE who prefer masturbation to partnered sex. Perelman [43] discussed the role of fantasy, as well as masturbation frequency, motivation, and idiosyncratic technique in the etiology and maintenance of RE. Many men with RE engage in stimulation that was striking in the speed, pressure, duration, and intensity necessary to produce an orgasm, and dissimilar to what they experienced with a partner. In this manner, they have preconditioned themselves to likely difficulty with a partner and experience secondary RE. Disparity between the reality of sex with the partner and the sexual fantasy (whether unconventional or not) used during masturbation is another cause of RE. This disparity takes many forms: body type, orientation, sex activity performed, and so on. Many men and women remain inhibited about using their masturbatory fantasies when with their partner. Yet like their female counterparts, when anorgasmic men integrate their masturbation fantasies into sex with their partner, orgasm is more likely [43].

It would seem that DED, like other sexual dysfunctions, is best understood as being caused by an interaction of both organic and psychogenic factors. A biologic set point for ejaculatory latency is affected by multiple organic and psychogenic factors in varying combinations over the course of a man's life cycle. Appropriate assessment requires an appreciation of how each of these factors determines the endpoint dysfunction for a particular individual, at a particular moment in time.

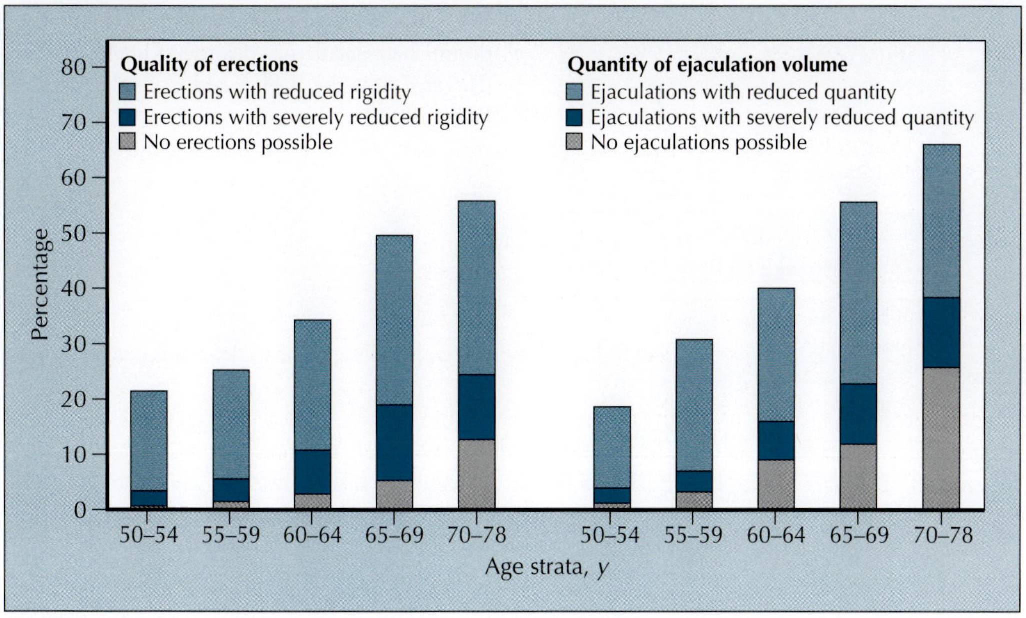

FIGURE 9-38. Ejaculatory dysfunction (ED) and diminished ejaculatory disorders (DED) in the aging man. While controversy exists regarding the labeling of normal age-related phenomena as pathologic, it is clear that increasing age is highly associated with diminished ejaculatory function. All types of DED show an age-related increase in prevalence. Although this may represent a normal aspect of aging, the applied definition factors in personal or relationship distress before the diagnosis is applied. (*Adapted from* Blanker *et al.* [44].)

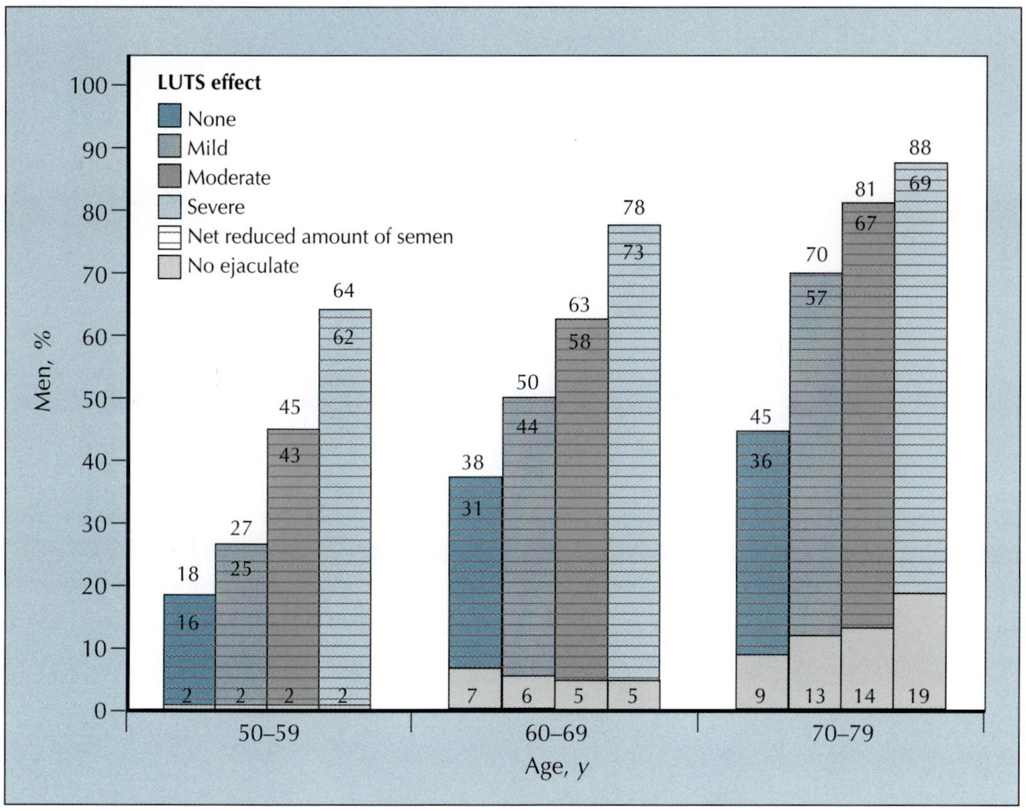

FIGURE 9-39. Prevalence of ejaculatory dysfunction increases with severity of lower urinary tract symptoms (LUTS) independent of age. As demonstrated in a large population-based study by Rosen (Presented at the Annual Meeting of the American Urological Association in Orlando, May 2002), there is an increase in the incidence of diminished ejaculation with increasing age. A validated questionnaire (DAN-PSSex) for determining diminished ejaculation or anejaculation in men with varying degrees of LUTS. Within each age group the number of men who experience diminished ejaculation increases significantly with increasing severity of identified LUTS. (*Adapted from* Rosen *et al.* [45].)

Evaluation and Assessment of Diminished Ejaculatory Disorders

Medical history, medication history
Global or situational, lifelong or acquired
Quality of desire, arousal, and orgasm
Patient's assessment of latency time in various sexual situations
Quantity and quality of semen volume and force
Partner's assessment
Overall relationship
Physical examination

FIGURE 9-40. Evaluation and assesment of diminished ejaculatory disorders (DED). Assessment begins by reviewing the conditions under which the man is able to ejaculate, *eg*, during sleep, with masturbation, with partner's hand or mouth stimulation, or infrequently with varying coital positions. The course of the problem is documented, and variables that improve or worsen performance are noted. Questions concerning the man's ability to relax, sustain, and heighten arousal and the degree to which he can concentrate on sensations are posed. If orgasmic attainment had been possible previously, the life events/circumstances temporarily related to orgasmic cessation are reviewed. The events in question may be pharmaceutical, illness, or a variety of life stressors and other psychologic factors previously highlighted in the section on etiology. This examination in conjunction with appropriate physical examination and laboratory results will provide understanding and determine an appropriate treatment path.

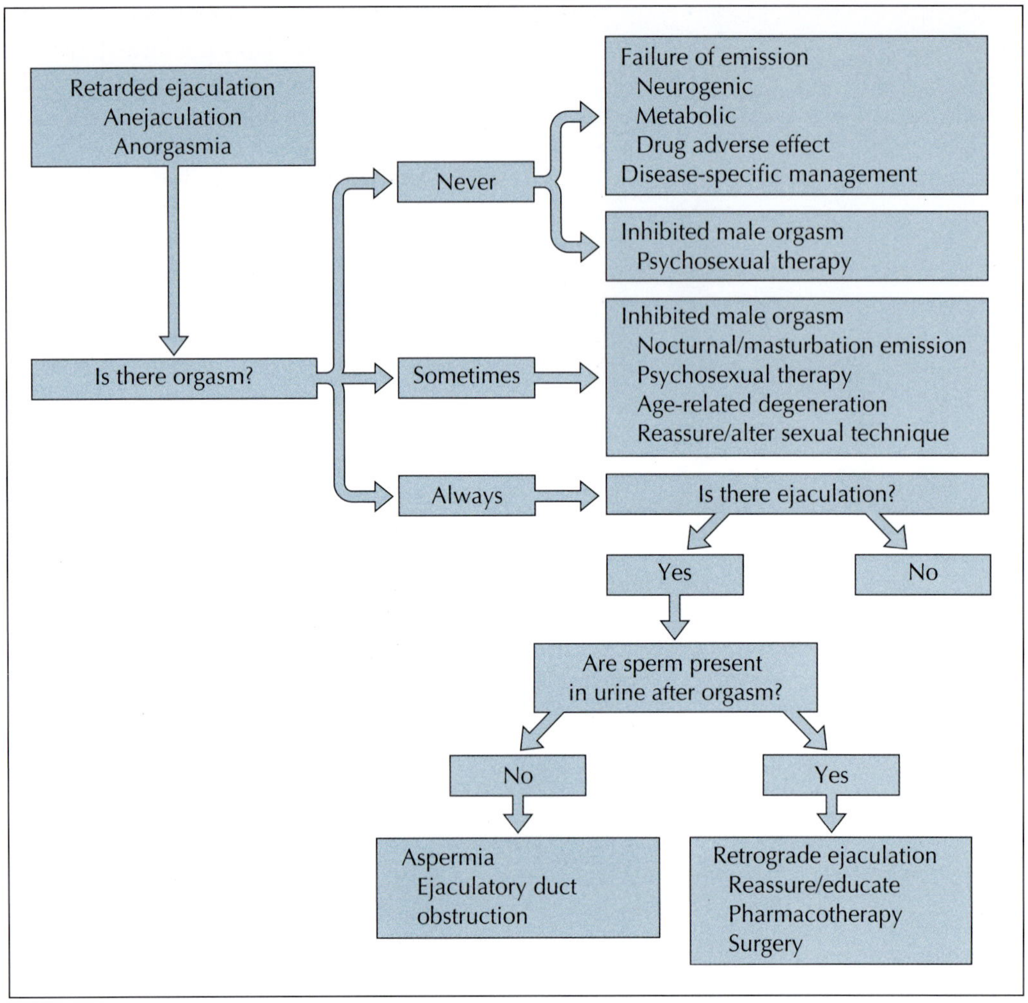

FIGURE 9-41. Diagnostic algorithm for diminished ejaculatory disorders (DED). (*Adapted from* the WHO 2nd Consultation, Paris, 2003.)

Adjunctive Drug Therapy for SSRI-Induced Sexual Dysfunction

			Dosage, mg	
Drug	***Mechanism***	***Symptom***	***As Needed***	***Daily***
Amantadine	Dopamine agonist	Anorgasmia Decreased libido Erectile dysfunction	100–400 (for 2 d prior to coitus)	75–100 bid/tid
Bupropion	Mixed 5-HT, NE, dopamine reuptake inhibitor	Anorgasmia	75–150	75 bid/tid
Buspirone	Partial 5-HT1A receptor agonist, dopamine adrenergic stimulant	Anorgasmia Decreased libido ED	15–60	5–15 bid
Cyproheptadine	Serotonin and histamine antagonist	Anorgasmia Decreased libido ED	4–12	Not applicable
Yohimbine	Central/peripheral α2 agonist	Anorgasmia Decreased libido ED	5.4–10.8	5.4 tid

FIGURE 9-42. Adjunctive drug therapy for selective serotonin reuptake inhibitor (SSRI)-induced sexual dysfunction. Sexual side effects are commonly seen with SSRI therapy. Decreased libido, erectile dysfunction, and ejaculatory disorders (ED) are seen with all of the current therapies and may be lead to treatment discontinuation, particularly in younger men. Treatment strategies take into account the underlying indication for therapy and the current or expected response. Early in the course of therapy, reassurance is necessary, because improvement may take 4 to 6 weeks. Continued difficulties and distress may prompt consideration of a treatment strategy to counteract the pharmacologic ejaculatory effects of SSRIs. Significant individual variegation in therapeutic response is seen with different drugs within the SSRI class and in a similar fashion, ejaculatory improvement may be seen with an alternative medication. Dosage adjustment, timing alteration, or brief (2 day) "holiday" may be of benefit. Recent interest in "SSRI antidotes" are primarily anecdotal and are based on activating proejaculatory dopaminergic pathways, while maintaining 5-HT neuromodulation. This table provides suggested medications and can be used with daily dosing or on demand 2 to 6 hours prior to anticipated sexual activity. PDE-5 inhibitors may also be of benefit as a durable erection may provide a "scaffold" for sufficient stimulation to achieve ejaculation/orgasm.

Treatment of Retarded Ejaculation

There is low-level evidence recommending sex therapy for RE
Numerous drugs, herbs, and medication dosing strategies exist for treatment of antidepressant-related RE (level 3)
Following the pattern seen in the treatment of ED—integration of pharmacotherapy and sex therapy—will become the likely treatment of choice

FIGURE 9-43. New optimism for using a combined sex therapy and pharmaceutical approach in treating ejaculatory disorders. Heiman and Meston's [46] summary of sex therapy treatments concluded that "inadequate data" on the topic of delayed orgasm in men prevented any conclusion regarding efficacy of treatment. However, many treatments for RE have been suggested in the psychotherapy literature, including early psychodynamic and sex therapy approaches. Masters and Johnson [3] reported a low failure rate of 17.6% using a treatment combination of sensate focus, vigorous noncoital penile stimulation, and modifications of intercourse technique. Apfelbaum [42] treated almost all of his RE cases with "body work" using sexual surrogates. Perelman [2] reported retrospective chart review success rates of over 80% in treating RE using a cognitive-behavioral sex therapy. However, these were uncontrolled case reports with treatment ranging from a few brief sessions of sex education to the nearly 2 years of multiple-modality treatment in more complex multiple etiologic cases.

Numerous drugs, herbs, and medication dosing strategies have been reported to offset an iatrogenic induced, antidepressant-related RE. Widespread use of selective serotonin reuptake inhibitors (SSRIs) in the last decade has triggered tremendous interest in the effect of these antidepressants on sexual function [47]. Additionally, case reports indicated successful use of sildenafil to treat SSRI-induced orgasmic latency problems in men and women, with clinical trials currently investigating this phenomenon. Recently, Nurnberg *et al.* [48] published a prospective, parallel-group, randomized, double-blind, placebo-controlled multicenter study to assess the efficacy of sildenafil citrate in men with sexual dysfunction associated with the use of selective and nonselective serotonin reuptake inhibitors. In this study, sildenafil effectively improved erectile function and other aspects of sexual function in men with sexual dysfunction associated with the use of SSRI antidepressants. Although the endpoints used were very limited, regarding the question of ejaculatory latency, this is one of the few randomized controlled trials to address this question and accordingly becomes important. It remains to be seen whether sildenafil will be shown to be an orgasmogenic agent; however, it is probable that multiple compounds will be developed to reduce orgasmic threshold and assist us in treating people who have difficulty reaching orgasm. Indeed, some speculate that a dopaminergic pathway might facilitate orgasm.

There is a need for integrated pharmacotherapy and sex therapy approaches. It seems likely that the most effective treatments for RE will follow the pattern seen in the treatment of ED, where an integration of pharmacotherapy and sex therapy is becoming the treatment of choice [18,43]. These recent articles by urologists and sex therapists have advocated a multidisciplinary approach for the treatment of ED, emphasizing the importance of follow-up in providing opportunity for necessary patient education and counseling. Additionally, the integration of sexual counseling and pharmacotherapy is likely to be of assistance to patients seeking adjustment and rehabilitation from multiple medical conditions (*eg*, retrograde ejaculation secondary to prostatic surgery). Further, couples presenting multiple sexual dysfunctions are likely to benefit from a model incorporating additional sex therapy with pharmacotherapy. An integrated model allows for resolving and balancing significant intra- and interpersonal psychologic issues that otherwise may destabilize treatment success. There are published case reports integrating sex therapy and pharmacotherapy when treating a couple's multiple dysfunctions (including RE), but large controlled prospective studies are needed in order to define an appropriate treatment algorithm [43]. The development of new pharmaceuticals will only refine such an algorithm and improve our opportunity for enhancing orgasmic function.

Sexual Dysfunction in Men with Lower Urinary Tract Symptoms

	Community > 40 y, % (n = 423)	*Community > 45 y, % (n = 1271)*
ED	53	60
Decreased ejaculation	47	62
Painful ejaculation	5	17
Sex life decreased by LUTS	8	46

FIGURE 9-44. Sexual dysfunction in men with lower urinary tract symptoms (LUTS). As shown previously, sexual function is adversely affected by LUTS. Frankel *et al.* [49] compared a community population with LUTS to those men presenting for LUTS to a urology clinic. The rate of erectile dysfunction (ED) was similar but a higher incidence of diminished ejaculatory disorders (DED) was identified in the clinic patients. It is commonly held that patients present for the bother of their voiding complaints, but may also consider the associated DED as a contributory reason for seeking therapy. A reduction in the enjoyment of sexual activity may be driven more by the DED than the underlying LUTS associated erectile dysfunction and should be considered carefully in treatment selection.

Arai *et al.* [50] evaluated 173 men with LUTs and normal ejaculatory function treated with four surgical modalities (transurethral resection of the prostate [TURP], transurethral microwave thermotherapy of the prostate, transurethral laser ablation of the prostate, and transurethral needle ablation). All therapies improved symptoms with a similar incidence of ED and no change in sexual desire. Postoperative DED (including retrograde ejaculation) was 48.6% in the TURP group and similar in the less invasive treatment groups (21%–28%). More importantly, 46% of men with postoperative DED reported deterioration in their sexual enjoyment compared to 3.5% with unchanged ejaculation. These data indicate that preoperative or surgically induced DED has an adverse impact on sexual activity and enjoyment.

10

Priapism

Ajay Nehra
Haluk Kulaksizoglu

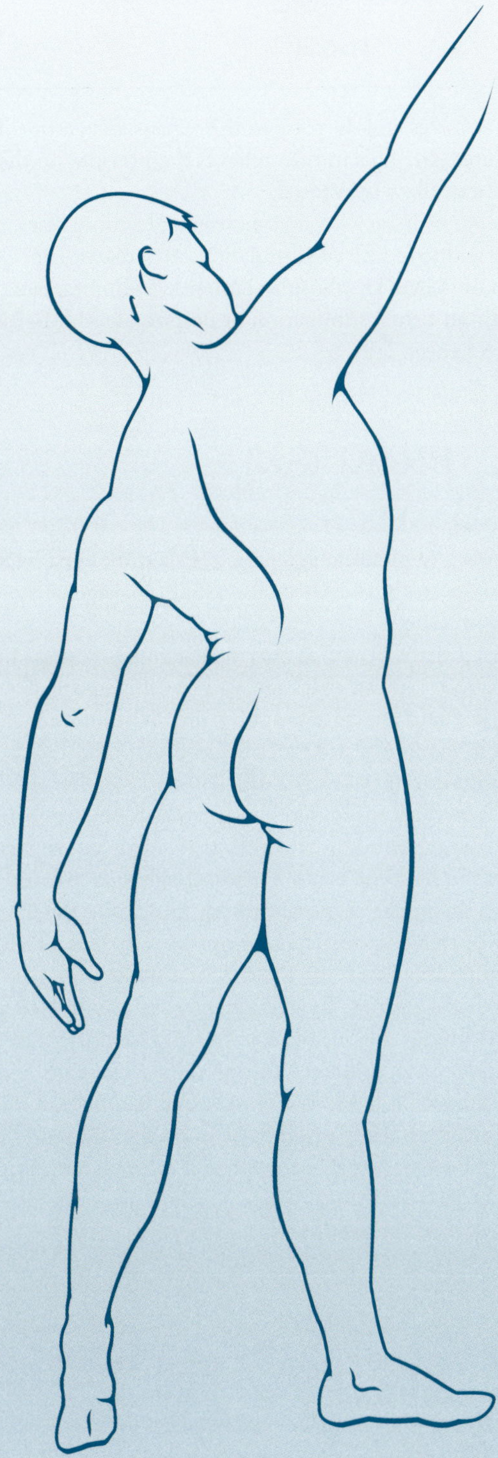

Priapism is a prolonged often painful erection that is not relieved by orgasm. It can be seen in all age groups, from newborns to the elderly. With the advent of intracavernosal pharmacotherapy, the incidence of priapism has been a more significant and common urologic emergency issue because delayed or inappropriate treatment may lead to irreversible penile functional loss.

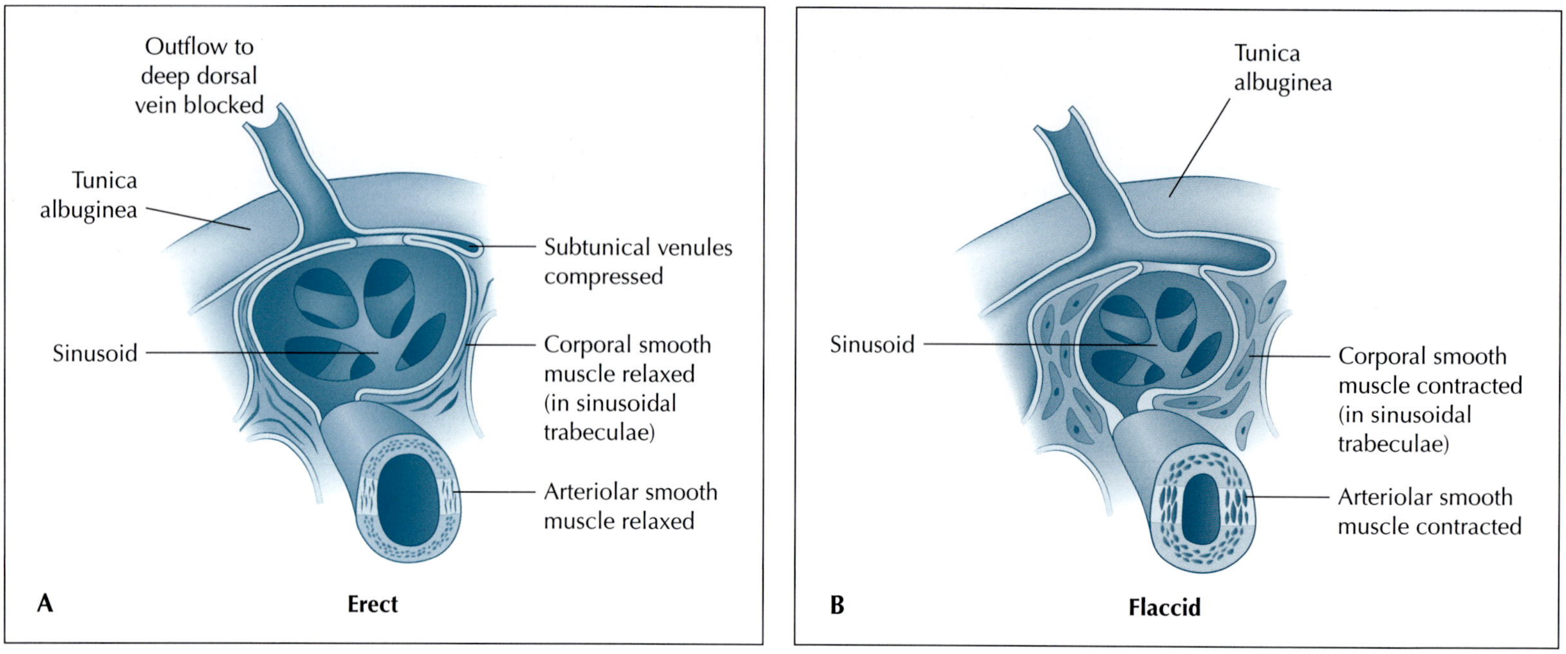

FIGURE 10-1. Priapism is possible because of the unique anatomic structure of the corpora cavernosa (see Fig. 8-1 in the chapter on penile vascular surgery). During erection with the relaxation of the corporal smooth muscles, inflowing blood results in volumetric expansion and thus compresses the subtunical venules under the less flexible tunica albuginea and blocks the backflow (**A**). With the increasing pressure in the corporal bodies, the inflowing arteries are also blocked and equilibrium is started. Following the orgasm, sympathetic discharge results in the contraction of the corporal smooth muscles and decrease in the expansive volume of the intracorporeal structures (**B**). This in turn relieves the pressure on the subtunical venules and outflow is restored.

Orgasm is not always necessary for detumescence. In some cases, the erection can detumesce due to lack of stimulation, NO release, or increased breakdown of cGMP by phosphodiesterase 5. In priapism, erection is prolonged without sexual stimulation or despite orgasm. In essence, the detumescence mechanism fails.

ISCHEMIC AND NONISCHEMIC PRIAPISM

Causes of Priapism

Ischemic priapism (low-flow, high-pressure venous priapism)
Inability of the corporal smooth muscles to contract (mostly due to pharmacotherapy)
Occlusion of the venules by blood clots (sickle cell disease, hematologic malignancies, parenteral hyperalimentation)
Nonischemic priapism (high flow, low-pressure arterial priapism)
The arteriovenous shunt* (mostly traumatic)

** Because of anatomic differences, the spongiosal body and glans penis are not involved in this procedure. This should be kept in mind because some of the salvage surgical interventions involve these structures.*

FIGURE 10-2. Ischemic and nonischemic priapism. *Ischemic priapism*, which is the most prevalent type, needs urgent medical attention. Since the inflow of oxygenated blood is ceased, prolonged erection results in decreased oxygen saturation in proportion to elapsed time. There is increased acidosis that in turn decreases the contractility of smooth muscle. Acidosis and hypoxia also decrease the synthesis and action of both prostaglandins and nitric oxide. These two molecules play an important role in the inhibition of platelet aggregation. In a prolonged hypoxic state, a vicious cycle of microthrombi formation and blockage of the vessels vicious circle is initiated.

All cells have protective antioxidative enzyme systems to protect themselves from the free oxygen radicals that may lead to cell damage. The concentrations of antioxidant enzymes are also dependent on the ischemic period length. When intervention and reperfusion is delayed, the protective enzyme concentration may not be sufficient to neutralize the free oxygen radicals. Reperfusion should be restored as soon as possible (preferably within a 4-hour period the most) to prevent tissue damage.

Nonischemic or *arterial priapism* is not a medical emergency, but it might be hazardous to the penile corporal smooth muscles in the long term and should also be treated properly. In most cases there is a history of blunt and rarely sharp trauma involving the corporal bodies. Because of the injury of the cavernosal arteries, an arteriocavernosal shunt is established and there is continuous uncontrolled inflow of blood. Because the trabecular smooth muscles are contracted during the flaccid state, a full erection is not established at all times, but with sexual stimulation the patient can still have erections (they may not be normal erections). In the acute phase, some of these cases have been reported to resolve within an 8- to 10-day period; and in some cases, patients lacking pain and discomfort might not seek medical attention for years.

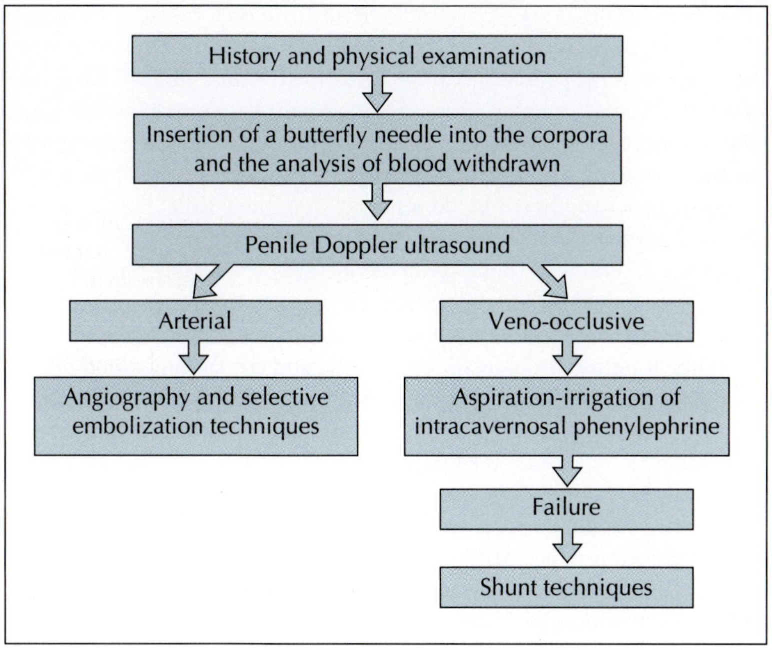

FIGURE 10-3. Diagnostic approach to priapism. Because of the deleterious effects of priapism, a correct diagnosis and prompt action is mandatory. A systematic approach might save time and unnecessary interventions. The history might give the clinician an 80% to 90% accuracy of diagnosis. (*Adapted from* Montague *et al.* [1].)

History

Timing of the episode
Past recurrences
Medications: intracavernosal pharmacotherapy, drug abuse (*eg,* cocaine)
Recent Doppler ultrasonographic evaluation
Any hematologic illnesses
Sexual act before incidence
Presence of pain

FIGURE 10-4. History. When talking to the patient it should be stressed that in addition to conservative approaches to reduce the erection, invasive procedures may be needed and, if not managed within 4 hours, the priapism itself may have deleterious effects on future erectile functions.

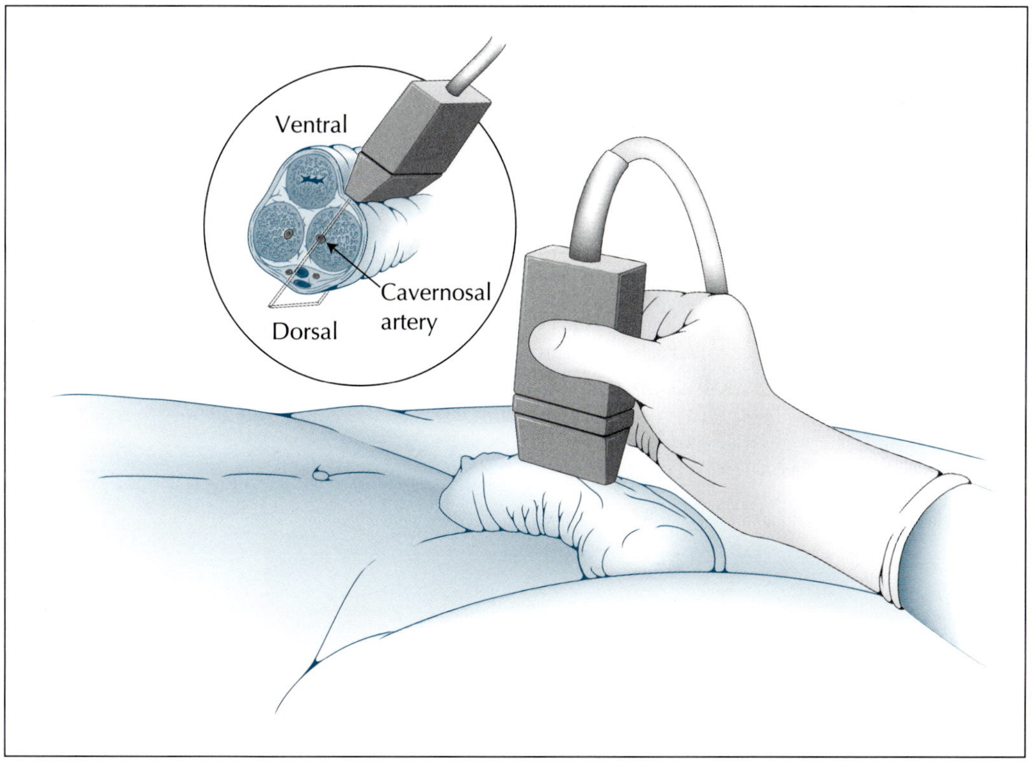

FIGURE 10-5. Penile Doppler ultrasonography. The use of penile color Doppler ultrasonography is now very common. It is the most reliable and noninvasive technique to evaluate priapistic patients. An absent arterial inflow suggests a veno-occlusive type of priapism. In the arterial nonischemic type, color Doppler ultrasound may be diagnostic and should also involve perineal scanning, which may uncover a localized flush of blood flow.

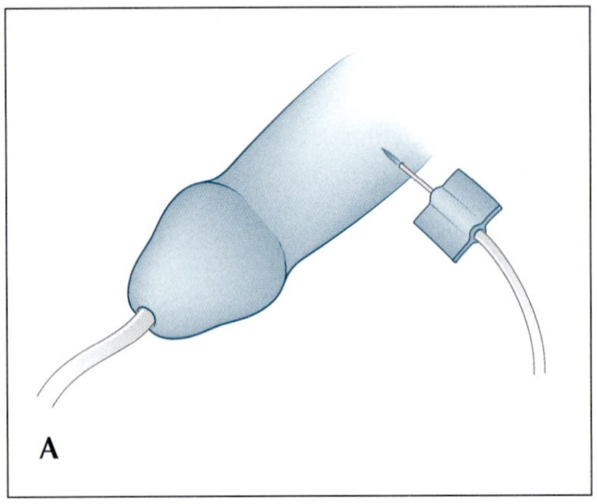

B. The α-adrenergic Drugs for Priapism and Their Dosages

Drug	*Recommended Dosage*
Epinephrine	10–20 μg
Phenylephrine	100–500 μg
Ephedrine	50–100 mg
Norepinephrine	10–20 μg

FIGURE 10-6. Aspiration. This approach is both therapeutic and diagnostic. Once the needle is inserted to the corpora, the pressure in the system should drop and thus break the vicious circle; arterial inflow may be reinitiated and corporal smooth muscles gain the ability to contract. The color of the aspirate would be dark red in an ischemic priapism and bright red in a nonischemic one. If uncertain about the cause, a pH and partial oxygen saturation (PO_2) might be evaluated in the aspirated blood sample.

Management of ischemic priapism should be performed in a stepwise fashion with an ideal goal to obtain complete detumescence as promptly as possible.

After insertion of a 19-G butterfly needle into each corpus cavernosum (**A**), laterally, aspiration of the stagnant blood might be enough to resolve the priapism if the procedure can be performed within 4 hours. After the initial aspiration, irrigation of the corpora might help to remove any small clots and decrease the concentration of any medication responsible for the situation. In cases where the underlying cause is intracavernosal pharmacotherapy, once bright red blood inflow is seen, the needle should not be removed immediately because the effect of medication might be persistent. An intracavernosal α-adrenergic drug (preferably phenylephrine) (**B**) should be administered if the pressure rises again after aspiration. Due to the cardiovascular effects of α-adrenergic drugs, patients should be monitored closely for tachycardia and elevation of blood pressure. Surgical intervention is recommended if ischemic priapism persists following aspiration/irrigation and repeated sympathomimetic injections.

If a hematologic cause is suspected, aspiration should again be initiated to decrease intracorporal pressure but also the oxygen tension in the circulating blood should be increased. Hydration, alkalinization, analgesia, and hypertransfusion to decrease hemoglobin S to less than 30% may be necessary in the case of a sickle cell–associated priapism. In this group of patients, several days to 2 weeks may be expected for full flaccidity. In recurrent cases, use of low-dose intracavernosal α-adrenergic drugs may be helpful to prevent recurrences.

There have also been reports of priapism due to oral intake of certain medications such as antihypertensives (hydralazine, guanethidine, prazosin, tamsulosin), phenothiazine-group antipsychotics (especially chlorpromazine), and antidepressants (trazadone). The shared pharmacologic action of all these drugs seems to be α-adrenergic blockage. Discontinuation of the drugs and administration of intracavernosal α-adrenergics only reverse the effects. A small subset of patients with ischemic priapism may present with recurrent episodes of priapism that are distinct from a single episode of priapism. These patterns of recurrent episodes known as "stuttering priapism" may present a significant challenge to the clinician that requires a management algorithm and counseling with the patient and partner to prevent future episodes of priapism. Each episode of ischemic and recurrent priapism should be managed in a step-wise fashion. (*Adapted from* Montague *et al.* [1].)

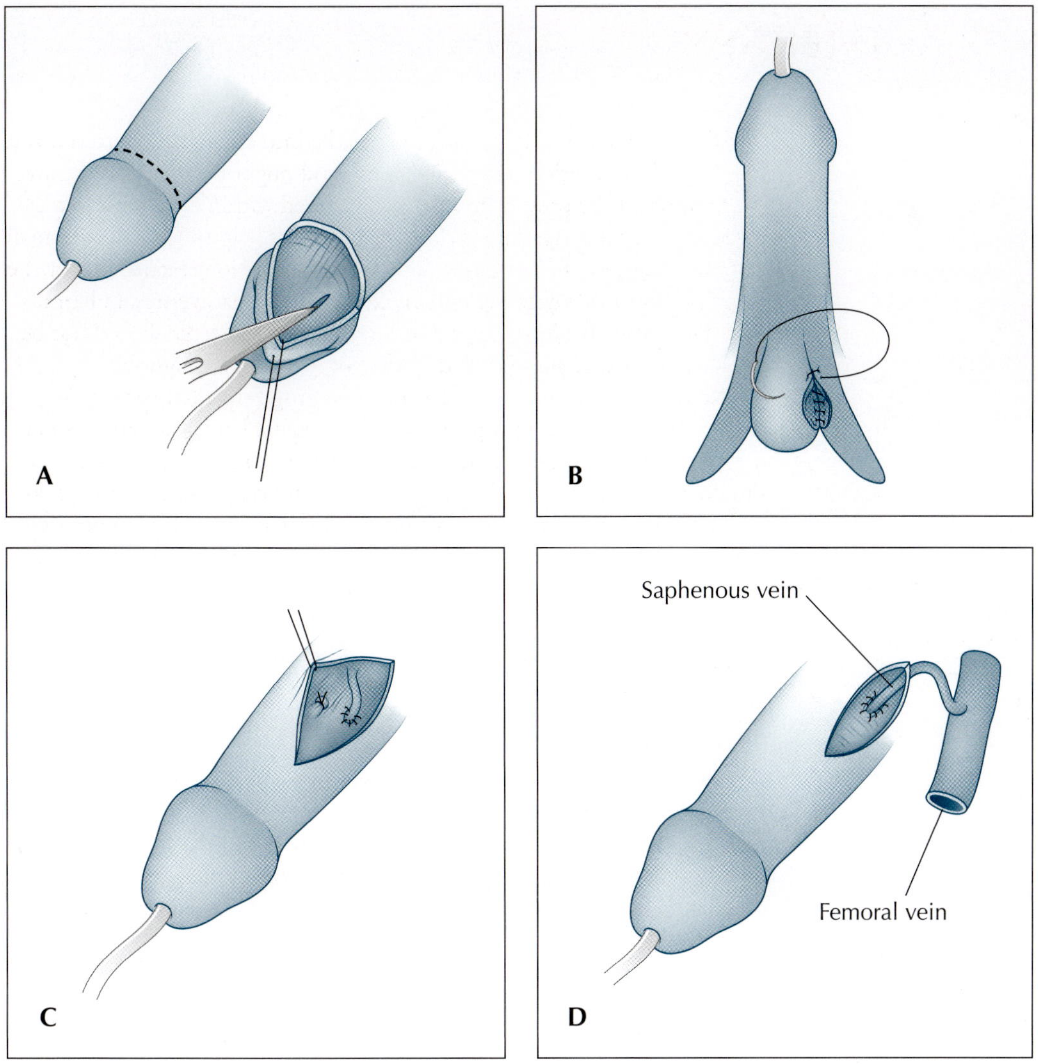

FIGURE 10-7. In adult patients, phenylephrine should be diluted with normal saline to a concentration of 1 to 500 μg/mL, and 1-mL injection made every 3 to 5 minutes for approximately 1 hour prior to deciding that this modality will not be successful. It should be noted that lower concentrations in patients with severe cardiovascular disease and in children should be used. After failure of medical therapy, a shunt procedure may need to be performed to protect penile structures. The shunt procedures may be performed in different ways but the idea is always to restore penile outflow. Because the spongiosal bodies and glans penis are not involved in priapism, the easiest way is to open a shunt between these. The main objective in such a procedure should be that it is reversible and the damage to the system should be minimal as the patient may need restoration of erection afterwards. The most well-known and practical shunt procedure is to disrupt the distal tip of the tunica albuginea and create a shunt between the glans penis and the corpora (**A**). This can be achieved by a trocar, a tru-cut biopsy needle, or a scalpel. **B,** A shunt can also be created by anastomosing the proximal corpora cavernosa to the spongiosum. **C** and **D,** More sophisticated methods involving corporavenous shunting procedure between dorsal vein or saphenous vein and the corpora have been described. However, in late presenting cases resistant to classic aspiration and irrigation techniques, there will be organized hematoma-like clots in the trabecular area, making it impossible to restore outflow just by opening a gate between the corpora and the systemic venous circulation.

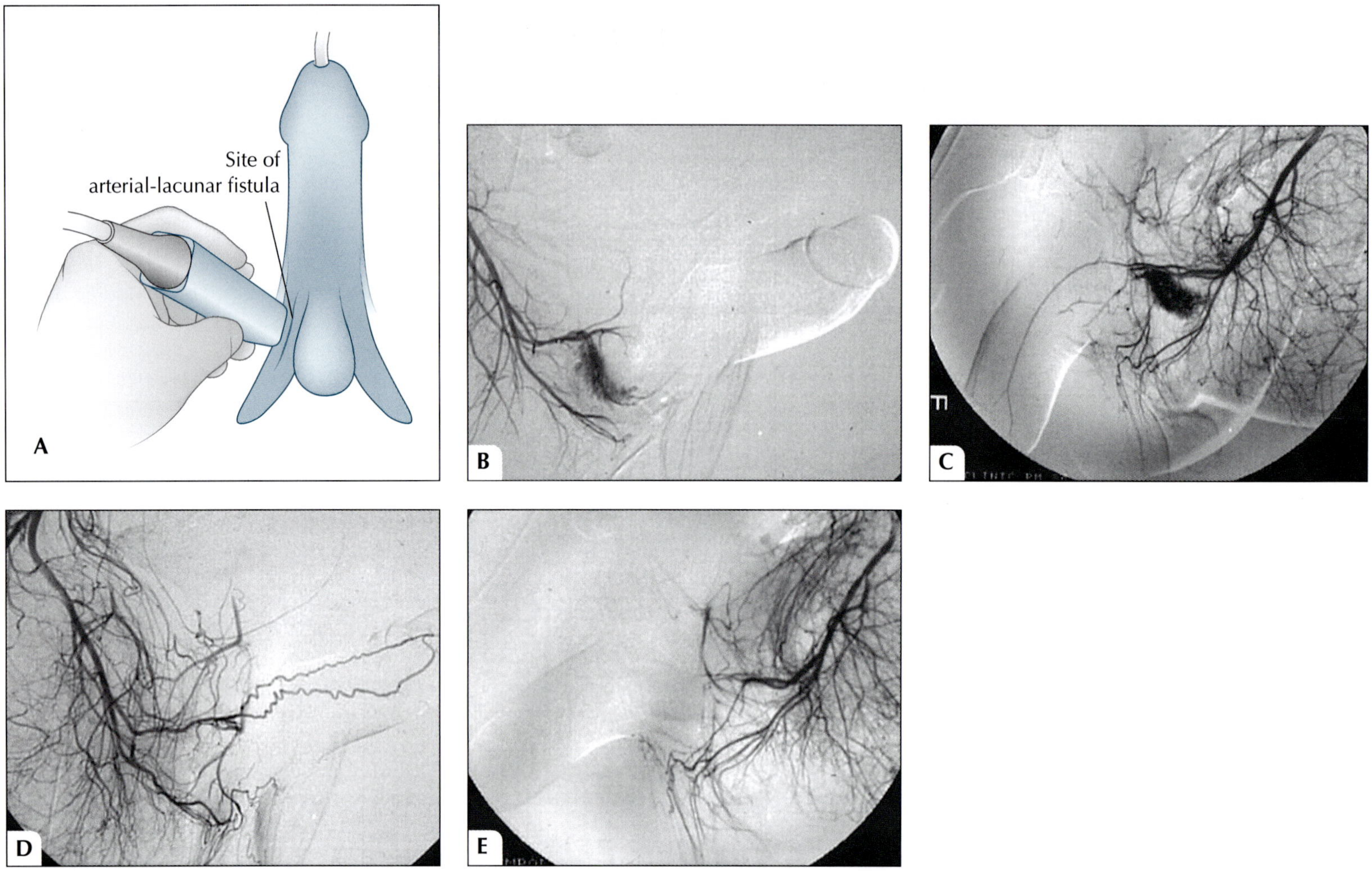

FIGURE 10-8. Power Doppler scanning. In traumatic arterial priapism, the timing of the trauma and the extensiveness of the fistula should be evaluated. This can be achieved through power Doppler ultrasound scanning of the penis including the perineal crura because most of the trauma tends to occur at this particular site (**A**). The patients' preference is of value here also. A small arteriovenous shunt that has recently been established must be closely monitored because of the chance of spontaneous recovery; if the patient is disturbed by continuous tumescence, a super- selective angiography together with embolization may be pursued. It should be stressed that long-term, high-flow pressure in the corpora cavernosa may lead to endothelial dysfunction and thus future erectile dysfunction. Any high-flow priapism would need an intervention if spontaneous recovery does not take place. The embolization should be performed in highly skilled centers and should not compromise future erectile function (**B–E**). Many agents have been suggested for embolization, including autologous blood clot, gelfoam, and minicoils. Autologous blood clot due to its resorption capacity does not compromise the arterial integrity. Cavernosal artery ligation procedures can also be an alternative treatment, but should be reserved as last resort because they are irreversible.

CONCLUSIONS

Conclusions

Priapism must be managed emergently
Best treatments are prevention and education of patients at risk
Importance of physician's role in treatment

FIGURE 10-9. Conclusions. Priapism is an important medical emergency in urologic practice, with detrimental effects if not acted on promptly and properly. The best treatment of priapism is prevention and education of the patients under risk, such as those with sickle cell disease and patients on intracavernosal pharmacotherapy. All patients using pharmacotherapy should be warned about priapism and early referral to their doctors in case of longer than expected erections (> 4 hours). With the advent of oral medications, uncontrolled use of concomitant phosphodiesterase inhibitors and intracavernosal drugs may lead to persistent priapism.

The physicians' role is to evaluate the situation and decide on the type of priapism. A low-flow high-pressure priapism is a urologic emergency. Patients should be informed about the reasons for their priapism, treatment choices, and associated morbidities. A systematic approach may result in prompt treatment with minimal morbidities.

REFERENCE

1. Montague DK, Jarow J, Broderick GA, *et al.*, for the Members of the Erectile Dysfunction Guideline Update Panel of the American Urological Association: American Urological Association guideline on the management of priapism. *J Urol* 2003, 170 (4 pt 1):1318–1324.

Peyronie's Disease: Pathophysiology and Medical Therapy

11

Jacob Rajfer
Nestor Gonzalez-Cadavid
Mark Jalkut

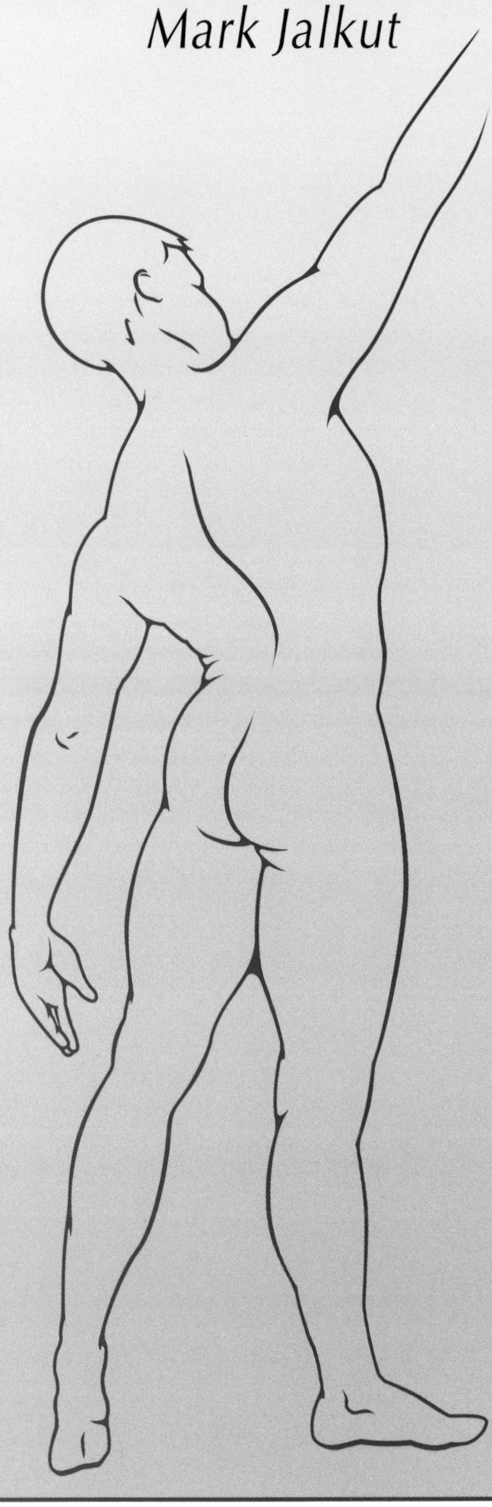

Peyronie's disease is an acquired benign condition with potential significant impact on quality of life that can include pain, penile deformity, and erectile dysfunction (ED). Modern studies have shown the disease to be prevalent. Once thought to resolve spontaneously, it is now known that the disease consists of an active phase and a mature phase, with resolution of pain and rarely resolution of penile deformity. The disease is now known to be caused by a "trapped" inflammatory response resulting from minor trauma, hematoma formation with fibrin deposition, and resultant cytokine activity. The cytokine transforming growth factor-β1 (TGF-β1) has demonstrated particular importance and is used in creating animal models to study the disease. This abnormal immune response may have a genetic predisposition. Modern molecular techniques, genomics, and proteomics are being applied to better understand the pathways that lead to Peyronie's disease.

The medical treatment of Peyronie's disease has a long history and has rarely been satisfactory. In evaluating a man with Peyronie's disease, it is most important to appreciate the progress of the disease, the presence of ED, and the degree of bother. Several modern medical treatments are used against Peyronie's disease and they may be either systemic or local. Few placebo-controlled, prospective, double-blind studies with objective measurements are available to evaluate the medical therapy for Peyronie's disease. A greater understanding of the pathophysiology that leads to the Peyronie's plaque will lead to the development of novel, directed medical treatments.

DEFINITION

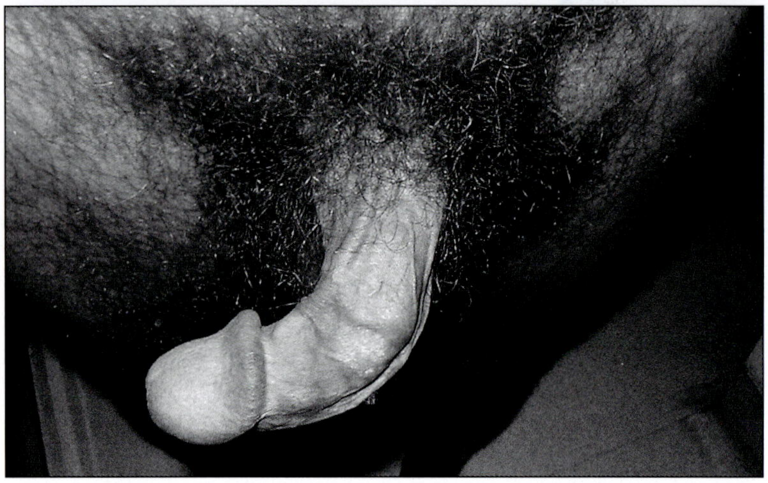

FIGURE 11-1. (*See Color Plate*) Francois de la Peyronie (1678–1747) first described the condition that bears his name in a 1743 paper entitled "Some Obstacles Preventing Normal Ejaculation of Semen." Men with Peyronie's disease present with a palpable plaque or induration and curvature or indentation of an erect penis. The erections may be painful and erectile dysfunction (ED) may be associated with the disease. Peyronie's disease is an acquired benign condition without known systemic sequelae.

NATURAL HISTORY

Incidence and Prevalence of Peyronie's Disease in Rochester, Minnesota, 1950–1984

Age Group	*Patients, n*	*Incidence Rate (Per 100,000 Men)*
20–29	5	4.3
30–39	5	4.6
40–49	24	30.2
50–59	42	66.0
60–69	21	46.3
70–79	2	7.6
80+	2	19.1
Age-adjusted	101	25.7
Prevalence (per 100,000)	388.6	
Mean age at diagnosis	53	

FIGURE 11-2. Incidence and prevalence of Peyronie's disease in Rochester, Minnesota, between 1950 and 1984. Lindsay *et al.* [1] completed a 35-year retrospective study that demonstrated the average age of onset of Peyronie's disease to be 53 years, with a prevalence of 388.6 per 100,000 (0.4%). A more recent questionnaire-based study of men in Germany revealed that 3.2% of respondents reported palpable penile plaques [2]. The true incidence of Peyronie's disease, however, remains unknown and may be higher, as an autopsy study demonstrated lesions of the tunica albuginea in 22 of 100 men with no known symptomatic disease [3]. In addition, the successful treatment of erectile dysfunction with phosphodiesterase therapy has increased the number of men who have had return of potency but remain with severe curvature. (*Adapted from* Lindsay *et al.* [1].)

Natural History of Peyronie's Disease

Study	*Symptom*	*Patients, n*	*Worse, %*	*Stable, %*	*Better, %*	*Resolved, %*
Dahl		19		18	1	
Ashworth		8	1		4	
Williams and Thomas		12		3	5	4
Bystrom *et al.*	Curvature	5		3	2	
	Plaque size	7		2	5	
	Pain	7				7
Gelbard		98	42	44	13	

FIGURE 11-3. Natural history of Peyronie's disease. This table compiles several studies on the natural history of Peyronie's disease. It was once thought that Peyronie's disease slowly and spontaneously resolved. In 1970, Williams and Thomas [4] reported on a series of 21 patients of whom greater than 50% had gradual resolution or improvement in their symptoms over a 4-year period. The resolution of pain was noted first, followed by plaque softening, then disappearance. In 1990, Gelbard *et al.* [5] reported on the natural history of Peyronie's disease in a study of 97 men with disease duration from 1 to 5 years. As outlined in the table, most men were found to have persistent or progressive symptoms. Current understanding of the disease recognizes that most men develop either stable or progressive disease with a rare few having spontaneous resolution within the first year.

The disease process can be divided into an active phase and a mature or stable phase. The onset of the disease is marked by painful erections, a changing configuration of plaque, and a dynamic curvature. Up to one third of patients, however, present with painless acquired curvature. Painful erections typically resolve over 6 months and plaques usually stabilize by 12 months, leaving a man with a bent erection of fixed degree. The stable phase consists of a painless, stable deformity with a mature scar and in many instances development or progression of erectile dysfunction. (*Adapted from* Ralph and Pryor [6].)

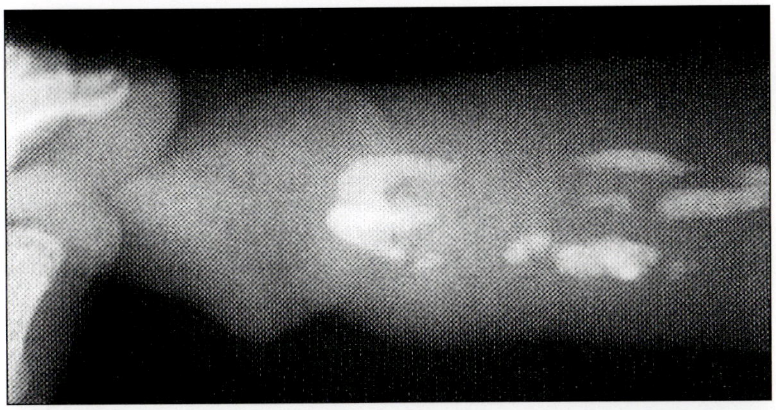

FIGURE 11-4. Calcificiation of Peyronie's plaque. This radiograph demonstrates calcification of penile plaques associated with Peyronie's disease. Patients with such calcification are unlikely to experience spontaneous improvement of their symptoms with the exception of painful erections, which is self-limiting in nearly all patients with Peyronie's disease. Other factors that suggest a patient's disease is less likely to resolve include plaque greater than 2 cm, bend more than 45°, and degrees and presence of Dupuytren's contractures [5]. (*From* Ralph and Pryor [6]; with permission.)

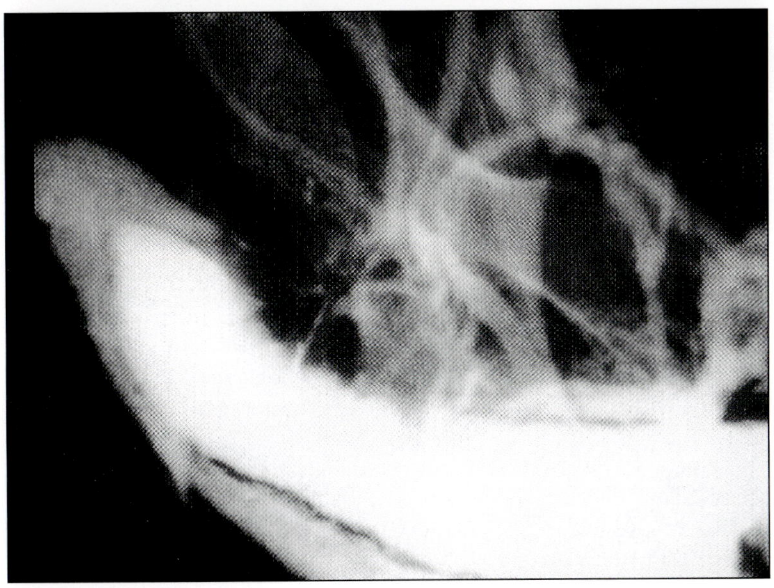

FIGURE 11-5. Venous leakage as a result of plaque in Peyronie's disease. Erectile dysfunction (ED) is estimated to be present in 30% of patients with Peyronie's disease [7]. In addition, in some cases the successful use of oral phosphodiesterase inhibitors has unmasked penile deformities, previously unknown by the patient, that are too severe to allow intercourse. Four factors contribute to ED in Peyronie's disease: penile deformity preventing intercourse, impaired vascular function, a flail penis due to circumferential plaque, and psychologic distress or anxiety due to the appearance of the penis [8]. Lopez and Jarow [9] reported that in a study of 76 men, 36% had arterial disease and 59% had veno-occlusive disease as a cause of ED [9]. Venous leakage, as demonstrated by the cavernosogram in Figure 11-4, is thought to occur when altered compliance prevents the passive transtunical occlusion of venous channels. ED is not only symptomatic of Peyronie's disease but also a dreaded complication of surgical reconstruction; thus careful documentation of its presence and degree is of utmost importance.

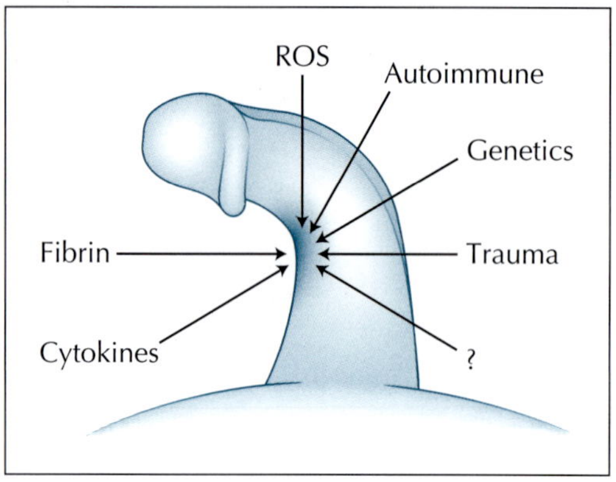

FIGURE 11-6. Proposed causes of Peyronie's disease. Over 250 years ago, Peyronie attributed the disease to chronic irritation resulting from a combination of sexual abuse, venereal diseases, and tuberculosis. Studies during the past decade have yielded a current model of pathophysiology whereby minor penile trauma from intercourse results in hematoma and fibrin deposition. Cytokines and reactive oxidative species (ROS) are then released and a "trapped" inflammatory response leads to aberrant wound healing. In addition, inheritable conditions associated with Peyronie's disease have been identified, suggesting a genetic role. In addition to the theorized genetic element, an autoimmune component may be present.

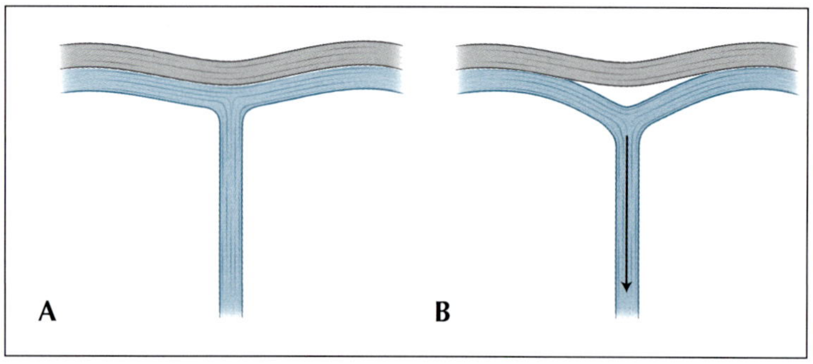

FIGURE 11-7. Tunical rupture with trauma resulting in delamination and hematoma. In 1957, Furey [10] first suggested, and most investigators now concur, that minor sexual trauma is the major cause of Peyronie's disease [11]. Subsequently, a survey of 732 men demonstrated an association between penile trauma and both Peyronie's disease and erectile dysfunction (ED)[12]. Devine *et al.* [12] in 1997 proposed a detailed model of trauma as a cause for the Peyronie's plaque. Deforming forces to the erect penis cause tears and delamination injuries within layers of the tunica albuginea. These injuries occur more commonly in older men as a result of lower intracavernosal pressures and age-associated elastic fiber fragmentation. Analysis of the tunica albuginea during erection reveals the dorsal midline area to experience distractive stress and to be surrounded by areas of shear stress. These areas of stress distribution correspond with plaque location with most plaques located in the dorsal midline. (*Adapted from* Devine *et al.* [12].)

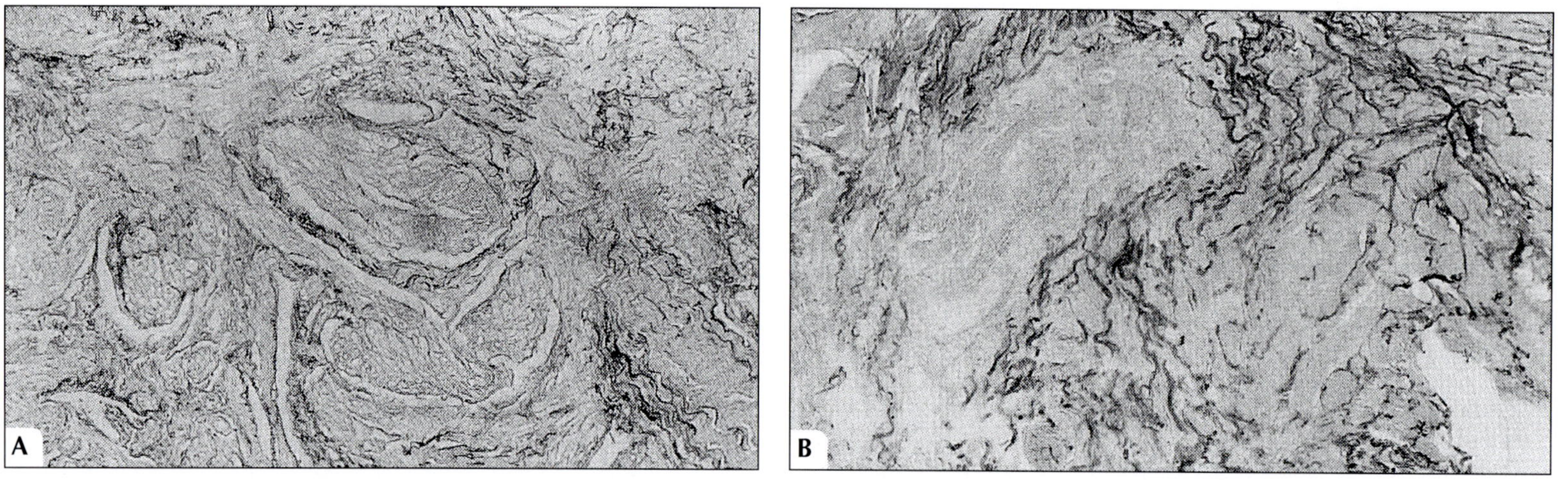

FIGURE 11-8. Histopathology of Peyronie's plaques. This figure demonstrates the end-stage aberrant wound healing. **A**, In normal tunica, woven undulating elastin fibers provide a network into which a frame of ordered collagen bundles insert. **B**, In Peyronie's disease, this normal arrangement is lost with elastin fibers severely fragmented and collagen-forming nodule-like clumps. (*Adapted from* Brock *et al.* [13].)

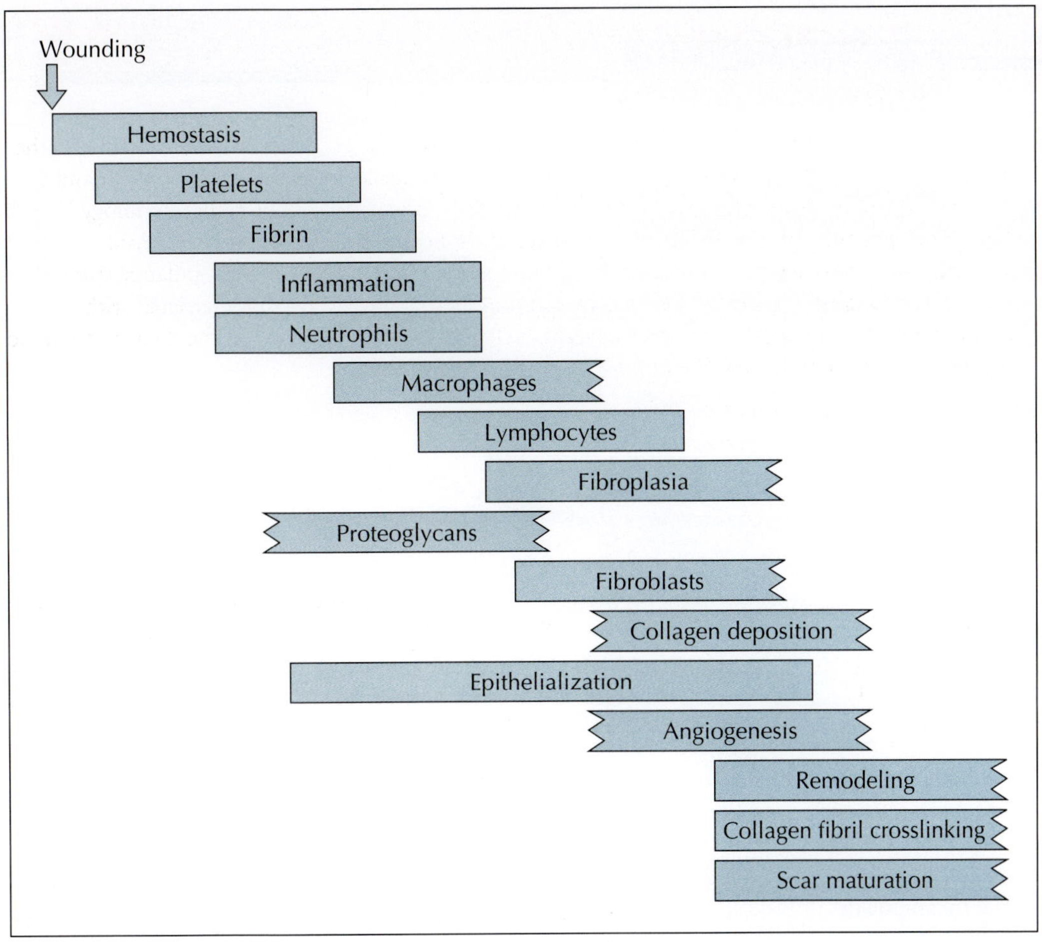

FIGURE 11-9. Cascade of normal wound healing comprising regulated, ordered, and self-limited steps. This figure demonstrates that normal wound healing is made up of an ordered sequence of events with transitions from one phase of healing into the next. Two key steps are fibrin activity and cytokine activity. Fibrin controls bleeding and binds various cytokines, initiating the healing process that leads to the recruitment of fibroblasts. Of the cytokines, transforming growth factor-β (TGF-β1) is a master control signal. (*Adapted from* Cohen *et al.* [14].)

Histologic Properties of Peyronie's Plaques Compared with Control Tissues

Tissue Source	Abnormal Collagen*	Abnormal Elastin	Fibrin Deposition	Ossification	Inflammatory Infiltrate
Peyronie's plaque	32/33 (97)	31/33 (91)	18/19 (95)	11/33 (33)	15/33 (45)
Dupuytren's contracture	7/8 (88)	5/8 (62)	7/8 (88)	0/8 (0)	1/8 (12)
Normal tissue	0/1	0/1	0/1	0/1	0/1
Penile scar	0/1	0/1	0/1	0/1	0/1
Invasive squamous cell carcinoma	0/1	0/1	0/1	0/1	0/1

Numbers in columns are given as n/n (%).

FIGURE 11-10. Histologic properties of Peyronie's plaques compared with control tissues. Simple injury with contractile scar formation is not enough to cause the plaque of Peyronie's disease. El-Sakka *et al.* [15] reported that trauma alone to the rat tunica does not produce the chronic phase of Peyronie's disease. As depicted in this figure, Peyronie's scars were compared with scar from Dupuytren's contractures, penile scar tissue, and normal tunica [16]. Peyronie's disease demonstrated abnormal collagen in 97% of plaques, disrupted elastin fibers in 91% of plaques, and fibrin deposition has been demonstrated in 95% of plaques as well as 88% of Dupuytren's lesions. Normal tunica and penile scar tissue had none of these findings. Fibrin deposition as a result of microvascular injury is thought to be a key initial step in the development of a Peyronie's plaque with subsequent aberrant wound healing. (*Adapted from* Somers and Dawson [16].)

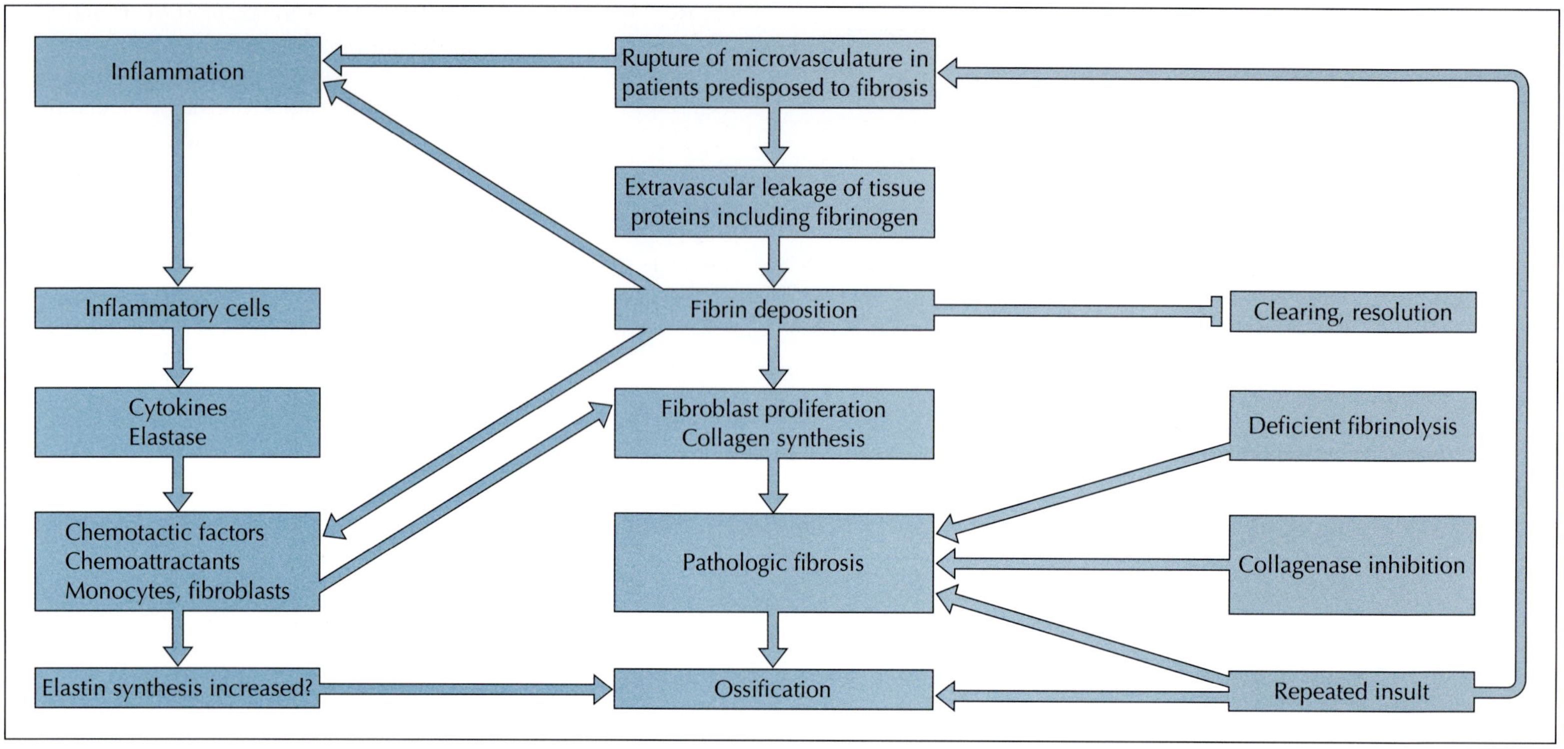

FIGURE 11-11. Role of fibrin deposition in the pathophysiology of plaque formation. This figure demonstrates the pathway through which aberrant wound healing may occur due to persistent fibrin. If fibrin is not cleared from the tunical injury, then a "trapped" inflammatory response results with fibrin acting as a chemoattractant, promoting the ingrowth of inflammatory cells and eliciting cytokine release. Persistent deposits of fibrin resulting from hematoma formation are a critical step in the pathway from minor trauma to plaque formation. (*Adapted from* Somers and Dawson [16].)

Expression of Transforming Growth Factor-β in Tunica Albuginea of Men with Peyronie's Disease

Tissue	*TGF-β1**	*TGF-β2†*	*TGF-β3‡*
Peyronie's disease	26/30 (86.7)	7/30 (23.3)	5/30 (16.7)
Control	1/6 (16.7)	1/6 (16.7)	1/6 (16.7)

**P=0.002.*
†P=0.858.
‡P=0.549.

FIGURE 11-12. Expression of transforming growth factor-β (TGF-β) in tunica albuginea of men with Peyronie's disease. With microvascular injury and subsequent deposition of fibrin, a change of events is initiated that results in aberrant wound healing. El-Sakka *et al.* [17] studied the expression of TGF-β1, a cytokine associated with multiple diseases of severe fibrosis, and found it to be elevated in 86% of Peyronie's patients in contrast to one of six normal control subjects [16]. The same group also studied the effects of surgical trauma on rat tunica and discovered that in normal healing, the levels of TGF-β1 were temporarily elevated but decreased to normal levels [17]. If rats were injected with a synthetic peptide with action similar to TGF-β1, however, they developed histologic changes similar to those seen in Peyronie's disease plaques [18].

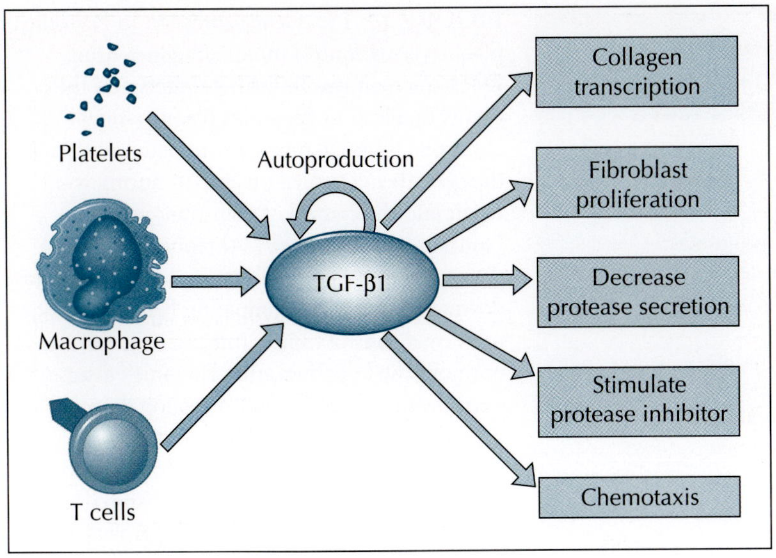

FIGURE 11-13. Role of transforming growth factor-β1 (TGF-β1) in wound healing. TGF-β1 is secreted by macrophages, activated platelets, and T lymphocytes. One of its unique abilities is to cause autosecretion. It is considered a master control signal with fibroblast activity and exerts three major effects. First, it increases transcription of genes that control collagen and proteoglycan deposition. Second, it decreases secretion of proteases, thus limiting the remodeling and termination of the inflammatory response. Finally, it secretes proteins that inhibit protease activity. In addition, TGF-β1 has been implicated in the generation of reactive oxidative species (ROS) and influences other chemokine activity. It is through this cytokine, along with ROS, that the result of trapped fibrin exerts the molecular effects that lead to plaque formation.

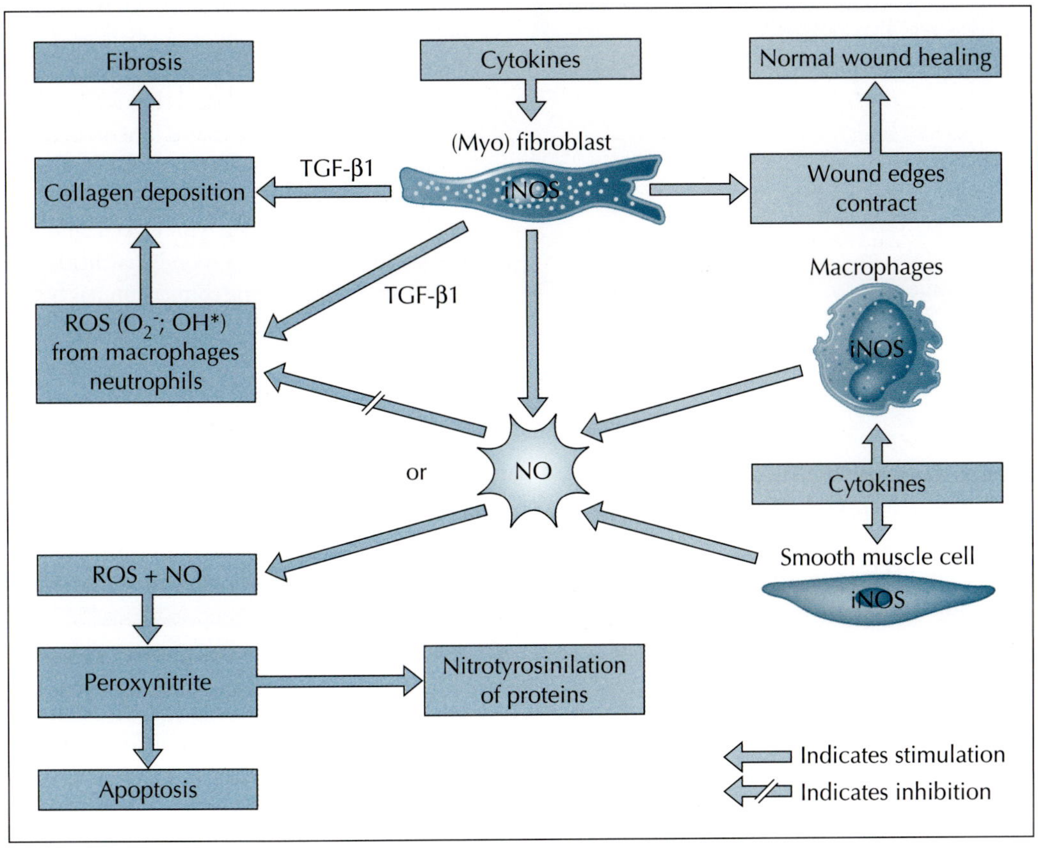

FIGURE 11-14. Reactive oxygenation species (ROS) and their role in fibrosis. ROS are hydroxyl radicals and superoxide anions that induce lipid peroxidation in cell membranes and increase vascular permeability and leakage of fibrinogen and other clotting factors. Transforming growth factor-β (TGF-β1) induces the production of ROS [19–22]. TGF-β1 also transcriptionally represses inducible nitric oxide synthase (iNOS), which may be an antifibrotic agent [22,23].

Gene Expression in Peyronie's Plaque Versus Control Tunica Albuginea Utilizing DNA Microarrays

	Genes	Action
Upregulated	Pleiotrophin	Osteoblast recruitment
	Monocyte chemotactic protein 1	Inflammation
	Early growth response protein	Fibroblast proliferation
	Elastase	Elastic fiber degradation
	α and γ smooth muscle actin	Myofibroblast marker
Downregulated		
	Ubiquitin	Tissue remodeling
	Id-2	Tissue remodeling
	Collagenase IV	Collagen breakdown
	TGF modulators	Limit TGF activity

FIGURE 11-15. Gene expression in Peyronie's plaque versus control tunica albuginea using DNA microarrays. To further understand the events that lead to Peyronie's plaque (and all abnormal fibrosis), one needs to better understand the genes being turned on and off during wound repair and the control of their transcription. Gonzalez-Cadavid *et al.* [24] reported on those genes, which have been found to be either up- or downregulated when comparing Peyronie's tissue to normal control tunica. Interestingly, this has born out the hypothesis that Peyronie's disease stems from abnormal wound healing. Future similar experiments will further our understanding of the pathophysiology that leads to Peyronie's disease and will provide inspired therapeutic targets. TGF—transforming growth factor.

Evidence for Genetic Determinants of Peyronie's Disease

Family history in 2% of cases
Discovery of multigenerational families with Peyronie's disease
HLA-B27 carries higher risk for developing Peyronie's disease
Dupuytren's contracture

FIGURE 11-16. Evidence for genetic determinants of Peyronie's disease. Minor penile trauma is ubiquitous and thus cannot fully explain the cause of Peyronie's disease. This observation has led some investigators to consider a genetic role in the development of Peyronie's disease. Peyronie's disease has not been linked to any predisposed populations; however, several conditions have been associated with Peyronie's disease. A family history can be elicited in 2% of cases [25]. In addition, Nyberg *et al.* [26] have reported on several multigenerational families with Peyronie's disease. HLA-B27, a class I human leukocyte antigen that is inherited, has been implicated in Peyronie's disease with a threefold increased risk over the general population [27]. HLA-B27 is associated with several autoimmune conditions, including spondyloarthritis. This potential autoimmune connection has been further suggested by studies demonstrating elevated levels of serum antielastin antibody in men with Peyronie's disease [28].

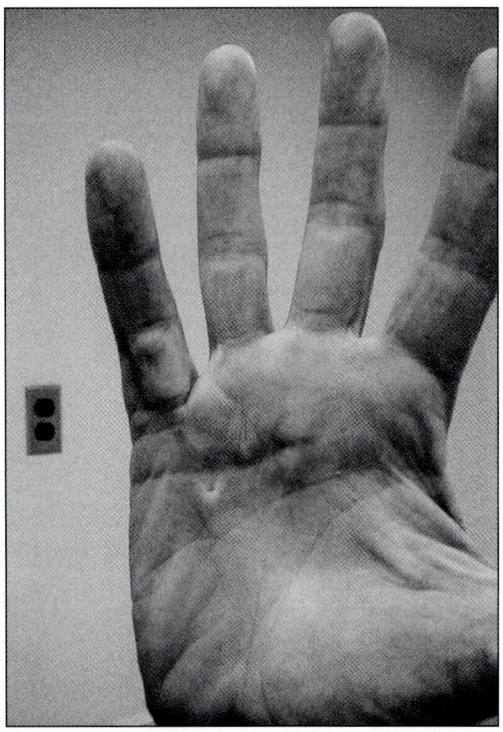

FIGURE 11-17. (*See Color Plate*) Dupuytren's contractures and Peyronie's disease. Dupuytren's contractures, or palmar fibromatosis, is a disease characterized by a thickened plaque overlying the flexor tendon of the ring finger and occasionally the little finger that develops into a thickened fibrotic cord. This condition is inherited in an autosomal dominant fashion and 16% to 20% of men with Dupuytren's contractures develop Peyronie's disease [29,30].

History and Physical Examination for the Patient with Peyronie's Disease

History
Degree of bother
Erectile dysfunction
  Risk factors
  Treatments used
Does degree of deformity prevent penetration?
Pain
  Duration
  Location
Physical examination
Number and location of plaques
Degree and direction of bend
Penile length

FIGURE 11-18. Relevant history and physical examination in a patient with Peyronie's disease. A review of the history and symptoms in a patient presenting with Peyronie's disease should focus on the factors as listed in this figure as they will be brought to bear on the timing and type of therapy initiated. The most important factors to assess are how the disease affects the lives of the patient and his partner and to determine the patient's expectations of therapy. Physical examination should focus on those findings that will aid in determining initial therapy and help to document disease progression versus resolution. Photographs taken by the patient while in an erect state or demonstration of penile curvature following office intracavernosal injection document the degree and angle of defect. Tracings of the erect penis can be placed into the patient chart for documentation and later reference. Rarely does sonography provide additional information regarding number, location, and size of plaques and extent of calcification.

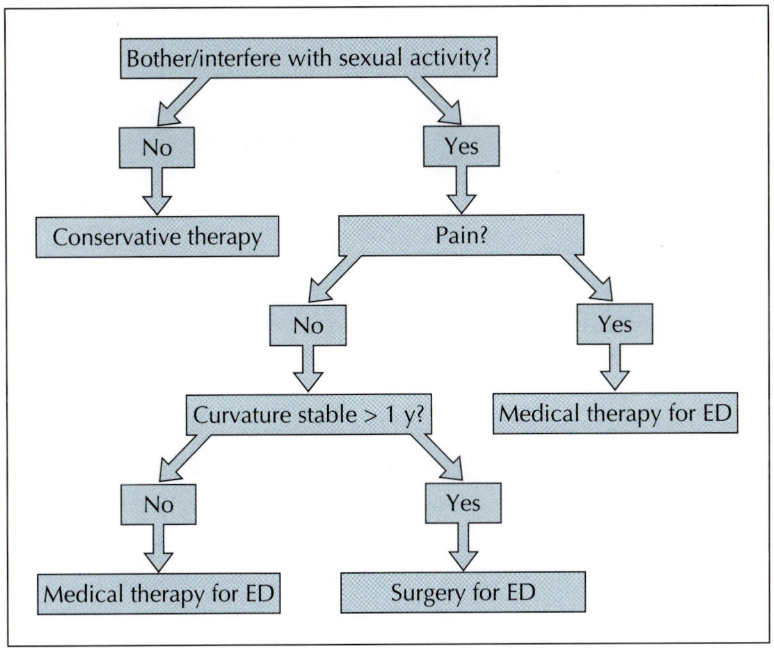

FIGURE 11-19. Treatment algorithm. Treatment should address each patient's specific problems and be based on agreeable objectives.

Conservative therapy is the standard treatment for Peyronie's disease. In a man with significant bother, who is able to maintain erections and in the acute phase of the disease, medical therapy may be initiated. A man who has long-standing Peyronie's disease and significant bother and is unable to penetrate or who has developed erectile dysfunction (ED) may be better suited for surgical intervention.

MEDICAL THERAPIES FOR PEYRONIE'S DISEASE

Contemporary Nonsurgical Therapies for Peyronie's Disease

Oral
- Vitamin E
- Potaba
- Colchicine
- Acetyl-L-carnitine

Intralesional
- Verapamil
- Collagenase
- Interferons

Iontophoresis

Extracorporeal shock-wave therapy

FIGURE 11-20. Contemporary nonsurgical therapies in the treatment of Peyronie's disease. The past decade has revealed more about the pathophysiology of Peyronie's disease; therefore, potential medical therapies can be understood in terms of halting or reversing the aberrant wound healing that follows penile trauma, bleeding, and fibrin deposition. This figure lists those therapies that are available and actively prescribed today. Widely available and actively prescribed therapies can be broadly divided into systemic (pills), intralesional (intraplaque injection), and topical (some relying on iontophoresis). The aim of iontophoresis is to take advantage of successful intralesional therapies. An electric current is used to force medicine into the plaque, thereby avoiding the painful and traumatic process of injection. In addition, limited studies have been reported on the use of extracorporeal shock-wave therapy on Peyronie's plaques.

ORAL THERAPY FOR PEYRONIE'S DISEASE

Results of Vitamin E Therapy for Peyronie's Disease

Study	*Patients, n*	*Improved Pain, %*	*Improved Plaque Size, %*	*Improved Angulation, %*
Scardino and Scott [31]	23	100	91	78
Chesney [34]	58	82	82	Not reported
Pryor [8]	40	35	Minimal	10
Devine and Horton [32]	107	99	20	33

FIGURE 11-21. Results of vitamin E therapy for Peyronie's disease. Vitamin E is actually a variety of the tocopherol family and a potent antioxidant. It has been hypothesized that vitamin E is protective against reactive oxygen species. This table shows the outcome of several reported experiences with vitamin E. In 1949, Scardino and Scott [31] reported on the use of vitamin E in 23 patients with a 2-year follow-up and then reported an additional 10 cases for overall improvement in pain, curvature, and plaque in 81%. In 1974, Devine and Horton [32] reported a 60% improvement in 30 patients treated with vitamin E. In 1990, however, a controlled study of vitamin E failed to demonstrate a significant difference in pain, bend, ability to have intercourse, and overall disease state with placebo [5]. Vitamin E is inexpensive and without any serious common side effect. It may, however, thin the blood, increase blood pressure, and interfere with prescribed anticoagulants or aspirin. Recommended dosage is 800 IU daily. (*Adapted from* Mynderse and Monga [33].

Recent Studies on Potaba Therapy

Study	Patients, n	Improved Pain, %	Improved Plaque Size, %	Improved Angulation, %
Zarafonetis [37]	21	100	76	82
Hasche-Klunder [36]	25	100	100	71
Riley	18	100	11	75
Carson [35]	32	44	56	58

FIGURE 11-22. Results with potaba (potassium aminobenzoate) therapy for Peyronie's disease. Potaba has been prescribed extensively for Peyronie's disease [35]. This figure shows the results of several noncontrolled subjective studies. In a larger noncontrolled study of 2653 patients, potaba was reported successful in 57% of treated patients [36]. The drug is prescribed at 12 g/d for 3 months and comes in 0.5-g tablets. This is a generally poorly tolerated treatment. The most frequent reported side effect is gastrointestinal upset. (*Adapted from* Mynderse and Monga [33].)

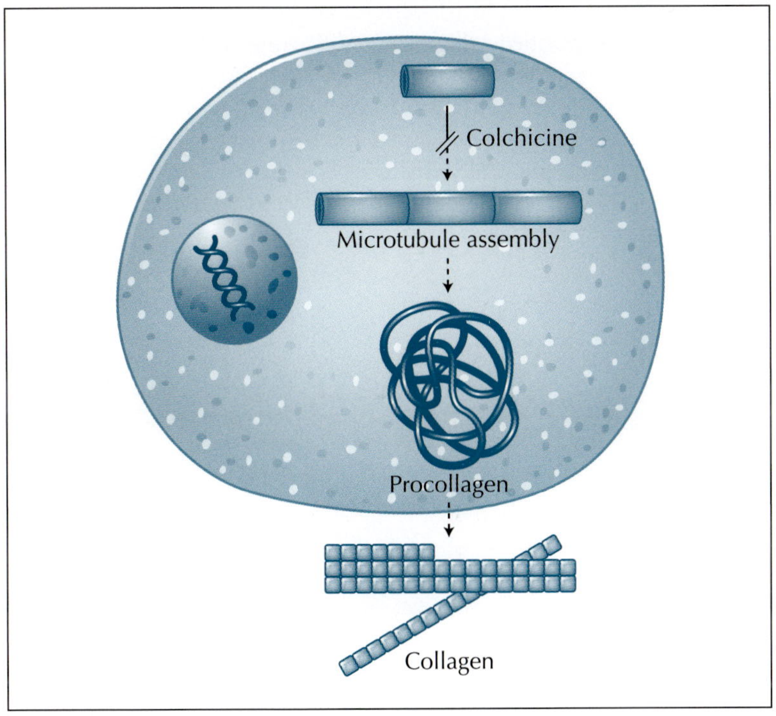

FIGURE 11-23. Colchicine's action as an anti-inflammatory agent. Colchicine is an oral antimicrotubular agent that inhibits collagen secretion by blocking the movement of procollagen within the cell. The drug also interferes with mitosis, binds microtubules inhibiting movement and leukocyte adhesion, and blocks the lipoxygenase pathway of arachidonic acid, which reduces chemotaxis and inflammation [38]. El-Sakka *et al.* [39] studied the use of colchicine in a rat model of tunical fibrosis. Peyronie's-like lesions were created by injecting transforming growth factor-β1 (TGF-β1) into the tunica of rats. Rats that were treated with colchicine early in the disease had less collagen deposition and elastin fragmentation than animals receiving water or colchicine later in the disease state. Molecular techniques demonstrated a downregulation of TGF-β1 in rats treated with colchicine.

Colchicine for the Treatment of Peyronie's Disease

Improved pain in 78%
Improved curvature in 26%
Smaller plaque in 42%
Major adverse effects include gastrointestinal upset/diarrhea
Other adverse effects include bone marrow suppression, myopathy, elevated liver function tests, edema

FIGURE 11-24. Effects of colchicine in the treatment of Peyronie's disease. A noncontrolled study treated 24 patients with 0.6 mg to 1.2 mg daily for 1 week then 2.4 mg daily in divided doses for 3 to 5 months [38]. Pain resolved in 78%, curvature improved in 26%, and plaque size decreased in 42%. The main adverse effect is gastrointestinal distress with pain, diarrhea, nausea, and vomiting in up to one third of subjects. These gastrointestinal side effects led to the early discontinuation of therapy in 17% of the subjects. Other potential and more severe adverse effects of colchicine therapy include agranulocytosis, aplastic anemia, myopathy, elevated liver enzyme levels, and angioneurotic edema.

Trial of Tamoxifen in 36 Men with Peyronie's Disease
Improved pain in 15/20 patients
Improved curvature in 1/31 patients
Improved plaque in 12/35 patients

FIGURE 11-25. Trial of tamoxifen in 36 men with Peyronie's disease. Tamoxifen has been shown to increase the release of transforming growth factor-β1 (TGF-β1) , the cytokine implicated in the aberrant wound healing of Peyronie's disease [40]. Elevated levels of TGF-β1 cause macrophage deactivation and inhibition of T lymphocyte activity. In a 1992 uncontrolled study of 36 patients, Ralph *et al.* [41] reported that treatment with 20 mg twice daily resulted in an overall response rate of 55%, with a better response seen in patients whose disease was present for less than 4 months [41]. A controlled study published in 1999, however, enrolling 25 patients, could not demonstrate any improvement in pain, curvature, or plaque size beyond that achieved by placebo [42]. Side effects of tamoxifen included gastrointestinal distress and alopecia.

INTRALESIONAL TREATMENT OF PEYRONIE'S DISEASE

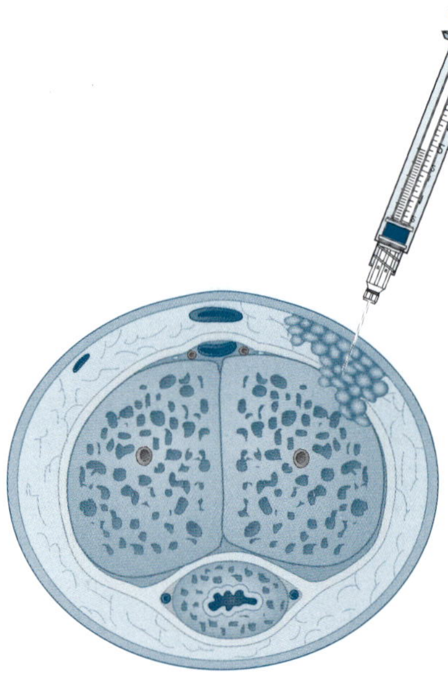

FIGURE 11-26. Injection into the Peyronie's plaque. Modern intralesional therapy can be credited to Gelbard *et al.* [43], who injected purified collagenase into Peyronie's plaque. They have also reported on the drug effect versus the hydraulic effect of injection [44]. The current technique recommended by Levine and Estrada [45] is to create a penile block, followed by grasping the plaque between index thumb and finger. A single skin puncture is made with a five-eighths-inch 25-G needle and then passed in and out of the plaque while dispensing drug into the needle tract. Pain and hematoma are common side effects. In the case of verapamil, blood pressure is monitored for 10 minutes after injection.

Intraplaque Verapamil Injection Outcome Based on the Kelami Classification

	Class/Grade I	*Class/Grade II*	*Class/Grade III*
Patients, *n*	33	68	38
Subjective, %			
Improved curvature	61	60	63
Improved distal rigidity	26	35	28
Improved sexual function	39	35	33
Improved girth	77	70	67
Objective, %			
Decreased curvature	41	68	62
Increased curvature	15	7	5
No change in curvature	44	25	32
Improved ED	14	18	15
Worse ED	3	5	18
No change in response	83	77	68

FIGURE 11-27. Intraplaque verapamil injection outcome based on the Kelami classification. Calcium antagonists have demonstrated an effect on scar formation, fibroblast activity, and collagen secretion. It was determined that the drug concentration required to retard extracellular matrix collagen synthesis was 10,000 times higher than that used for hypertension [46]. This figure represents Levine's experience with injecting verapamil (10 mg/10 mL) in 156 men [47,48]. He reports his data based on the Kalemi classification, a pretreatment grading of the severity of the Peyronie's disease. According to the scale, grade 1 is plaque 2 cm or less, curve of 30° or less; grade 2, plaque 2 to 4 cm and 30° to 60° curve; grade 3, plaque greater than 4 cm and curve greater than 60° with degree of curvature taking precedence. Of note in this series, even men with long-term and severe Peyronie's disease noted both subjective and objective improvement.

Experience with Intralesional Injection of Interferon Alfa-2b in the Treatment of Peyronie's Disease

Study	*Patients, n*	*Improved Pain, %*	*Improved Curvature, %*	*Smaller Plaque, %*
Benson [51]	10	100	50	80
Ahuja [50]	20	90	65	85

FIGURE 11-28. Experience with intralesional injection of interferon alfa-2b (IFN-alfa 2b) and Peyronie's disease. Duncan *et al.* [49] first demonstrated the potential use of interferons with their report on the in vitro effect of interferons against collagen production from human fibroblasts cultured from Peyronie's tissue. In addition, they reported that IFN alfa-2b also stimulated production of collagenase. Furthermore, Ahuja *et al.* [50] demonstrated that IFN alfa-2b protects against reactive oxygen species stimulation of collagen production by fibroblasts. This figure shows two reports on the use of intralesional IFN alfa-2b on Peyronie's plaques. There currently exists some controversy over whether to inject into the plaque or adjacent to the plaque. The major side effects of this exciting new therapy include "flu-like" symptoms and more rarely anorexia, rash, hypotension, and cardiac arrhythmias.

EXTRACORPOREAL SHOCK-WAVE THERAPY

Extracorporeal Shock-wave Therapy and the Treatment of Peyronie's Disease

Number of sessions: ≥ 3
Dose: 3000 shocks, 0.11–0.17 mJ/mm^3

FIGURE 11-29. Extracorporeal shock-wave therapy (ESWT) and the treatment of Peyronie's disease. ESWT is an investigative treatment of Peyronie's disease that was first described in 1997 [52]. To date, several small, uncontrolled studies have reported subjective improvements with the use of ESWT. Experts have not been able to postulate a mechanism of action in this therapy, which itself results in the trauma thought to cause Peyronie's disease. It is possible that local heating or alternate inflammatory pathways may occur. No basic science data exist on the effect of ESWT on normal tunica nor on Peyronie's plaque. In a recent study by Manikandan *et al.* [53], there was no relationship between resolution of plaque size on ultrasonography and symptomatic improvement. The treatment protocol used in that study is demonstrated in this figure. Fourteen percent of 42 patients reported an excellent outcome with respect to pain and curvature, and 50% of men claimed symptomatic improvement. Of men who had pain, 84% claimed complete or significant resolution on completion of treatment. Complications were limited to minor penile pain, severe penile pain in one patient, and hematoma formation in two patients. This investigational therapy has yet to be tested in a controlled, prospective study with defined and measurable outcomes.

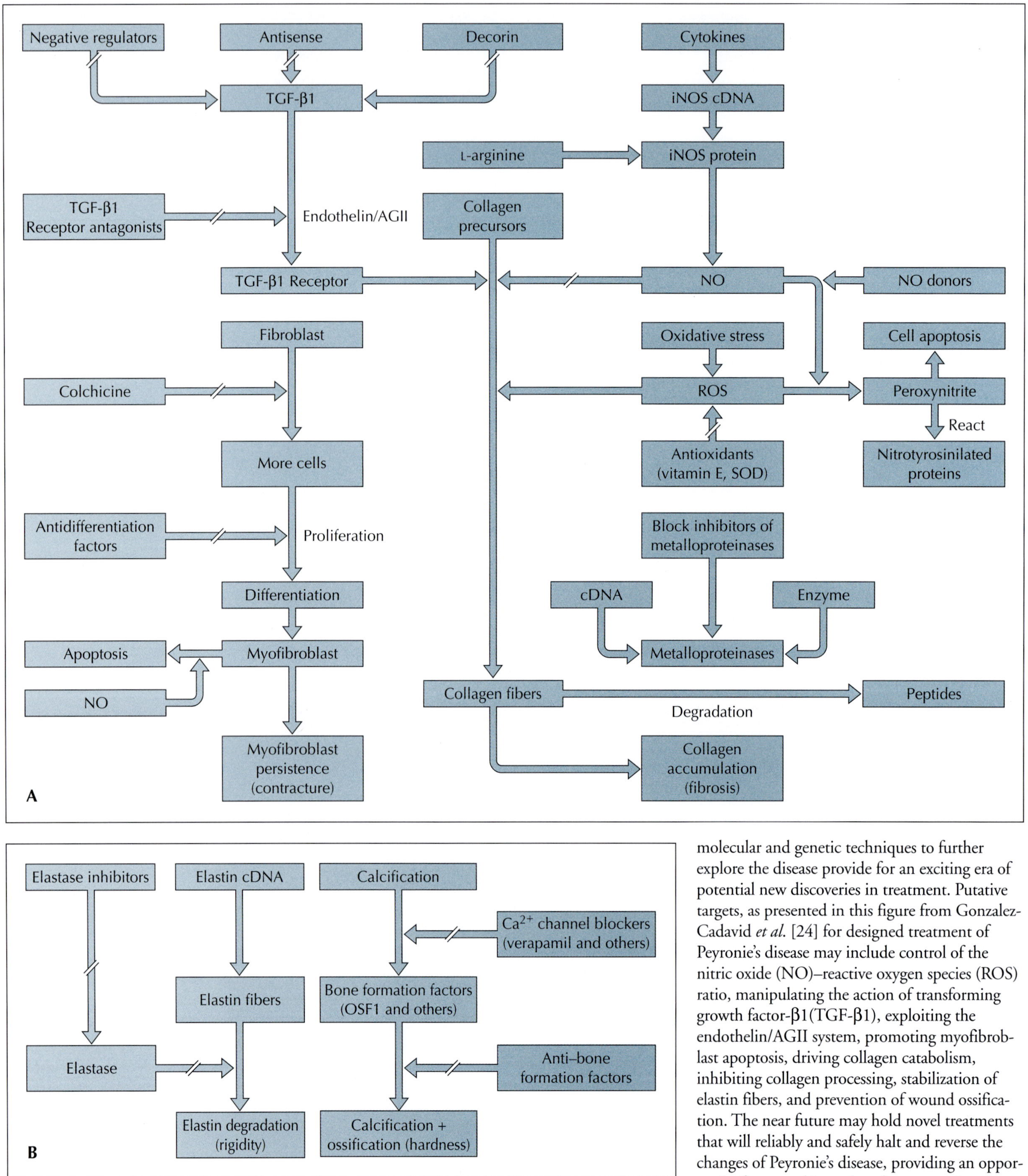

FIGURE 11-30. New potential pathways in the treatment of Peyronie's disease. **A**, Myofibroblast and collagen accumulation. **B**, Elastin degradation and ossification. The current understanding of the pathophysiology of Peyronie's disease together with animal models that recreate the disease and novel molecular and genetic techniques to further explore the disease provide for an exciting era of potential new discoveries in treatment. Putative targets, as presented in this figure from Gonzalez-Cadavid *et al.* [24] for designed treatment of Peyronie's disease may include control of the nitric oxide (NO)–reactive oxygen species (ROS) ratio, manipulating the action of transforming growth factor-β1(TGF-β1), exploiting the endothelin/AGII system, promoting myofibroblast apoptosis, driving collagen catabolism, inhibiting collagen processing, stabilization of elastin fibers, and prevention of wound ossification. The near future may hold novel treatments that will reliably and safely halt and reverse the changes of Peyronie's disease, providing an opportunity for something other than preserving the status quo hoped for with medical therapy or the risk of surgery. iNOS—inducible nitric oxide synthase; SOD—superoxide dismutase.

REFERENCES

1. Lindsay MB, Schain DM, Grambsch P, *et al.*: The incidence of Peyronie's disease in Rochester, Minnesota, 1950 through 1984. *J Urol* 1991, 146:1007–1009.
2. Schwarzer U, Sommer F, Klotz T, *et al.*: The prevalence of Peyronie's disease: results of a large survey. *BJU Int* 2001, 88:727–730.
3. Smith BH: Subclinical Peyronie's disease. *Am J Clin Pathol* 1969, 52:385–390.
4. Williams JL, Thomas GG: The natural history of Peyronie's disease. *J Urol* 1970, 103:75–76.
5. Gelbard MK, Dorey F, James K: The natural history of Peyronie's disease. *J Urol* 1990, 144:1376–1379.
6. Ralph DJ, Pryor J: Peyronie's disease. In *Textbook of Erectile Dysfunction.* Edited by Carson C, Kirby R, Goldstein I. Oxford, UK: Isis; 1999:515–528.
7. Weidner W, Schroeder-Printzen I, Weiske WH, Vosshenrich R: Sexual dysfunction in Peyronie's disease: an analysis of 222 patients without previous local plaque therapy. *J Urol* 1997, 157:325–328.
8. Pryor JP: Peyronie's disease and impotence. *Acta Urol Belg* 1988, 56:317–321.
9. Lopez JA, Jarow JP: Penile vascular evaluation of men with Peyronie's disease. *J Urol* 1993, 149:53–55.
10. Furey CA: Peyronie's disease: a treatment by the local injection of meticortelone and hydrocortisone. *J Urol* 1957, 55:251–266.
11. Jarow JP, Lowe FC: Penile trauma: an etiologic factor in Peyronie's disease and erectile dysfunction. *J Urol* 1997, 158:1388–1390.
12. Devine CJ, Jr., Somers KD, Jordan SG, Schlossberg SM: Proposal: trauma as the cause of the Peyronie's lesion. *J Urol* 1997, 157:285–290.
13. Brock G, Hsu GL, Nunes L, *et al.*: The anatomy of the tunica albuginea in the normal penis and Peyronie's disease. *J Urol* 1997, 157:276–281.
14. Cohen IK, Diegelmann RF, Crossland MC: Wound care and wound healing. In *Principles of Surgery*, edn 6. Edited by Schwartz SI, *et al.* New York: McGraw-Hill, Inc.; 1994:279–303.
15. El-Sakka AI, Selph CA, Yen TS, Dahiya R, Lue TF: The effect of surgical trauma on rat tunica albuginea. *J Urol* 1998, 159:1700–1707.
16. Somers KD, Dawson DM: Fibrin deposition in Peyronie's disease plaque. *J Urol* 1997, 157:311–315.
17. El-Sakka AI, Hassoba HM, Pillarisetty RJ, *et al.*: Peyronie's disease is associated with an increase in transforming growth factor-beta protein expression. *J Urol* 1997, 158:1391–134.
18. El-Sakka AI, Hassoba HM, Chui RM, *et al.*: An animal model of Peyronie's-like condition associated with an increase of transforming growth factor beta mRNA and protein expression. *J Urol* 1997, 158:2284–2290.
19. Casini A, Ceni E, Salzano R, *et al.*: Neutrophil-derived superoxide anion induces lipid peroxidation and stimulates collagen synthesis in human hepatic stellate cells: role of nitric oxide. *Hepatology* 1997, 25:361–367.
20. Poli G: Oxidative damage and fibrogenesis. *Free Radic Biol Med* 1997, 22:287–305.
21. Poli G: Pathogenesis of liver fibrosis: role of oxidative stress. *Molecular Aspects of Medicine* 2000, 21:49–98.
22. Geller DA, Billiar TR: Molecular biology of nitric oxide synthases. *Cancer Metast Rev* 1998, 17:7–23.
23. Nathan C: Inducible nitric oxide synthase: what difference does it make? *J Clin Invest* 1997, 100:2417–2423.
24. Gonzalez-Cadavid NF, Magee TR, Ferrini M, *et al.*: Gene expression in Peyronie's disease. *Int J Impot Res* 2002, 14:361–374.
25. Chilton CP, Castle WM, Westwood CA, Pryor JP: Factors associated in the aetiology of Peyronie's disease. *Br J Urol* 1982, 54:748–750.
26. Nyberg LM, Jr., Bias WB, Hochberg MC, Walsh PC: Identification of an inherited form of Peyronie's disease with autosomal dominant inheritance and association with Dupuytren's contracture and histocompatibility B7 cross-reacting antigens. *J Urol* 1982, 128:48–51.
27. Ralph DJ, Schwartz G, Moore W, *et al.*: The genetic and bacteriological aspects of Peyronie's disease. *J Urol* 1997, 157:291–294.
28. Stewart S, Malto M, Sandberg L, Colburn KK: Increased serum levels of anti-elastin antibodies in patients with Peyronie's disease. *J Urol* 1994,152:105–106.
29. Bystrom J, Rubio C: Induratio penis plastica Peyronie's disease: clinical features and etiology. *Scand J Urol Nephrol* 1976, 10:12–20.
30. Ling RS: The genetic factor in Dupuytren's disease. *J Bone Joint Surg Am* 1963, 45:709–718.
31. Scardino P, Scott WW: The use of tocopherols in the treatment of Peyronie's disease. *Ann N Y Acad Sci* 1949, 52:390.
32. Devine CJ, Jr., Horton CE: Surgical treatment of Peyronie's disease with a dermal graft. *J Urol* 1974, 111:44–49.
33. Mynderse LA, Monga M: Oral therapy for Peyronie's disease. *Int J Impot Res* 2002, 14:340–344.
34. Chesney J: Peyronie's disease. *Br J Urol* 1975, 47:209–219.
35. Carson CC: Potassium para-aminobenzoate for the treatment of Peyronie's disease: is it effective? *Tech Urol* 1997, 3:135–139.
36. Hasche-Klunder R: Treatment of Peyronie's disease with para-aminobenzoacidic potassium (POTOBA). *Urologe A* 1978, 17:224–227.
37. Zarafonetis CJ, Horrax TM: Treatment of Peyronie's disease with potassium para-aminobenzoate (potaba). *J Urol* 1959, 81:770–772.
38. Akkus E, Carrier S, Rehman J, *et al.*: Is colchicine effective in Peyronie's disease? A pilot study. *Urology* 1994, 44:291–295.
39. El-Sakka AI, Bakircioglu ME, Bhatnagar RS, *et al.*: The effects of colchicine on a Peyronie's-like condition in an animal model. *J Urol* 1999, 161:1980–1983.
40. Colletta AA, Wakefield LM, Howell FV, *et al.*:. Anti-oestrogens induce the secretion of active transforming growth factor beta from human fetal fibroblasts. *Br J Cancer* 1990, 62:405–409.
41. Ralph DJ, Brooks MD, Bottazzo GF, Pryor JP: The treatment of Peyronie's disease with tamoxifen. *Br J Urol* 1992, 70:648–651.
42. Teloken C, Rhoden EL, Grazziotin TM, *et al.*: Tamoxifen versus placebo in the treatment of Peyronie's disease. *J Urol* 1999, 162:2003–2005.
43. Gelbard MK, Walsh R, Kaufman JJ: Collagenase for Peyronie's disease experimental studies. *Urol Res* 1982, 10:135–140.
44. Gelbard MK, James K, Riach P, Dorey F: Collagenase versus placebo in the treatment of Peyronie's disease: a double-blind study. *J Urol* 1993, 149:56–58.
45. Levine LA, Estrada CR: Intralesional verapamil for the treatment of Peyronie's disease: a review. *Int J Impot Res* 2002, 14:324–328.
46. Lee RC, Ping JA: Calcium antagonists retard extracellular matrix production in connective tissue equivalent. *J Surg Res* 1990, 49:463–466.
47. Levine LA, Goldman KE, Greenfield JM: Experience with intraplaque injection of verapamil for Peyronie's disease. *J Urol* 2002, 168:621–625.
48. Kelami A: Classification of congenital and acquired penile deviation. *Urol Int* 1983, 38:229–233.
49. Duncan MR, Berman B, Nseyo UO: Regulation of the proliferation and biosynthetic activities of cultured human Peyronie's disease fibroblasts by interferons-alpha, -beta and -gamma. *Scand J Urol Nephrol* 1991, 25:89–94.
50. Ahuja S, Bivalacqua TJ, Case J, *et al.*: A pilot study demonstrating clinical benefit from intralesional interferon alpha 2B in the treatment of Peyronie's disease. *J Androl* 1999, 20:444–448.
51. Benson RC Jr, Knoll LD, Furlow WL: Interferon alpha 2 b in the treatment of Peyronie's disease [abstract]. *J Urol* 1991, 145 (suppl):1342.
52. Colombo F, Baroni P, Serrago M, *et al.*: Shock waves in Le Peyronie's disease: two years experience. *Eur Urol* 1997, 35(suppl 2):124.
53. Manikandan R, Islam W, Srinivasan V, Evans CM: Evaluation of extracorporeal shock wave therapy in Peyronie's disease. *Urology* 2002, 60:795–799.

12

Peyronie's Disease: Surgical Treatment

Derek Bochinski
Rafael Carrion
Nadeem Rahman
Tom F. Lue

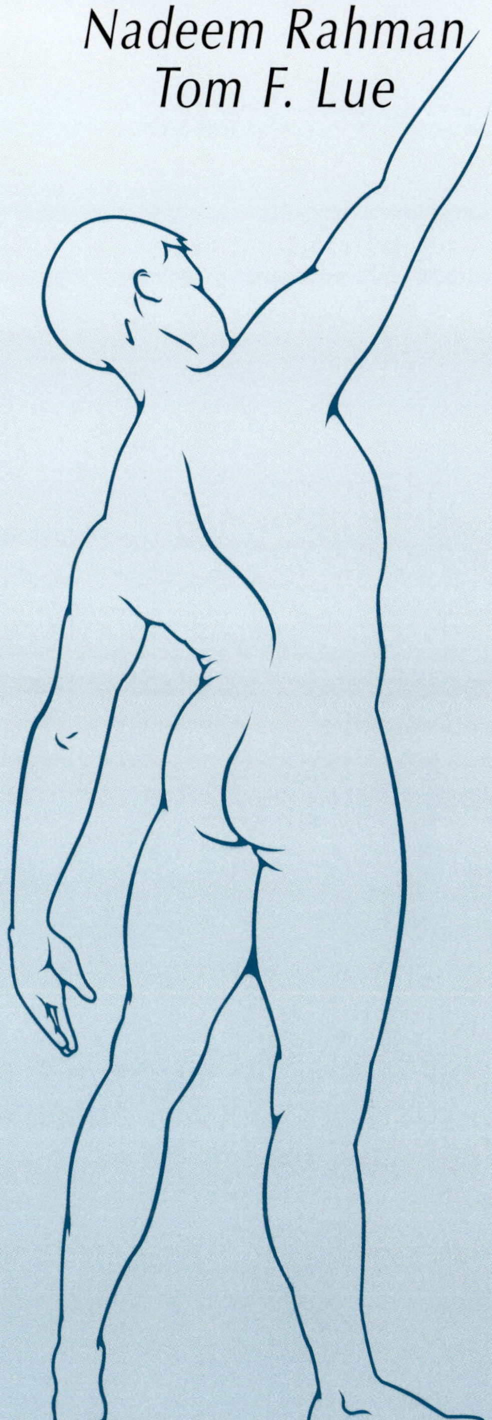

A detailed medical and psychosexual history of the patient with Peyronie's disease should include information about the duration and progression of the symptoms, penile rigidity, ability to have sexual intercourse, history of penile trauma or surgery, history of medication, and family history of Peyronie's disease or Dupuytren's contracture.

Physical examination consists of palpation of the penis to outline the location and extent of the plaque, the circumcision status, and the size of the saphenous vein. There is no special blood test for Peyronie's disease. In addition to routine blood chemistry, however, obtaining a testosterone level and lipid profile is advised for impotent men.

In office consultation, a photograph taken by the patient may be adequate for documentation. If surgery is contemplated, however, we prefer photographs or drawings of the deformed penis (dorsal and side views) after intracavernous injection of prostaglandin E_1. We also document the length of both the shorter and the longer side of the penis in the patient's chart. The patient is informed that the postoperative length of the penis will be the same as the shorter side for plication and the longer side for grafting. (We have received no more complaints about "shortened penis after surgery" since this policy was instituted.) We also perform color duplex ultrasound (after prostaglandin E_1 injection) to evaluate vascular function and to locate any communication between the cavernous, dorsal, and spongiosal arteries. Injury to a major communicating artery may render a man impotent if the function of the cavernous artery is marginal.

EVALUATION OF THE PATIENT WITH PEYRONIE'S DISEASE

Preoperative Evaluation for Penile Deformity

History: duration, penile rigidity, progression, sexual difficulty (painful erection, penile deformity, psychosexual history)
Physical examination: extent of plaque, Dupuytren's contracture, circumcision status, size of lower saphenous vein
Blood chemistry: not routinely performed (may add serum testosterone if libido is low)
Combined injection and stimulation test: examine curvature and narrowing, record penile length (both long and short side), document deformity with photograph or drawing
Duplex ultrasound: evaluate penile circulation and collateral arteries, assess number and site of plaques and calcifications

FIGURE 12-1. Preoperative evaluation for penile deformity. The patient should be informed that the goal of surgery is to correct the deformity and provide a straight penis for sexual relations but that surgery will not, in most cases, improve penile length or rigidity. This will avoid postoperative dissatisfaction and frustration due to unrealistic expectations.

INDICATIONS FOR MEDICAL AND SURGICAL TREATMENT

Therapeutic Strategy

Reassurance
- Minimal deformity not interfering with sexual function
- No pain
- No discomfort
- No erectile dysfunction

Nonsurgical treatment
- Pain or sexual difficulty for less than 1 year
- Recent onset or progression of plaque

Surgical treatment*
- Persistent pain for more than 12 mo
- Sexual difficulty because of deformity
- Stable condition (unchanged for more than 3 mo)
- Severe penile shortening
- Severe curvature, narrowing, or indentation
- Various combinations of the above

** At least 12 months after onset.*

FIGURE 12-2. Our therapeutic strategy for Peyronie's disease. Not every patient with Peyronie's disease needs medical or surgical treatment.

Nonsurgical Treatments

Counseling
Education
Reassurance
Systemic treatments
- P-amino benzoic acid
- Tamoxifen
- Acetyl-L-carnitine
- Colchicine (1.2 mg twice daily for 3 mo; watch for possibility of bone marrow depression and diarrhea)
- Vitamin E

Intralesional treatments
- Steroids
- Calcium channel blockers
- Interferons
- Purified clostridial collagenase
- Metalloprotein orgotein

Topical treatments
- Orgotein, dexamethasone, and lidocaine
- Local penile shock wave
- Verapamil cream

FIGURE 12-3. Nonsurgical treatments. Although the efficacy of medical treatment is unpredictable, patients with shorter duration, smaller plaque, and less angulation seem to respond better.

Surgical Procedures

Plication
Wedge resection
Incision and grafting
Excision and grafting
Implantation of a penile prosthesis

FIGURE 12-4. Surgical procedures. Surgical correction involves either shortening the longer side of the penis (plication, wedge resection) or lengthening the shorter side (incision or excision with grafting).

Recommended Selection Criteria for Surgery

Plication
- Potent
- Impotent, but has good response to oral agent ICI, intraurethral medication, or VCD
- Adequate penile length

Incision and venous grafting
- Potent
- Impotent, but has good response to oral agent, ICI, intraurethral medication, or VCD
- Short penis
- Hourglass deformity
- Persistent pain for more than 1 year

Implantation of prosthesis
- Impotent and has poor response to or refuses oral agent, ICI, intraurethral medication, and VCD

FIGURE 12-5. Our selection criteria for surgical correction of penile deformity. In the past, penile prosthesis was the only treatment for patients with both erectile dysfunction and Peyronie's disease. With advances in treatment of erectile dysfunction, we now routinely offer reconstructive surgeries to patients who respond well to nonsurgical impotence therapy. ICI—intracavernous injection; VCD—vacuum constriction device.

SURGICAL PROCEDURES

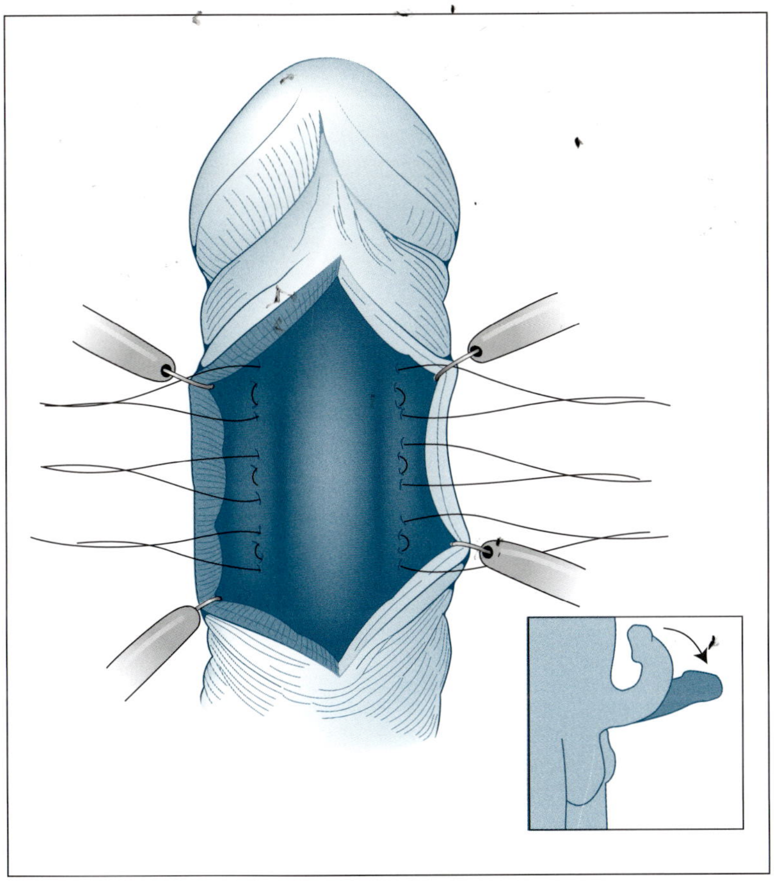

FIGURE 12-6. Plication of the tunica albuginea. We performed plication without removing an ellipse of the tunica or dissecting the neurovascular bundles or corpus spongiosum in the following manner. First, inject 1.5 to 2 mL of papaverine into the corpus cavernosum with a 212-gauge needle. Then, surgically scrub and prepare the genital area. Assess the curvature and deformity. If the patient's erection is not rigid, compress the crura of the penis or insert a 21-gauge scalp-vein needle into the cavernosum for saline infusion if needed. Locally infiltrate approximately 10 mL of 0.25% bupivacaine hydrochloride at the base of penis and toward the dorsal nerves. For dorsal curvature, make a ventral longitudinal incision down to Buck's fascia. Identify the corpus spongiosum. It is not necessary to dissect and free the spongiosum from the cavernosum. Place two to three pairs of deep plication sutures onto the tunica at the center of the curvature, 2 to 3 mm from the spongiosum on both sides [1]. (*Adapted from* Carrier and Lue [2].)

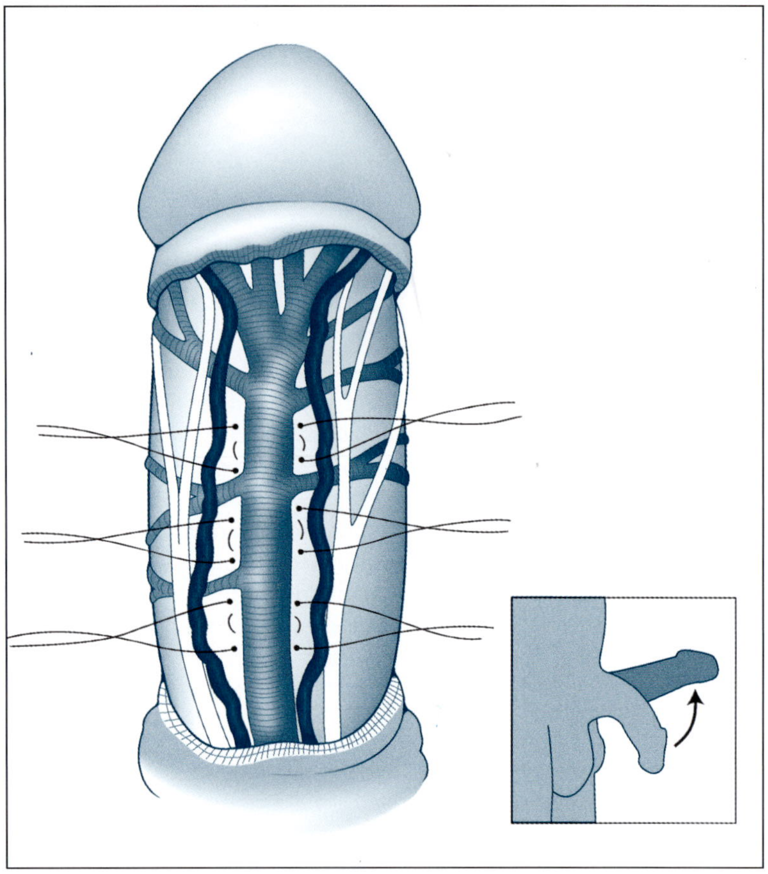

FIGURE 12-7. For ventral curvature, make a circumcision incision, then dissect and reflect the skin and subcutaneous tissue to the base of the penis. Identify the deep dorsal vein and arteries by incising Buck's fascia in the midline. It is not necessary to dissect and free the neurovascular bundle. Place two to three pairs of deep plication sutures onto the tunica at the center of the curvature between the deep dorsal vein and arteries. Using only nonabsorbable braided sutures (2-0 Ticron), tie the sutures with surgical knots slowly until the penis is straight. If lateral curvature is noted, place lateral sutures between branches of the dorsal nerves. If the penis remains rigid after completion of plication, insert a 21-gauge scalp-vein needle and aspirate 10 to 15 mL of blood. Inject 500 µg of phenylephrine solution every 3 to 5 minutes until detumescence is achieved. Close the wound with 4-0 chromic absorbable sutures. Wrap the penis with a light dressing. Check the dressing 2 to 3 hours later to ensure that the dressing is not tight. Change the dressing the next day, and instruct the patient to abstain from sexual intercourse for 4 to 6 weeks. (*Adapted from* Carrier and Lue [2].)

Complications of Tunical Plication

Encapsulated hematoma
Plaque progression
Recurrence
Prolonged painful erection, pain lasting for 5 mo
Shortened penis (all)
Palpable nodule

FIGURE 12-8. Complications of tunical plication. Although plication is a less invasive procedure, a number of complications have occurred in our experience.

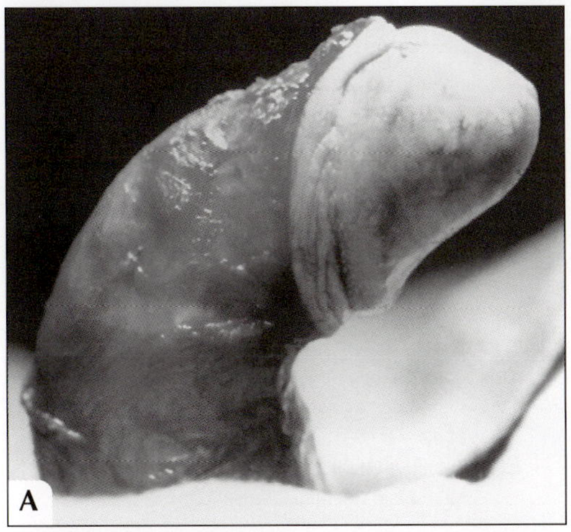

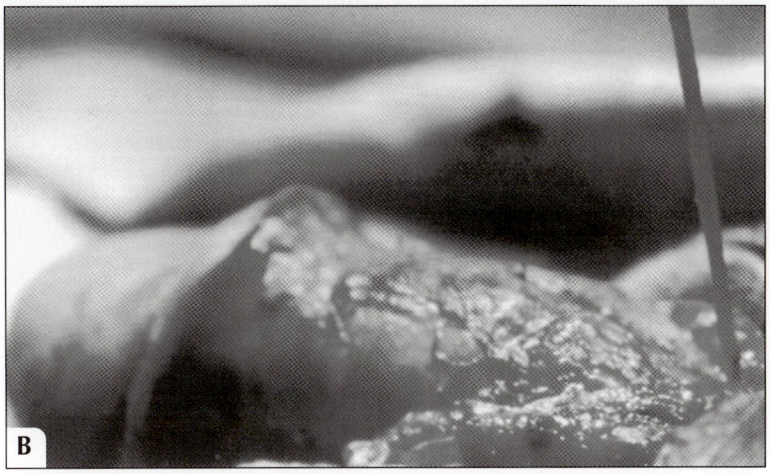

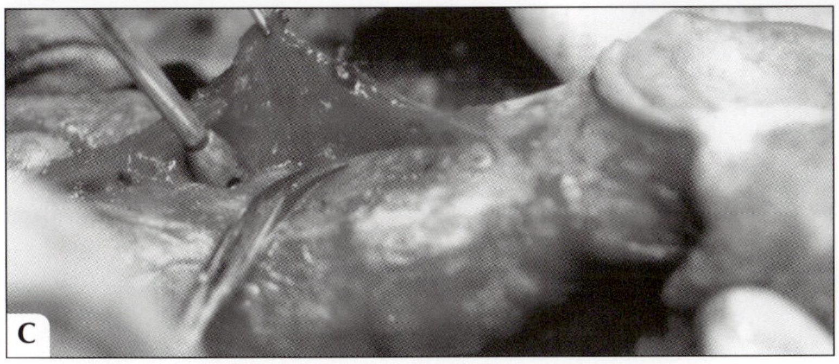

FIGURE 12-9. Degloving of the penis and dissection of blood vessels and nerves. First, prepare genital area and upper leg. Mark a circumcision incision. Dissect and reflect the skin and subcutaneous tissue to the base of the penis. For dorsal curvature (**A**), first resect the deep dorsal vein (**B**), then dissect the dorsal arteries and the nerves off the tunica albuginea (**C**). Surgical loupes are very helpful in preventing the dorsal arteries and dorsal nerves from injury and removing scar tissue from the neurovascular bundle to restore its length. For ventral curvature, dissect the corpus spongiosum off the tunica.

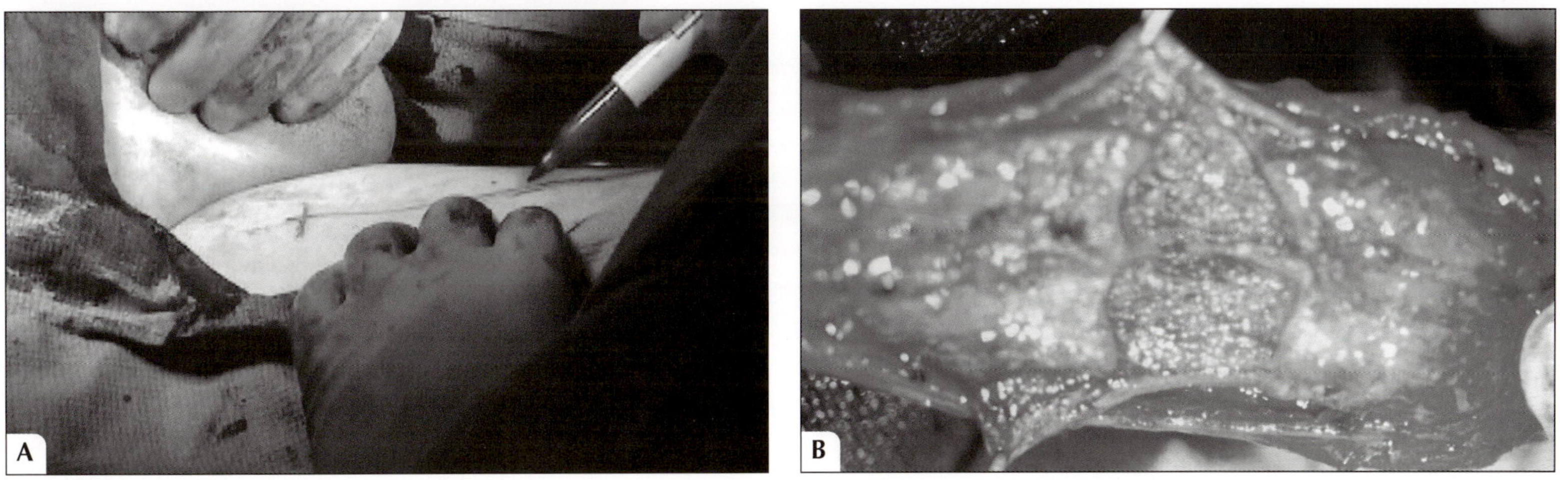

FIGURE 12-10. Incisions. Make an incision in the inner thigh to isolate a segment of the saphenous vein (**A**). Make a relaxation incision: transverse for curvature, longitudinal for hourglass deformity (**B**). Then stretch the penis to measure the size of the defect. Different configurations, sizes, and numbers of the tunical incisions can be used depending on the size and shape of the penile deformity. We have found that an H-shaped incision can suit most deformities.

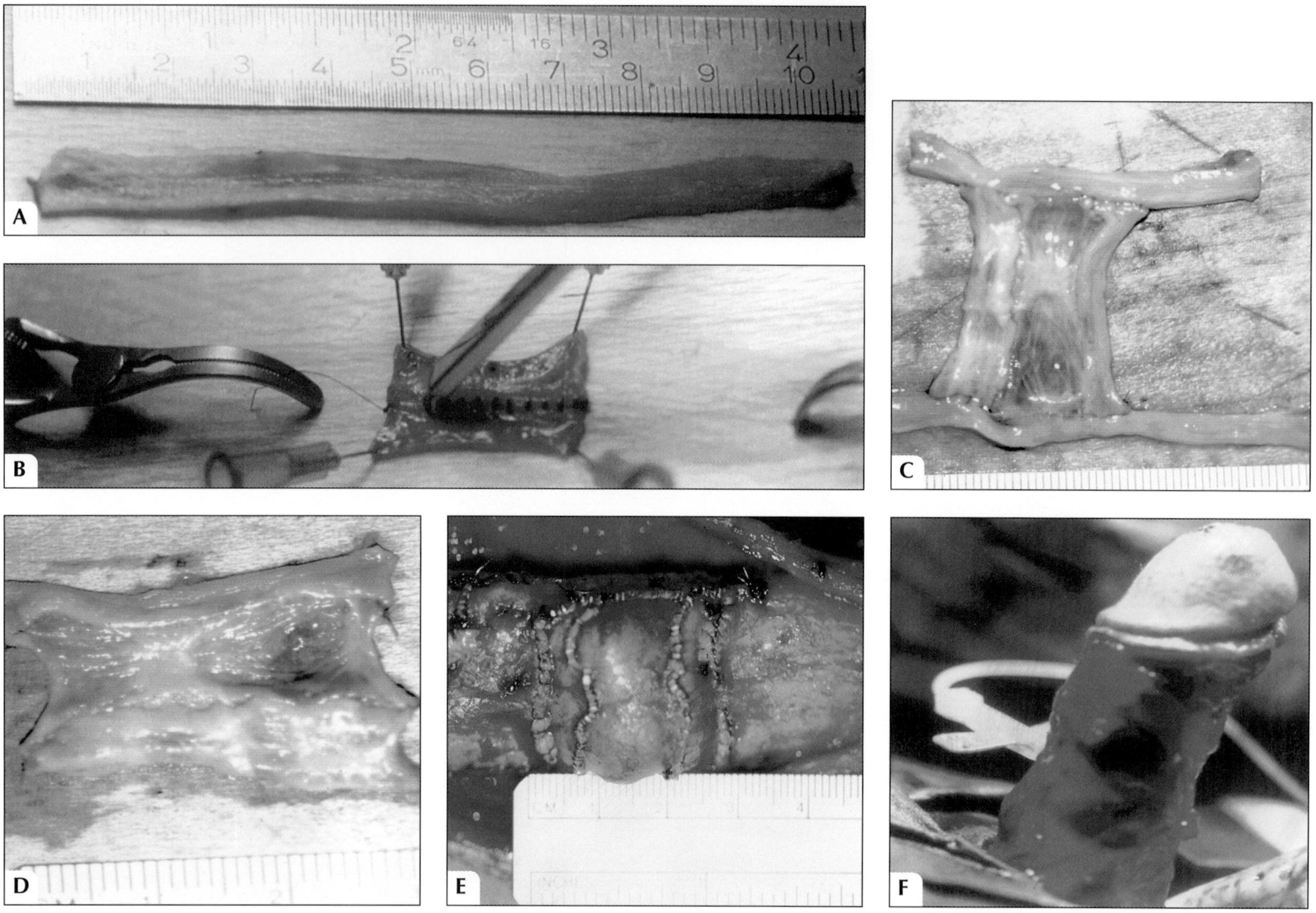

FIGURE 12-11. Saphenous vein grafting and closure. A segment of saphenous vein adequate to cover the tunical defect is excised. The harvested vein is opened, divided into several segments, and assembled using the autosuture clip applicator (**A** and **B**). Suture the preassembled saphenous patch grafts (**C** and **D**) to the defect with endothelial side down (**E**) [3]. We prefer continuous 4-0 Maxon sutures (Sherwood-Davis & Geck, St. Louis, MO). Inject saline to induce an erection and assess deformity (**F**). If necessary, repeat the last three steps. Do so until the penis is straight. If you repeat these steps and minor correction is still needed, place 2-0 Ticron plication sutures to compensate for overcorrection or undercorrection or to correct for lateral curvature. Close the penile wound with absorbable 4-0 chromic sutures; the leg wound is closed with 4-0 polyglycolic acid suture subcuticularly and sterile dressing is placed over the incision. Wrap the penis with a light dressing and check it 2 to 3 hours later to ensure adequate blood supply to the glans. A scrotal support is then placed over the dressing. The following day, the penile dressing and urinary catheter are removed. The patient is discharged home with instructions to change the dressing once a day for 10 days and to abstain from sexual intercourse for 6 weeks.

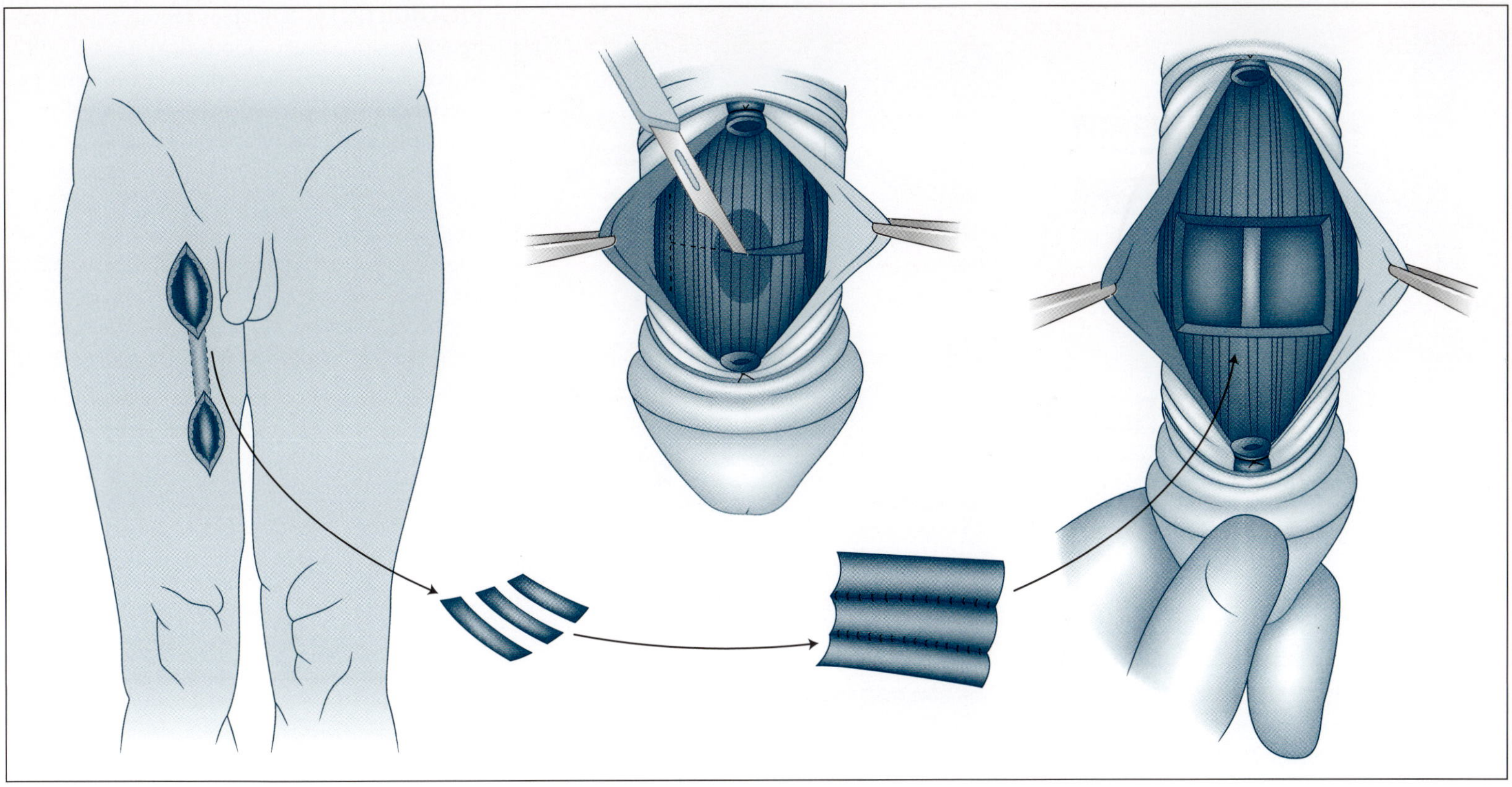

FIGURE 12-12. Summary of the incision and venous grafting procedure. First, resect the deep dorsal vein and restore the length of the neurovascular bundle. Then make an H-shaped incision onto the contractured tunica saphenous vein graft. (*Adapted from* Lue [4].)

Complications of Plaque Incision and Grafting

Ischemic necrosis of foreskin
Inadequate correction
Less rigidity during erection
Prolonged painful erection, pain lasting more than 6 mo
Prolonged induration at base of penis
Numbness lasting longer than 6 mo
Shortened penis
Recurrence (none at graft site)

FIGURE 12-13. Complications of plaque incision and grafting. Plaque incision and grafting procedures result in a variety of complications owing to the complexity of the procedure and the need to dissect the neurovascular bundles.

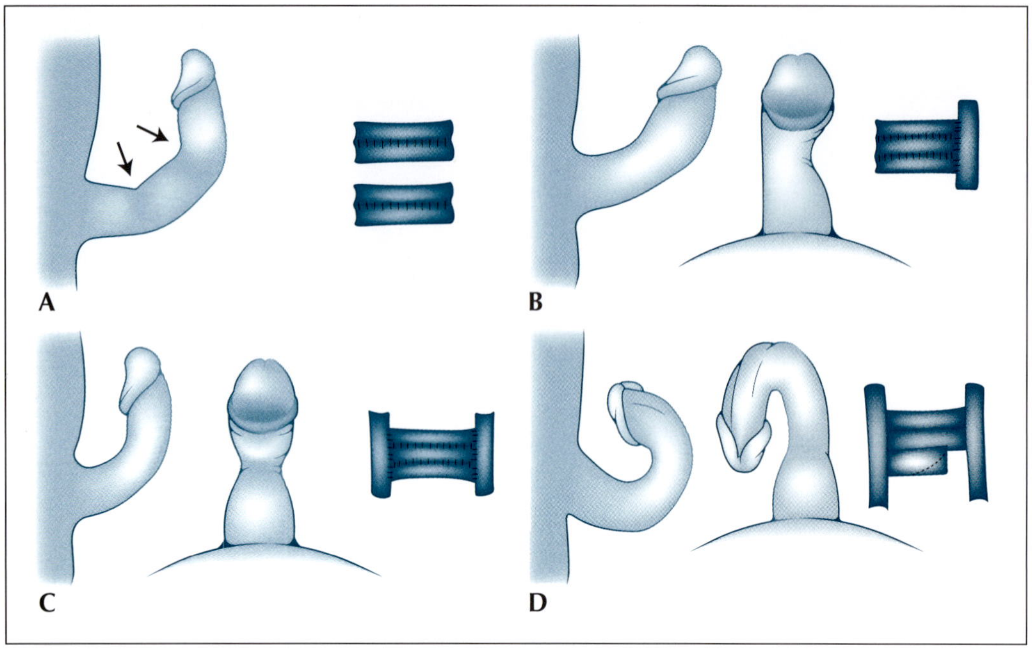

FIGURE 12-14. Different venous patch configurations to correct various deformities. **A**, For dorsal curvature with no lateral bending, a rectangular graft is sufficient. If there are two angulation sites, two grafts can be used. **B**, For a dorsal curvature associated with unilateral narrowing, a T-shaped graft is suitable. **C**, For an hourglass deformity, an H-shaped graft is important for correcting the deviation as well as the penile indentation. **D**, For a complex deformity, tailoring of a suitable graft shape is important for a satisfactory postoperative result.

Graft Materials Used for Peyronie's Disease

Saphenous vein
Dermis
Tunica vaginalis
Temporalis fascia
Dura mater
Fascia lata
Dacron
Gortex
Cadaveric pericardium

FIGURE 12-15. Graft materials used for Peyronie's disease. Various graft materials both autologous and synthetic have been used in the treatment of Peyronie's disease. Morbidity associated with harvesting and the ultimate surgical outcome are important determinants as to the type of graft used [5].

REFERENCES

1. Gholami SS, Lue TF: Correction of penile curvature using the 16-dot placation technique: a review of 132 patients. *J Urol* 2002, 167:2066–2069.
2. Carrier S, Lue TF: Peyronie's disease. *Contemp Urol* 1994, 6:54.
3. Lue TF, El-Sakka AI: Venous patch graft for Peyronie's disease: part I. Technique. *J Urol* 1998, 160(6 pt 1):2047–2049.
4. Lue TF: A conservative approach to Peyronie's disease. *AUA News* 1996, 1:1–3.
5. Leungwattanakij S, Bivalacqua T, Reddy S, Hellstrom WJ: Long term follow-up on use of pericardial graft in the surgical management of Peyronie's disease. *Int J Impot Res* 2001, 13:183–186.

INDEX

R

S

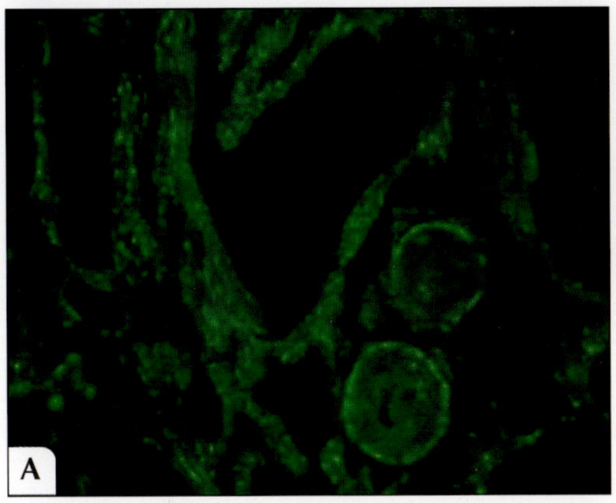

FIGURE 1-29A.

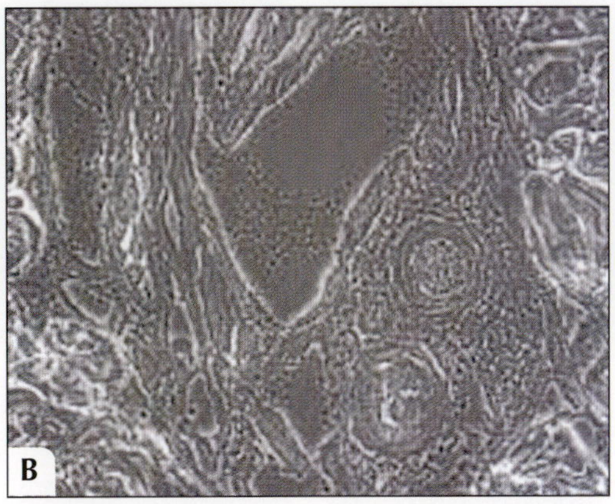

FIGURE 1-29B.

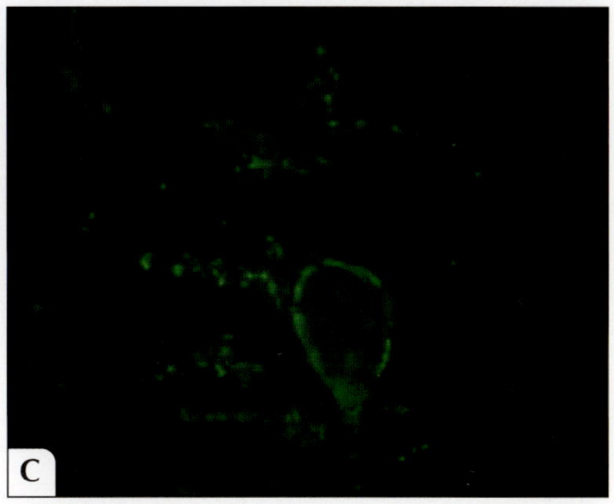

FIGURE 1-29C.

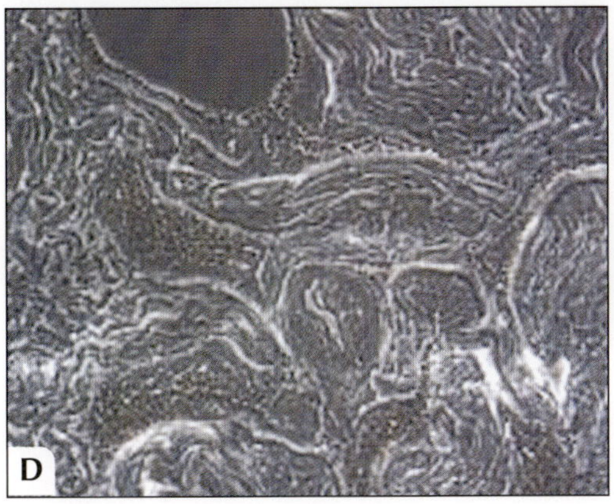

FIGURE 1-29D.

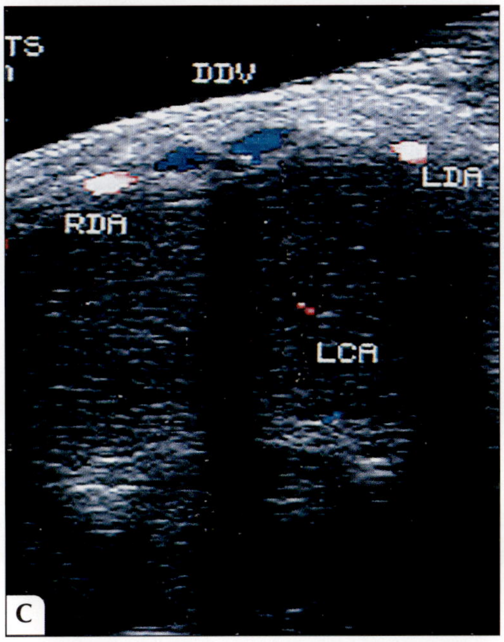

FIGURE 3-10C.

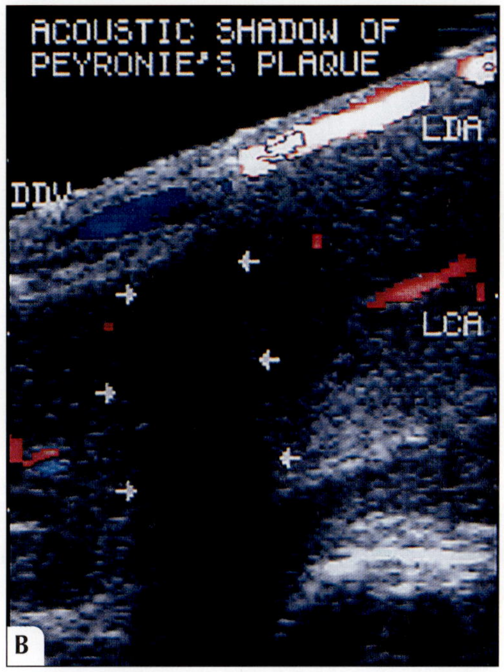

FIGURE 3-11B.

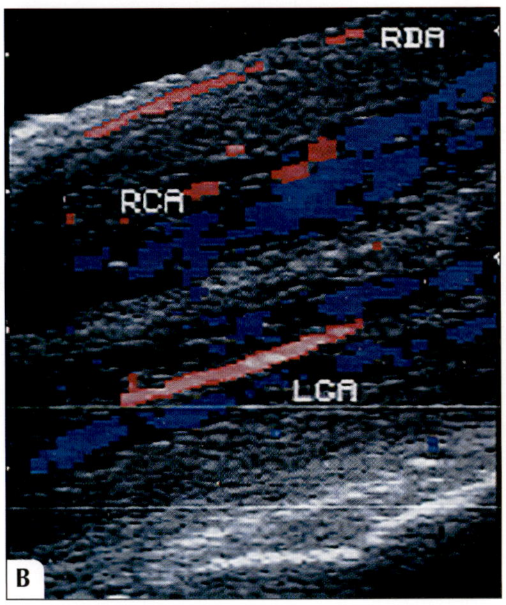

FIGURE 3-13B.

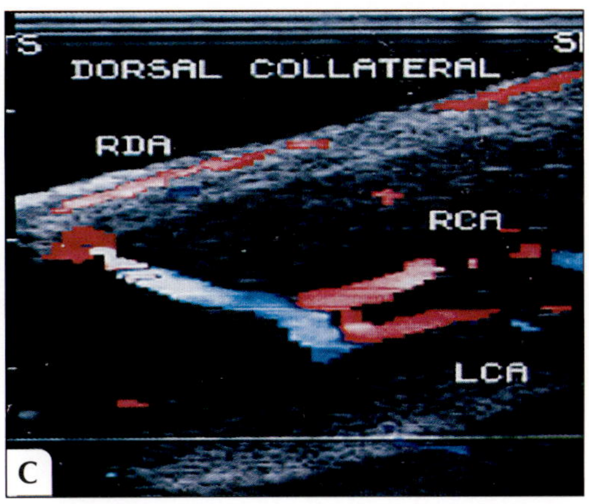

FIGURE 3-13C.

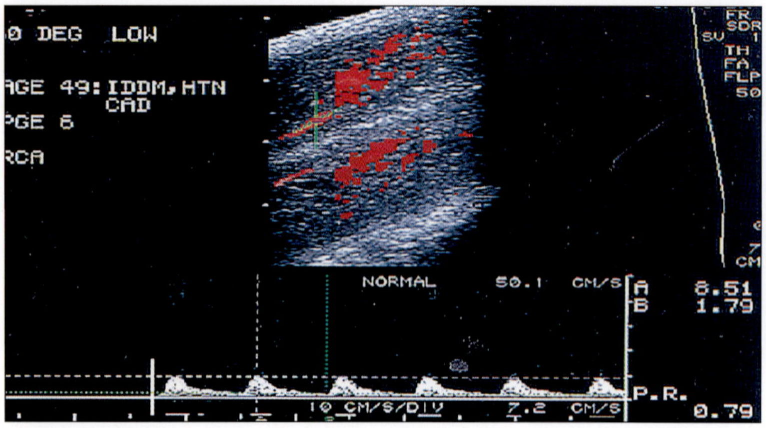

FIGURE 3-15.

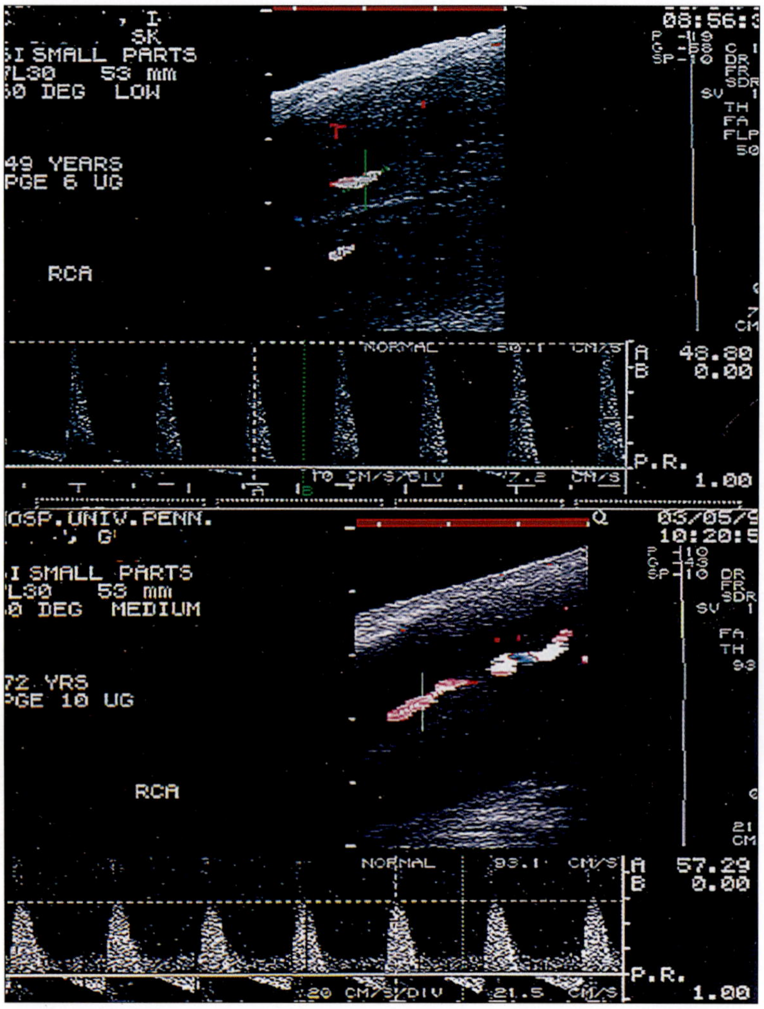

FIGURE 3-16.

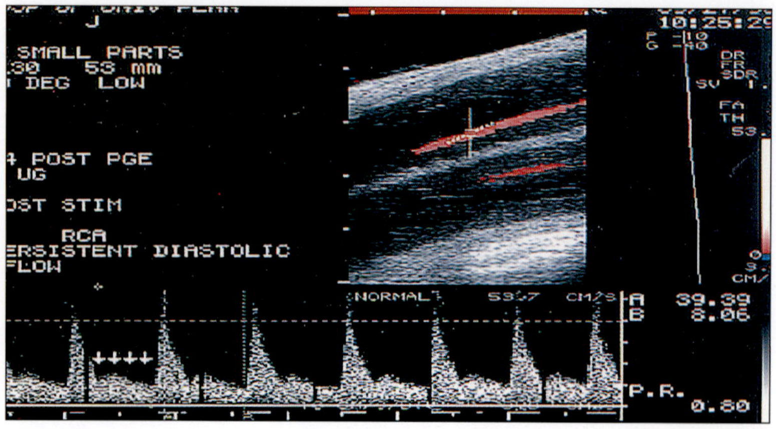

FIGURE 3-17.

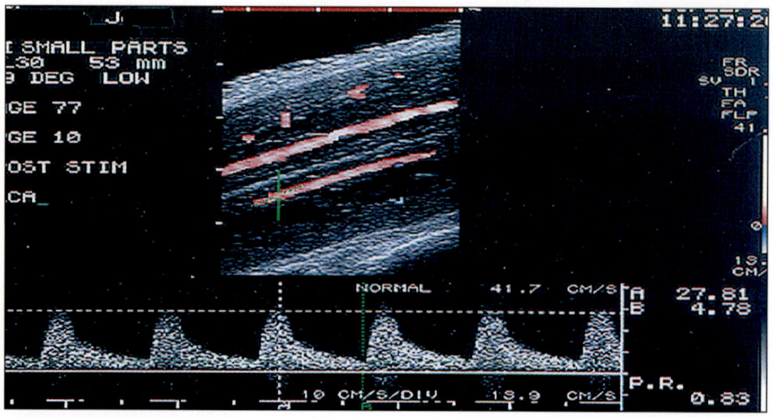

FIGURE 3-18.

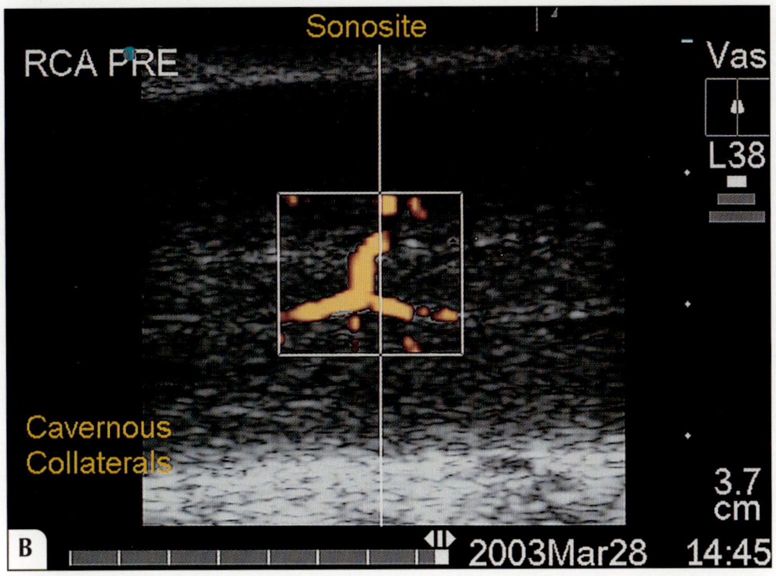

FIGURE 3-19B.

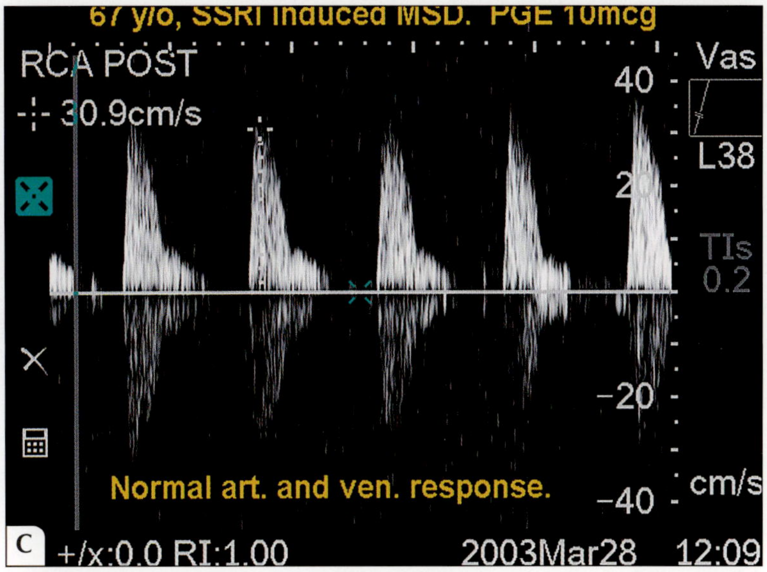

FIGURE 3-19C.

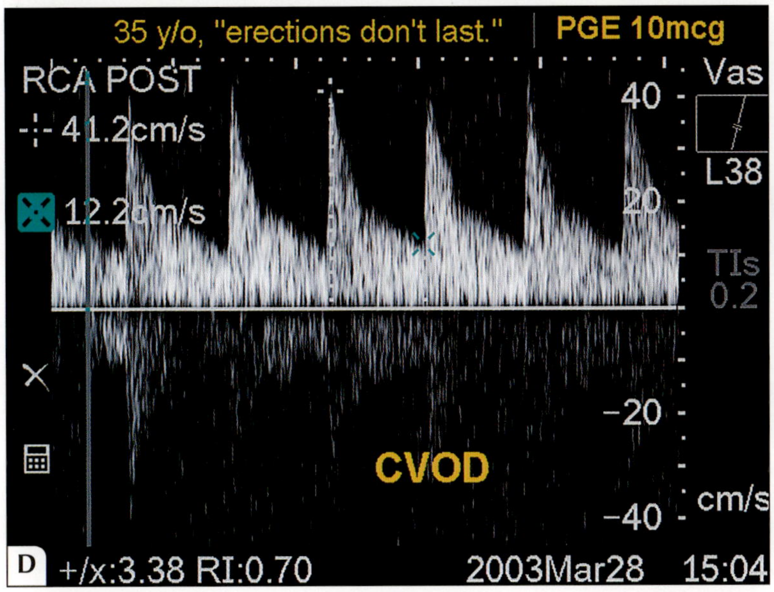

FIGURE 3-19D.

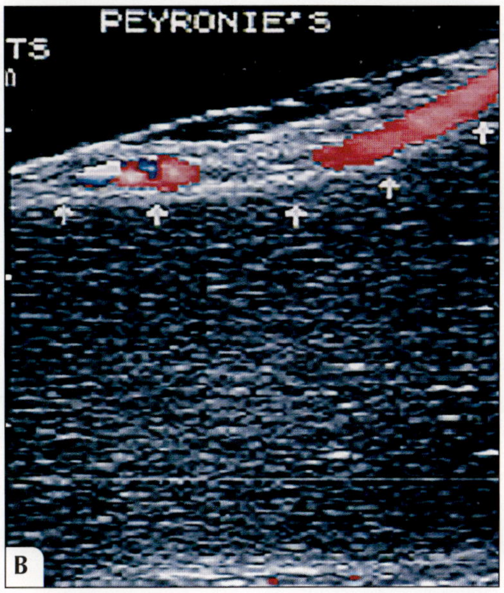

FIGURE 3-21B.

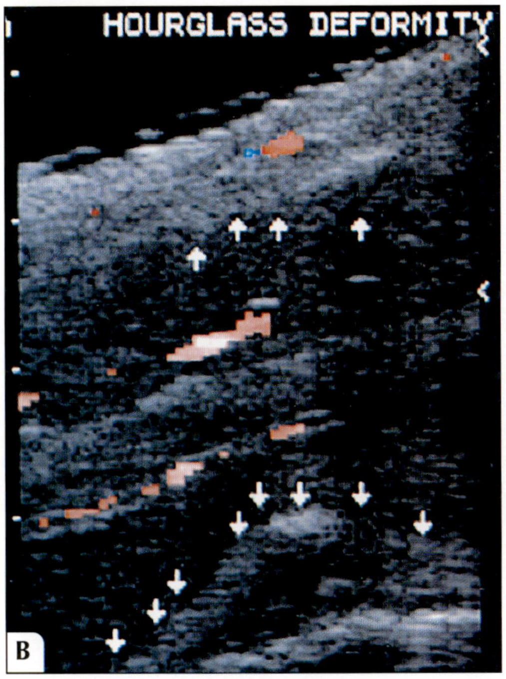

FIGURE 3-22B.

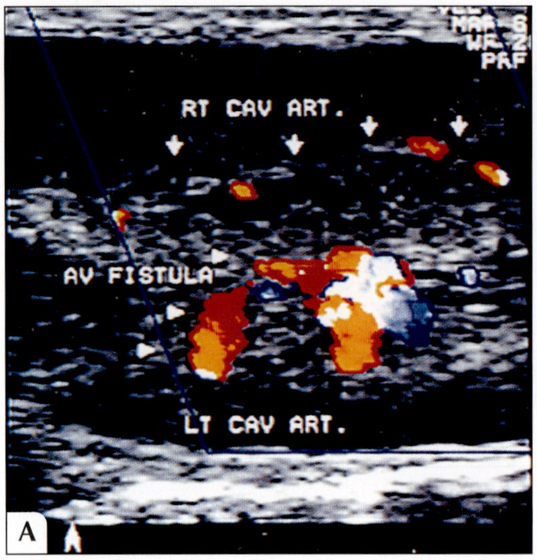

FIGURE 3-24A.

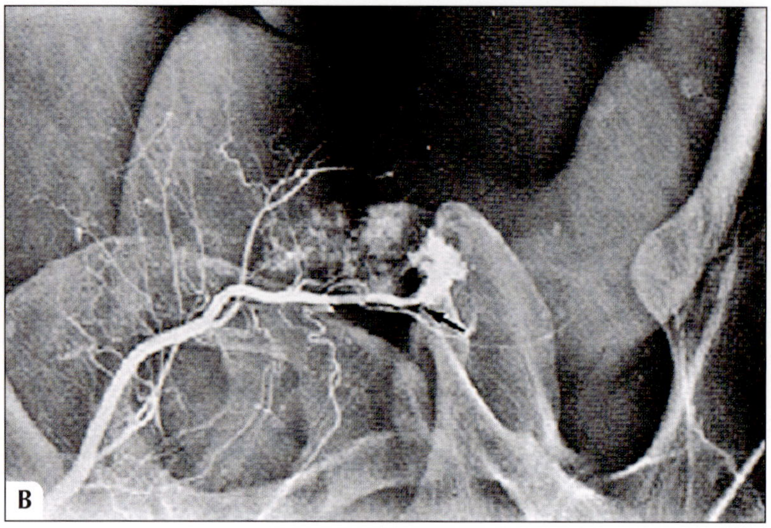

FIGURE 3-24B.

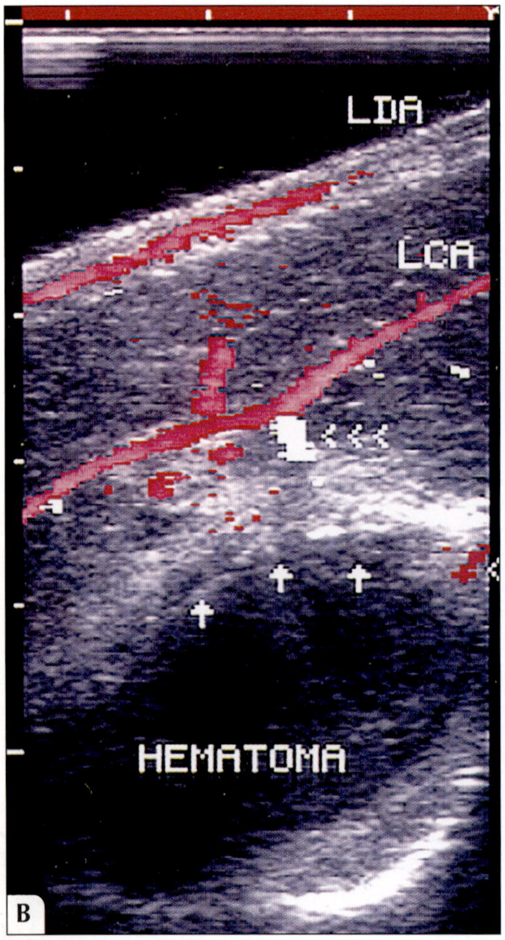

FIGURE 3-25B.

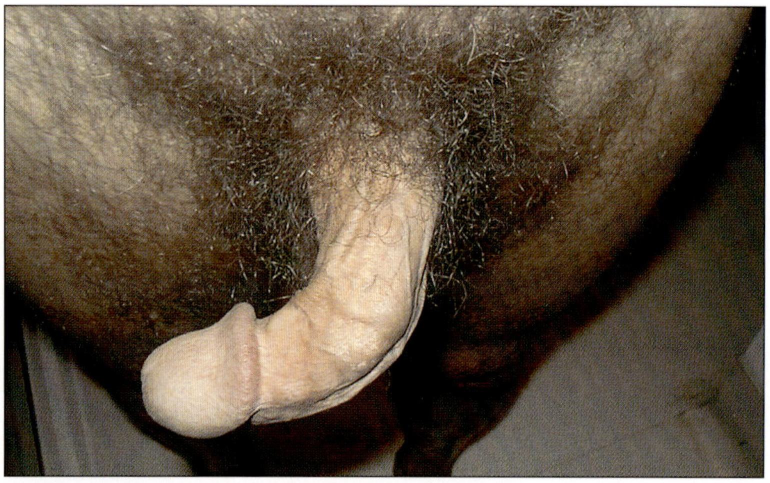

FIGURE 11-1.

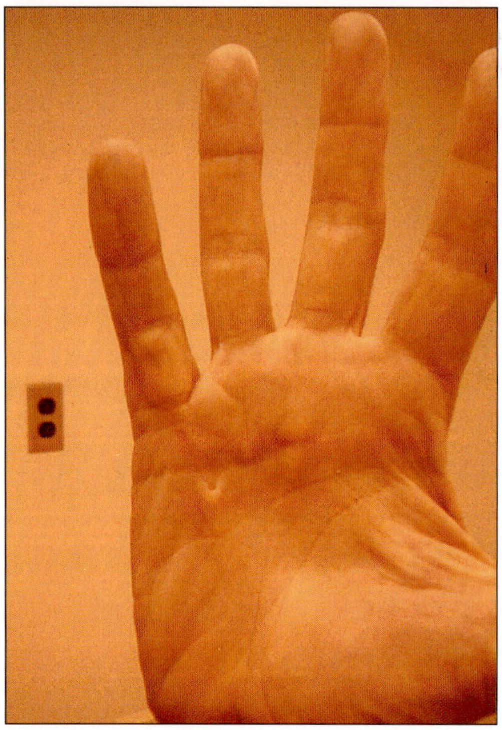

FIGURE 11-17.